ENDOCRINE EMERGENCIES

ELSEVIER

1600 John F. Kennedy Blvd.
Ste 1800
Philadelphia, PA 19103-2899

ENDOCRINE EMERGENCIES

ISBN: 978-0-323-76097-3

Notice

Practitioners and researchers must always rely on their own experience and knowledge in evaluating and using any information, methods, compounds or experiments described herein. Because of rapid advances in the medical sciences, in particular, independent verification of diagnoses and drug dosages should be made. To the fullest extent of the law, no responsibility is assumed by Elsevier, authors, editors or contributors for any injury and/or damage to persons or property as a matter of products liability, negligence or otherwise, or from any use or operation of any methods, products, instructions, or ideas contained in the material herein.

Library of Congress Control Number: 2021932737

Senior Content Strategist: Nancy Duffy
Content Development Specialist: Beth LoGiudice
Content Development Manager: Ellen M. Wurm-Cutter
Publishing Services Manager: Shereen Jameel
Senior Project Manager: Umarani Natarajan
Design Direction: Patrick C. Ferguson

Printed in India

Last digit is the print number: 9 8 7 6 5 4 3 2 1

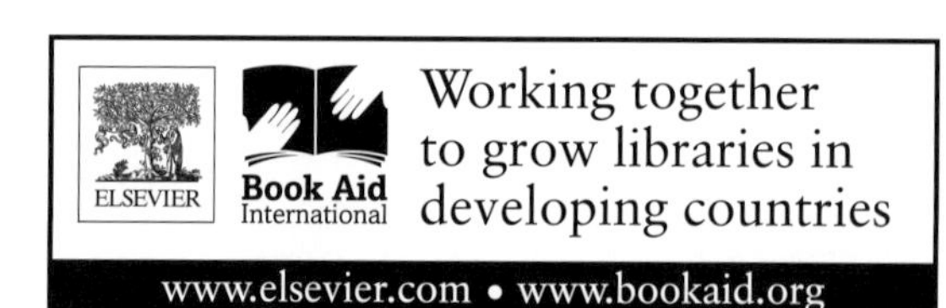

ENDOCRINE EMERGENCIES

ALEXANDER L. SHIFRIN, MD, FACS, FACE, ECNU, FEBS (ENDOCRINE), FISS

Clinical Associate Professor of Surgery
Rutgers Robert Wood Johnson Medical School
New Brunswick, New Jersey

Associate Professor of Surgery
Hackensack Meridian School of Medicine
Nutley, New Jersey
Director of Endocrine Oncology
Hackensack Meridian Health of Monmouth and Ocean Counties
Nutley, New Jersey

Surgical Director
Center for Thyroid, Parathyroid, and Adrenal Diseases
Department of Surgery
Jersey Shore University Medical Center
Neptune, New Jersey

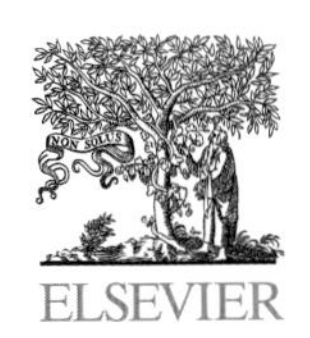

ELSEVIER

In memory of my father, Leonid Shifrin, medical engineer, the inventor of thromboelastographs; and my uncle, pediatric surgeon, Vadim Shifrin, MD.

To my mother, Margarita Shifrina, for her love and endless support.

To my beloved children, Michael, Daniel, Benjamin, Julia, Christian, and Liam, who continue to provide perspective on what is truly important in life.

To the love of my life, Svetlana L. Krasnova, for her love, patience, and encouragement.

To my teachers and mentors, who dedicated their lives and efforts to the science of surgery. Those who made me into a surgeon and inspired me to produce this book: Ali Bairov, MD, Steven Raper, MD, William Inabnet, MD, John Chabot, MD, and Jerome Vernick, MD.

ACKNOWLEDGMENTS

The creation of this book, covering the entire scope of endocrine emergencies, was dependent on a team effort, which was possible only with the support and enthusiasm of many individuals who contributed to this book, my colleagues, who trusted me and dedicated their time and effort to make it happen, and without whom this book would have never come to life!

Special thanks to Nancy Duffy, Senior Content Strategist at Elsevier, who believed in me, and to the entire staff at Elsevier, who were very supportive from the first idea of this book and maintained their enthusiasm until the end.

PREFACE

Endocrine Emergencies is an up-to-date guide for endocrinologists, endocrine surgeons, surgical oncologists, ENT surgeons, head and neck surgeons, emergency physicians, internists and primary care physicians, critical care physicians and trauma surgeons, neurosurgeons, obstetricians and gynecologists, neurologists, advanced practice providers, residents, and medical students. The book covers the most common and serious emergencies related to endocrine metabolic conditions of the pituitary gland, thyroid, parathyroid, adrenal glands, pancreas, and neuroendocrine tumors. It also includes separate chapters on endocrine responses in critically ill and trauma patients, use of potassium iodide ingestion in a nuclear emergency, endocrine emergencies during pregnancy, and postoperative endocrine emergencies after thyroid and parathyroid surgeries. It covers up-to-date information and serves as a guide on how to recognize, diagnose, and treat each condition using modern diagnostic techniques and modern therapeutics.

We hope that this book will provide an indispensable source of knowledge to all practitioners, those who just started their career and those who are in the more advanced stages of their practice.

Alexander L. Shifrin, MD, FACS, FACE, ECNU, FEBS (Endocrine), FISS
February 2021

CONTRIBUTORS

Sara Ahmadi, MD, ECNU
Endocrine Faculty
Department of Medicine
Division of Endocrinology
Brigham and Women's Hospital
Harvard Medical School
Boston, Massachusetts

Monika S. Akula, MD
Endocrinology, Diabetes and Metabolism Fellow
Department of Endocrinology and Metabolism
Jersey Shore University Medical Center
Neptune, New Jersey

Erik K. Alexander, MD
Chief, Thyroid Section & Professor of Medicine
Department of Medicine
Division of Endocrinology
Brigham Women's Hospital
Harvard Medical School
Boston, Massachusetts

Trevor E. Angell, MD
Assistant Professor of Clinical Medicine
Department of Endocrinology and Diabetes;
Associate Director of the Thyroid Center
Keck School of Medicine
University of Southern California
Los Angeles, California

Maureen McCartney Anderson, DNP, CRNA/APN
Assistant Professor
Division of Advanced Nursing Practice
Rutgers School of Nursing Anesthesia Program
Rutgers, The State University of New Jersey
Newark, New Jersey

John P. Bilezikian, MD
Dorothy L. and Daniel H. Silberberg Professor of Medicine and Professor of Pharmacology
Vice Chair, Department of Medicine for International Education and Research
Chief (Emeritus), Division of Endocrinology
Department of Medicine
Vagelos College of Physicians and Surgeons
Columbia University, New York

Stefan Richard Bornstein, MD, PhD
Division of Internal Medicine and Division of Endocrinology and Metabolism
University Hospital Carl Gustav Carus
Technical University of Dresden
Dresden, Germany

Jan Calissendorff, MD, PhD
Senior Consultant
Department of Endocrinology, Metabolism and Diabetes
Karolinska University Hospital
Department of Molecular Medicine and Surgery
Karolinska Institutet
Stockholm, Sweden

Stuart Campbell, MD, MSc
Resident
Division of Endocrine Surgery, Department of Surgery
Jersey Shore University Medical Center
Neptune, New Jersey

Tariq Chukir, MD
Assistant Professor
Department of Medicine, Division of Endocrinology, Diabetes, and Metabolism
Weill Cornell Medicine and New York Presbyterian Hospital
New York, New York

Tara Corrigan, MHS, PA-C
Physician Assistant
Division of Endocrine Surgery, Department of Surgery
Jersey Shore University Medical Center
Neptune, New Jersey

Henrik Falhammar, MD, PhD, FRACP
Department of Endocrinology, Metabolism and Diabetes
Karolinska University Hospital;
Associate Professor
Department of Molecular Medicine and Surgery
Karolinska Institutet
Stockholm, Sweden

Azeez Farooki, MD
Attending Physician
Endocrinology Service
Department of Medicine
Memorial Sloan Kettering Cancer Center
New York, New York

Chelsi Flippo, MD
Pediatric Endocrinology Fellow
Eunice Kennedy Shriver National Institute of Child Health and Human Development
National Institutes of Health
Bethesda, Maryland

Lane L. Frasier, MD, MS
Fellow, Surgery
Division of Traumatology, Surgical Critical Care & Emergency General Surgery
Department of Surgery
University of Pennsylvania
Philadelphia, Pennsylvania

Vincent Gemma, MD
Major Health Partners
Department of Surgery
Shelbyville Hospital
Shelbyville, Indiana

Monica Girotra, MD
Associate Clinical Member
Endocrine Service, Department of Medicine
Memorial Sloan Kettering Cancer Center;
Assistant Clinical Professor
Endocrine Division
Weill Cornell Medical College
New York, New York

Ansha Goel, MD
Endocrinology Fellow
Division of Endocrinology and Metabolism
Georgetown University Hospital
Washington, District of Columbia

Christopher G. Goodier, BS, MD
Associate Professor
Division of Maternal Fetal Medicine
Department of Obstetrics and Gynecology
Medical University of South Carolina
Charleston, South Carolina

Heidi Guzman, MD
Assistant Professor of Medicine
Columbia University Irving Medical Center
New York, New York

Makoto Ishii, MD, PhD
Assistant Professor
Department of Neurology
Feil Family Brain and Mind Research Institute
Weill Cornell Medicine
New York Presbyterian Hospital
New York, New York

Yasuhiro Ito, MD, PhD
Kuma Hospital
Department of Surgery
Kobe, Japan

Michael Kazim, MD
Clinical Professor
Oculoplastic and Orbital Surgery
Edward S. Harkness Eye Institute
Columbia University Irving Medical Center
New York-Presbyterian Hospital
New York, New York

Jane J. Keating, MD
Division of Traumatology, Surgical Critical Care & Emergency General Surgery
Department of Surgery
University of Pennsylvania
Philadelphia, Pennsylvania

Anupam Kotwal, MD
Assistant Professor of Medicine
Division of Diabetes, Endocrinology, and Metabolism
University of Nebraska Medical Center
Omaha Nebraska;
Research Collaborator
Division of Endocrinology, Diabetes, Metabolism and Nutrition
Mayo Clinic
Rochester, Minnesota

Svetlana L. Krasnova, APRN, FNP-C, RNFA
Advanced Practice Registered Nurse
Department of Otolaryngology, Head and Neck Surgery
Rutgers Robert Wood Johnson Medical School
New Brunswick, New Jersey

David W. Lam, MD
Assistant Professor
Division of Endocrinology, Diabetes, and Bone Disease
Icahn School of Medicine at Mount Sinai
New York, New York

Melissa G. Lechner, MD, PhD
Assistant Professor of Medicine
Division of Endocrinology, Diabetes, and Metabolism
David Geffen School of Medicine
University of California at Los Angeles
Los Angeles, California

Aundrea Eason Loftley, MD
Assistant Professor
Division of Endocrinology, Diabetes and Metabolic Diseases
Department of Internal Medicine
Medical University of South Carolina
Charleston, South Carolina

Sara E. Lubitz, MD
Associate Professor
Department of Medicine
Rutgers Robert Wood Johnson Medical School
New Brunswick, New Jersey

Louis Mandel, DDS
Director
Salivary Gland Center;
Associate Dean, Clinical Professor (Oral and Maxillofacial Surgery)
Columbia University College of Dental Medicine
New York, New York

Hiroo Masuoka, MD, PhD
Department of Surgery
Kuma Hospital
Kobe, Japan

Jorge H. Mestman, MD
Professor of Medicine and Obstetrics & Gynecology
Division of Endocrinology, Diabetes and Metabolism
Department of Medicine and Obstetrics and Gynecology
Keck School of Medicine
University of Southern California
Los Angeles, California

Akira Miyauchi, MD, PhD
Department of Surgery
Kuma Hospital
Kobe, Japan

Caroline T. Nguyen, MD
Assistant Professor of Clinical Medicine, Obstetrics and Gynecology
Division of Endocrinology
Diabetes & Metabolism
Department of Medicine
Keck School of Medicine
University of Southern California
Los Angeles, California

Raquel Kristin Sanchez Ong, MD
Endocrinologist, Fellowship Assistant Program Director
Division of Endocrinology and Metabolism
Jersey Shore University Medical Center
Neptune, New Jersey;
Assistant Professor
Department of Internal Medicine
Hackensack Meridian School of Medicine
Nutley, New Jersey

Randall P. Owen, MD, MS, FACS
Chief, Section of Endocrine Surgery
Division of Surgical Oncology
Program Director, Endocrine Surgery Fellowship
Department of Surgery Mount Sinai Hospital
Icahn School of Medicine
New York, New York

Rodney F. Pommier, MD
Professor of Surgery
Division of Surgical Oncology, Department of Surgery
Oregon Health & Science University
Portland, Oregon

Jason D. Prescott, MD, PhD
Chief, Section of Endocrine Surgery
Director of Thyroid and Parathyroid Surgery
Assistant Professor of Surgery and of Oncology
Department of Surgery
Johns Hopkins School of Medicine
Baltimore, Maryland

Ramya Punati, MD
Clinical Assistant Professor of Medicine
Division of Endocrinology and Metabolism
Pennsylvania Hospital
University of Pennsylvania Health System
Pennsylvania, Philadelphia

Gustavo Romero-Velez, MD
Chief Resident
Department of Surgery
Montefiore Medical Center
Albert Einstein School of Medicine
Bronx, New York

Arthur B. Schneider, MD, PhD
Professor of Medicine (Emeritus)
Department of Medicine
University of Illinois at Chicago
Chicago, Illinois

Alison P. Seitz, MD
Resident
Department of Neurology
Weill Cornell Medicine
New York Presbyterian Hospital
New York, New York

Alexander L. Shifrin, MD, FACS, FACE, ECNU, FEBS (Endocrine), FISS
Clinical Associate Professor of Surgery
Rutgers Robert Wood Johnson Medical School
New Brunswick, New Jersey;
Associate Professor of Surgery
Hackensack Meridian School of Medicine
Nutley, New Jersey;
Director of Endocrine Oncology
Hackensack Meridian Health of Monmouth and Ocean Counties
Hackensack, New Jersey;
Surgical Director, Center for Thyroid, Parathyroid, and Adrenal Diseases
Department of Surgery
Jersey Shore University Medical Center
Neptune, New Jersey

Adam Michael Shiroff, MD, FACS
Associate Professor of Surgery
Division of Traumatology, Surgical Critical Care & Emergency Surgery
University of Pennsylvania
Penn Presbyterian Medical Center
Pennsylvania, Philadelphia

Marius N. Stan, MD
Associate Professor of Medicine
Division of Endocrinology, Diabetes, Metabolism and Nutrition
Mayo Clinic
Rochester, Minnesota

Constantine A. Stratakis, MD, D(med)Sci
Senior Investigator
Eunice Kennedy Shriver National Institute of Child Health and Human Development
National Institutes of Health
Bethesda, Maryland

Christina Tatsi, MD, PhD
Staff Clinician, Pediatric Endocrinologist
Eunice Kennedy Shriver National Institute of Child Health and Human Development
National Institutes of Health
Bethesda, Maryland

Daniel J. Toft, MD, PhD
Assistant Professor
Division of Endocrinology, Diabetes and Metabolism
Department of Medicine
University of Illinois at Chicago
Chicago, Illinois

Arthur Topilow, MD, FACP
Department of Hematology Oncology
Jersey Shore University Medical Center
Neptune, New Jersey

Ann Q. Tran, MD
Oculoplastic and Orbital Surgery
Edward S. Harkness Eye Institute
Columbia University Irving Medical Centery
New York-Presbyterian Hospital
New York, New York

Joseph G. Verbalis, MD
Professor of Medicine
Georgetown University;
Chief, Endocrinology and Metabolism
Georgetown University Medical Center
Washington, District of Columbia

Leonard Wartofsky, MS, MD, MPH
Director, Thyroid Cancer Research Center
MedStar Health Research Institute;
Professor of Medicine
Department of Medicine
Georgetown University School of Medicine
Washington, District of Columbia

Sarah M. Wonn, MD
Resident
Department of Surgery
Oregon Health & Science University
Portland, Oregon

Dorina Ylli, MD, PhD
Thyroid Cancer Research Center
MedStar Health Research Institute
Washington, District of Columbia

William F. Young, Jr, MD, MSc
Professor of Medicine, Tyson Family Endocrinology Clinical Professor
Division of Endocrinology, Diabetes, Metabolism, and Nutrition
Mayo Clinic
Rochester, Minnesota

CONTENTS

PART 1

Thyroid

CHAPTER 1

Severe Thyrotoxicosis and Thyroid Storm

Melissa G. Lechner ■ Trevor E. Angell

CHAPTER OUTLINE

Introduction

Thyroid hormone excess, also known as thyrotoxicosis, encompasses a wide range of signs and symptoms. Thyrotoxicosis and hyperthyroidism may have semantic distinctions but are often used interchangeably. Patients with clinical manifestations of severe thyrotoxicosis need urgent evaluation and may require hospitalization and emergency intervention. Therefore it is important to be able to recognize the presence of thyrotoxicosis, know the causative factors, evaluate its severity, and, when necessary, know the critical aspects of management for patients with life-threatening disease.

Thyroid storm is a clinical syndrome of decompensated thyrotoxicosis in which the compensatory physiologic mechanisms have been overwhelmed. It is considered an endocrine emergency due to its high morbidity and mortality, and prior to the availability of advanced intensive care and multimodality therapeutic interventions, this condition was uniformly fatal.[1–5] Outcomes remain very poor for patients not quickly identified and treated. Historically, cases of thyroid storm were associated with surgical interventions, but the majority of recognized cases are now medical, related to underlying infections, cardiovascular events, or other conditions. Not all patients will have a previous diagnosis of hyperthyroidism, and thyroid storm may occur in many circumstances with myriad precipitants. Despite its rarity, thyroid storm has been estimated to represent 1%–16% of hospital admissions for thyrotoxicosis, with estimates varying across studies depending upon methodology.[1,6–9] Providers should be vigilant in identifying patients who may have thyroid storm and initiating appropriate care.

This chapter provides a summary of the evaluation and management of patients with severe thyrotoxicosis and thyroid storm, with emphasis on the latter given the importance of recognizing and treating this condition.

Pathophysiology of Thyrotoxicosis and Thyroid Storm

Thyroid hormone exerts effects throughout the body. During thyrotoxicosis, the influences of excess thyroid hormone, particularly upon energy expenditure and the cardiovascular system, result in altered metabolism and hemodynamics for which the body may compensate but lacks the reserve capacity to adapt to additional stresses.

Excess thyroid hormone, predominantly through the nuclear actions of triiodothyronine (T3) on gene transcription and posttranslational modification, causes increased cardiac contractility and cardiac output (CO). Upregulated cardiac genes include myosin heavy chain, voltage-gated potassium channels, and sarcoplasmic reticulum calcium ATPase.[10] T3 also directly induces vascular smooth muscle relaxation and vasodilation that is further augmented by the need to remove excess heat generated by upregulation of uncoupling protein-3, Na^+/K^+ ATPase, and increased energy expenditure. Vasodilation in thyrotoxicosis causes relative underperfusion of renal and splanchnic circulation, resulting in increased activation of the renin-angiotensin-aldosterone system (RAAS) and subsequent increased blood volume and cardiac preload.[11] This new compensated steady state puts a chronic workload on the cardiovascular system. Due to these changes, patients with thyrotoxicosis will typically demonstrate increased resting heart rate (HR) and respiratory rate. In compensated thyrotoxicosis, the skin is often warm and sweating may be present to dissipate heat, but fever is absent. Cardiovascular findings include reduced systemic vascular resistance (SVR), increased CO and ejection fraction, and increased pulmonary artery pressure. Systolic blood pressure is increased whereas diastolic and mean arterial pressure are reduced, leading to a widened pulse pressure. Thyrotoxic patients experience exercise intolerance due to the inability to further augment HR, CO, or SVR, as would occur in the euthyroid state.[12] Additionally, weakness results from T3-mediated protein catabolism and skeletal muscle loss, including the diaphragm.

What differentiates thyroid storm from thyrotoxicosis is hemodynamic decompensation. Although an exact pathophysiology is unknown, the close association with precipitating physiologic stresses provides some clues. Events such as infection, acute coronary syndromes (ACS), hypovolemia, or trauma upset the tenuous hemodynamic balance created by the aforementioned physiologic changes, and there is an inability by the body to augment cardiovascular function further. Loss of effective circulation results in heat retention and organ hypoperfusion leading to the classic findings of hyperthermia and altered mental status.[4,13]

Evaluation of Patients for Thyrotoxicosis

SIGNS AND SYMPTOMS OF THYROID STORM

The acute evaluation of a patient with thyrotoxicosis should proceed similarly to other patients, with emergent evaluation of cardiopulmonary, hemodynamic, and neurologic status. The initial secondary survey should seek to identify not only the presence of thyrotoxicosis but its most severe manifestations. These would include hyperthermia, altered mentation (e.g., confusion, lethargy, seizures, coma), tachyarrhythmia, or congestive heart failure (CHF; e.g., elevated jugular venous pressure, lower extremity swelling, pulmonary edema, congestive hepatopathy), and the presence of jaundice. Other manifestations may be evident but do not necessarily indicate thyroid storm.

The presentation of thyrotoxicosis may include classic symptoms or be atypical in nature. The influence of excess thyroid hormone on the body leads to a number of predictable symptoms. Heat intolerance, tachycardia and/or palpitations, fine bilateral tremor, weight loss, muscle weakness or fatigue, and dyspnea on exertion or shortness of breath are all symptoms of moderate to severe thyrotoxicosis regardless of the etiology. On physical examination, patients without thyroid storm are usually afebrile but their skin is warm to the touch from cutaneous vasodilation. The resting heart rate may be modestly elevated (80–100 beats per minute [bpm]) or tachycardic (>100 bpm). More significant cardiac effects include supraventricular tachyarrhythmias (SVT), particularly atrial fibrillation (AF) with rapid ventricular rate, or manifestations of heart failure. Not all patients with signs of heart failure will have reduced systolic function, but cardiomyopathy with markedly reduced ejection fraction can occur in a small percentage. In patients with preexisting arrhythmias or heart failure, these may be nonspecific findings or may demonstrate an acute worsening. In one retrospective cohort analysis, patients with a history of coronary artery disease, AF, peripheral vascular disease, renal failure, pulmonary circulation disorders, or valvular disease were more likely to have cardiogenic shock with thyroid storm. Additionally, 45% of patients with thyroid storm complicated by cardiogenic shock had a preexisting diagnosis of CHF.[14]

Less commonly, these overt symptoms of thyrotoxicosis are absent. Symptoms may be limited, particularly in older individuals. Termed *apathetic hyperthyroidism*, in these individuals symptoms might only include weight loss, failure to thrive, fatigue, or lethargy. In patients already taking medications blocking the β-adrenergic system, classic symptoms of palpitations, tremor, or agitation may also be blunted. Rare manifestations of thyrotoxicosis include paroxysmal periodic paralysis, related to changes in potassium channel function, affecting the lower before the upper extremities, proximal more than distal muscle groups, and usually sparing the diaphragm.

CAUSES OF THYROTOXICOSIS AND THYROID STORM

Historical information, or specific signs or symptoms, may suggest an underlying cause of thyrotoxicosis. Common and significant etiologies are shown in Table 1.1. A diffusely enlarged nontender thyroid gland suggests Graves' disease, and the presence of a thyroid bruit is pathognomonic. Similarly, the presence of proptosis or other aspects of ophthalmopathy (periorbital edema, chemosis, optic nerve compression) are seen only in Graves' disease.[15] Exquisite thyroid tenderness and recent onset of symptoms suggest subacute thyroiditis; recent pregnancy may indicate postpartum thyroiditis; and the presence of a large nodule may represent an autonomously functioning nodule. Iatrogenic causes of thyroiditis include iodine exposure (including iodinated contrast agents), amiodarone-induced thyrotoxicosis (AIT), lithium, tyrosine kinase inhibitors, and immune therapy agents such as programmed death receptor (PD)-1 and cytotoxic T-lymphocyte–associated protein (CTLA)-4 inhibitors.[16–18] The absence of thyroid pathology in the appropriate clinical setting may suggest accidental or surreptitious patient use of thyroid hormone, often exogenous T3 if symptoms are severe. Lastly, patients presenting with thyroid storm may not have a prior known diagnosis of thyroid disease (up to 30% of patients in one series[19]), and therefore clinician suspicion for underlying hyperthyroidism as a cause of clinical manifestations is paramount.

The most common events precipitating thyroid storm are infections, ACS, venous thromboembolism or pulmonary embolism, trauma, surgery, childbirth, diabetic ketoacidosis (DKA), or discontinuation of medical treatment of Graves' disease, with many other potential causes possible.[4,13,15,20] Unusual causes of thyroid storm reported in the literature include strangulation,[21] stew containing marine neurotoxin,[22] and thyroid impaction by a fishing trident.[23] In short, any stressful event or concurrent medical condition may be a destabilizing force to push a patient with thyrotoxicosis into thyroid storm.

LABORATORY FINDINGS

If thyrotoxicosis in the hospital is suspected clinically, serum thyrotropin (thyroid stimulating hormone; TSH) is the most important test to establish this diagnosis definitively. In patients without a previous diagnosis of thyroid disease, obtaining a free thyroxine (T4) is also a practical

TABLE 1.1 ■ **Common and Significant Causes of Thyrotoxicosis**

Increased Thyroid Hormone Production	
Diagnosis	Mechanism
Graves' disease	Stimulatory TSH receptor antibody
Inappropriate TSH secretion	TSH-secreting pituitary adenoma or pituitary resistance to thyroid hormone
Solitary or multiple thyroid nodule(s)	Autonomous thyroid hormone production by one or more adenoma(s)
Trophoblastic tumor or choriocarcinoma	HCG stimulation of the TSH receptor
Hyperemesis gravidarum	
Familial gestational hyperthyroidism	Mutant TSH receptor with increased sensitivity to HCG
Stuma ovarii	Ovarian teratoma with functional thyroid tissue[a]
Increased Thyroid Hormone Without Increased Production	
Diagnosis	Mechanism
Subacute thyroiditis (de Quervains', granulomatous)	Release of preformed stored hormone
Postpartum and sporadic silent thyroiditis	
Medication induced thyroiditis (e.g., amiodarone, immune checkpoint inhibitor, tyrosine kinase inhibitor)	
Acute (infectious) thyroiditis	
Surgical manipulation	
Thyroid hormone ingestion	Excess exogenous thyroid hormone administration (particularly T3 containing)

[a]Increased hormone not by the thyroid itself but by extra-thyroidal tissue.
HCG, Human chorionic gonadotropin; *T3,* triiodothyronine; *TSH,* thyroid stimulating hormone.

and helpful test to demonstrate the presence and degree of thyroid hormone excess. However, the degree of thyroid hormone excess is not helpful in determining which patients simply have severe thyrotoxicosis and which have thyroid storm.[3,24,25]

When thyroid storm is suspected, other biochemical testing will help to determine the existence of organ system failure and/or presence of other acute conditions. Although laboratory information can be helpful in the evaluation of these patients, there is no test that confirms or excludes the diagnosis of thyroid storm.[4,26] Many laboratory abnormalities, including mild hyperglycemia, hypercalcemia, normocytic anemia, and elevation in alkaline phosphatase, are commonly seen in thyrotoxicosis.[26] Because serum creatinine levels are lowered in the thyrotoxic state, providers should recognize that acute kidney injury may be underestimated. Despite frequently exhibiting mildly increased international normalized ratio (INR), studies have indicated relative hypercoagulability and increased risk of thrombosis in thyrotoxic patients. Elevated transaminase levels may be present in thyroid storm complicated by hepatic dysfunction, and elevated bilirubin is a particularly important finding, as it has been correlated with adverse outcomes in thyroid storm.[8,27]

It is critical to identify concurrent illnesses that may be precipitants of thyroid storm. In addition to a thorough physical examination, sources of infection may be identified through urinalysis, blood cultures, chest and abdominal imaging, or lumbar puncture as clinically indicated. Evaluations should include looking for potential ACS, hyperglycemia and ketosis consistent with DKA, and drug use (especially cocaine and methamphetamines).

DIAGNOSIS OF THYROID STORM

Thyroid storm is a clinical diagnosis. Hospitalized patients with suspected or confirmed thyrotoxicosis should be evaluated for the severity of disease to identify those with clinical decompensation who would be defined as having thyroid storm. Coming to absolute agreement on the diagnosis of thyroid storm is less important than identifying the subset of thyrotoxic patients with the features of thyroid storm, because these patients are at the highest risk of morbidity or mortality and should receive emergent and directed therapy.

Traditionally, thyroid storm has been recognized as a clinical syndrome involving thyrotoxicosis, hyperthermia, alerted mentation, and a precipitating event.[13,28,29] These findings, along with clinical evidence of congestive heart failure, identify patients at greatest risk for adverse hospital-based outcomes and mortality.[8] Biochemical confirmation of thyrotoxicosis is not necessary to diagnose thyroid storm and treatment of suspected thyroid storm should not be delayed awaiting test results. However, in unclear cases, TSH concentration should be suppressed, confirming the presence of clinically significant thyroid hormone excess. TSH levels will most often be at the lower limit of detectability (e.g., 0.01 mIU/L) or undetectable.[8] Mildly reduced TSH concentrations (0.1–0.5 mIU/L) frequently seen in patients with nonthyroidal illness, or the "euthyroid-sick syndrome," are less suggestive of thyroid storm. The absolute level of thyroid hormone elevation is not predictive of the presence or absence of thyroid storm.[8]

Any elevated temperature should be considered consistent with thyroid storm, but fevers will frequently be pronounced (>102°F). Additional clinical manifestations of thyrotoxicosis will frequently be present, but are less specific and often present in patients with severe thyrotoxicosis without thyroid storm. Because of the subjectivity of these assessments, the variability of patient presentations, and significant overlap between these features and other acute medical conditions in hospitalized patients,[4,8,13] more objective diagnostic criteria have been published.

The Burch-Wartofsky Score (BWS) (Table 1.2) assigns points for dysfunction of the thermoregulatory, central nervous, gastrointestinal-hepatic, and cardiovascular systems, with increasing points given for greater severity of dysfunction.[30] A score of greater than 45 is considered highly suspicious, and very sensitive, for thyroid storm, but this cut-off is not specific, indicating thyroid storm in patients for whom this label is likely not appropriate.[8] Furthermore, a patient with a score below 45 may still clinically be considered to have thyroid storm for which treatment should be given. Although potentially useful in quantifying disease severity, the numerical score should not supplant physician judgment. Other reported diagnostic criteria have not been clinically validated. Regardless of the precise criteria used, once a diagnosis of thyroid storm is confirmed or highly suspected, treatment should be initiated without delay.

TREATMENT OF THYROID STORM

The treatment of thyroid storm should be initiated as early as possible after recognition of the diagnosis. The essential elements of treatment (Table 1.3) involve: (1) intensive supportive care; (2) decreasing β-adrenergic receptor stimulation; (3) decreasing thyroid hormone production and release; (4) decreasing the peripheral availability of T3; and (5) the treatment of precipitating or intercurrent medical conditions. Multimodality treatment addressing these aspects of thyrotoxic decompensation is crucial. Advances in intensive care practices and specific therapy have been

TABLE 1.2 ■ **Burch-Wartofsky Diagnostic Criteria for Thyroid Storm**

Parameter	Score	Parameter	Score
Thermoregulatory		Cardiovascular	
• Temperature (°F)		• Heart Rate (bpm)	
99.0–99.9	5	100–109	5
100.0–100.9	10	110–119	10
101.0–101.9	15	120–129	15
102.0–102.9	20	130–139	20
103.0–103.9	25	>=140	25
>=104.0	30	• Atrial Fibrillation	
		Absent	0
Central Nervous System		Present	10
Absent	0	• Congestive Heart Failure	
Mild (agitation)	10	Absent	0
Moderate (delirium, psychosis, extreme lethargy)	20	Mild (pedal edema)	5
Severe (seizure, coma)	30	Moderate (bibasilar rales)	10
		Severe (Pulmonary edema)	15
Precipitant History			
Negative	0	Gastrointestinal–Hepatic	
Positive	10	Absent	0
		Moderate (diarrhea, abdominal pain, nausea/vomiting)	10
		Severe (jaundice)	20
Total Score	Diagnosis of Thyroid Storm		
>45	Likely		
25–45	Impending		
<25	Unlikely		

driving forces in reducing the mortality of thyroid storm from 100% to approximately 8% to 25% in recent series.[8,31,32] Notably, for patients with severe thyrotoxicosis who are considered to have "impending" thyroid storm based on clinical evaluation or a BWS of 25 to 45, similar treatment to thyroid storm may be considered.

Supportive Care

Hemodynamic stabilization is critical in cases of thyroid storm as it is for all unstable patients, but warrants specific consideration because of differences in the underlying physiology of

TABLE 1.3 ■ **Essential Treatment of Thyroid Storm**

Supportive Therapy			
Hemodynamic Support			
	Intensive care unit admission		
	IV fluid resuscitation		
	Consider invasive hemodynamic monitoring		
	Intubation and mechanic ventilation		
	Vasopressor agents		
Reduce Hyperthermia			
	Cooling blankets, ice packs		
	Acetaminophen, chlorpromazine		
Treat Underlying Conditions			
	Appropriate management for concurrent illnesses (may include broad spectrum antibiotics, medication or interventions for acute coronary syndromes, continuous glucose infusion for diabetic ketoacidosis, blood products and analgesia for trauma)		
Disease-Specific Therapy			
Treatment	Mechanism	Intervention	Dosing
β-adrenergic blockade[a]	Inhibit β-adrenergic receptor stimulation Inhibit T4→T3 conversion	Propranolol Esmolol	IV: 0.5–1.0 mg every 4 h; continuous infusion 5–10 mg/h PO: 60–80 mg every 4 h continuous infusion 0.05–0.1 mg/kg per min
Antithyroid Drugs	Inhibit thyroid hormone production Inhibit T4→T3 conversion (PTU)	PTU Methimazole	PO[b]: Loading dose 500–1000 mg, 250 mg every 4 h PO[b]: 60–80 mg daily
Iodines	Inhibit thyroid hormone release from the thyroid	SSKI	5 drops (50 mg/drop, 250 mg) every 6 h
Glucocorticoids	Inhibit T4→T3 conversion Treat possible concurrent adrenal insufficiency	Hydrocortisone	IV: Loading dose 300 mg, 100 mg every 8 h

[a]Other beta-blockers (e.g., metoprolol, carvedilol) have not been specifically studied, but may be appropriate based on clinical circumstances.
[b]In patients unable to take PO medications, nasogastric tube administration can be considered. IV and per rectum dosing has been reported in the literature (see text).
IV, Intravenous; *PO,* per os (orally); *PTU,* propylthiouracil; *SSKI,* saturated solution of potassium iodine.

thyrotoxicosis. Because of the frequent need for invasive therapies and close monitoring, management in the intensive care unit (ICU) is most appropriate for cases of thyroid storm.

Optimization of volume status is a paramount consideration in the initial management of thyroid storm.[13,26] Insufficient volume status may be due to absolute volume depletion from diaphoresis or gastrointestinal losses, or inadequate volume to maintain perfusion due to vasodilation or reduced cardiac function. The etiology of shock may be multifactorial, and invasive hemodynamic monitoring with pulmonary artery catheterization is often appropriate. When hypotension is not responsive to fluid resuscitation, vasopressor agents may be required for hemodynamic support. Care should be taken when using sedatives, narcotics, and diuretics that may lower blood pressure and worsen hypoperfusion.[4]

The treatment of hyperthermia may be accomplished through cooling measures such as cooling blankets or ice packs. Medical treatment with acetaminophen is preferred because salicylates inhibit thyroid hormone binding to serum proteins, thereby increasing free hormone levels.[33] Treatment of the central mechanisms of increased thermogenesis can be addressed by intravenous (IV) chlorpromazine 25 to 50 mcg or meperidine.[4]

Finally, addressing underlying illnesses is a vital aspect in the treatment of thyroid storm.[15] Appropriate management will necessarily depend on the etiology. Broad-spectrum empiric antibiotics should be considered given the frequency with which infections are implicated.

Beta-Blockers

Blocking of β-adrenergic receptor activity is one of the most important aspects of therapy of thyroid storm. Mazzaferri et al.[1] demonstrated a significant reduction in thyroid storm mortality after introduction of therapy reducing β-adrenergic stimulation. Decreased β-adrenergic activity may improve tachycardia, cardiac workload, oxygen demand, agitation, tremor, fever, and diaphoresis. Propranolol inhibits the type 1 deiodinase enzyme that converts T4 to T3 at doses above 160 mg per day, and therefore can additionally contribute to reducing the availability of active thyroid hormone.

Regimens include initial IV propranolol doses of 0.5 to 1.0 mg, followed by continuous infusions of 5 to 10 mg/hour.[4] Oral propranolol may be given at 60 to 80 mg every 4 hours. The short-acting β-adrenergic blocker esmolol is an alternative used as a 0.25- to 0.50-mg/kg loading dose followed by continuous infusion rates of 0.05 to 0.1 mg/kg per minute.[34,35] Fluid resuscitation should be utilized to support blood pressure during use of beta-blockade. Therapy should be titrated to achieve heart rates of 90 to 110 bpm in afebrile patients rather than slower rates.[4] Several case reports have raised concerns regarding the use of beta-blockers in thyroid storm due to cardiovascular collapse suffered after initiation of therapy.[36–40] This may have been due to the over-vigorous applications of beta-blockade and/or insufficient volume replacement. Careful monitoring and use of shorter-acting agents aim to attenuate this risk. Some have considered beta-blockers relatively contraindicated in patients with CHF or reactive airway disease,[41] but given the fundamental role of beta-blockade in the management of thyroid storm, use should not be omitted unless absolutely necessary.

Antithyroid Drugs

Antithyroid drugs (ATD), methimazole and propothyouracil (PTU), inhibit the enzymatic steps necessary for thyroid hormone production. PTU is favored in the treatment of thyroid storm because it decreases peripheral conversion of T4 to T3, and has been shown to reduce serum thyroid hormone levels more rapidly than methimazole.[42,43] Though the absolute risks are very small, vasculitis and hepatic failure are more frequent side effects of PTU compared with methimazole.[44] Other adverse reactions of ATD therapy include agranulocytosis, transaminase elevation, cholestasis, or urticarial rash. A previous significant adverse reaction such as agranulocytosis is a contraindication to ATD use. If other adverse reactions occur with PTU use, treatment with methimazole can be attempted. Recommended PTU treatment is a loading dose of 500 to 1000 mg, then 250 mg every 4 hours. Alternatively, methimazole is administered at 60 to 80 mg daily.[15] ATD should be given at least 1 hour before iodine preparations in the treatment of thyrotoxicosis to prevent iodine from being used to produce additional thyroid hormone.

Only oral formulations of ATD are available in the United States, but patients with vomiting, altered mental status, or critical illness may have barriers to enteric administration or absorption of medications. Rectal and intravenous formulations of ATD have been employed to address this.[45] Per rectum administration of PTU and methimazole has been reported, but requires specially made suppository or enema formulations. One study made an IV preparation of PTU dissolving tablets in isotonic saline with an alkaline pH of 9.25 to create a dose of 50 mg/mL. Perhaps because it is more readily soluble, IV methimazole has been more frequently reported, with reconstitution in 0.9% saline solution and given as a slow IV push.[46,47]

Iodine

Inorganic iodine produces rapid decreases in thyroidal hormone release and circulating thyroid hormone levels near normal within 4 to 5 days.[48] This may be given as saturated solution of potassium iodide (SSKI) 250 mg every 6 hours. Iodine treatment should not be started until 1 hour after administration of ATD in order to prevent iodine incorporation and increased production of thyroid hormone.[13] The benefit of iodine treatment is likely limited to 72 hours of treatment.

Lithium

Lithium causes inhibition of thyroid hormone release from the thyroid and has been utilized in the treatment of thyroid storm.[49] Data regarding the efficacy of lithium are limited, but expert guidance for dosing recommends 300 mg lithium carbonate given every 6 hours with titration to serum lithium levels of 0.8 to 1.2 mEq/L.[15,26] Although not a component of standard therapy, lithium is occasionally used in cases where ATD are contraindicated.

Steroids

The use of glucocorticoids in the treatment of thyroid storm acts to reduce conversion of T4 to T3, as well as addressing the possibility of concurrent adrenal insufficiency that may exist, particularly in autoimmune etiologies of thyrotoxicosis. An initial dose of hydrocortisone 300 mg followed by 100 mg every 8 hours is considered adequate therapy.[15] Glucocorticoids may worsen hyperglycemia. Animal and human studies have raised concern that glucocorticoid use post–myocardial infarction is associated with ventricular thinning and free wall rupture,[50] but a metaanalysis of the limited data available did not find an increased risk.[51] Glucocorticoid therapy should still be considered carefully in this population. Another population where the use of steroids should be considered on an individual basis is patients with thyroid storm due to checkpoint inhibitor immunotherapy (e.g., PD-1, CTLA-4 inhibitors). These drugs mediate a destructive thyroiditis, the severity and duration of which were not significantly decreased by glucocorticoid use in one retrospective analysis,[18] and it remains unclear whether steroids may decrease the effectiveness of cancer immunotherapy.

Adjunct Treatments

In cases where patients remain critically ill despite therapy for thyroid storm, or when aspects of therapy are contraindicated, adjunctive therapies have been employed, including plasmapheresis, L-carnitine, and thyroidectomy. Perhaps the most common situation when these adjuncts are considered is in the face of life-threatening thyrotoxicosis in a patient with contraindications to ATD (e.g., agranulocytosis, hepatocellular injury). The evidence for these measures remains largely anecdotal or retrospective, but may be considered when standard therapy is insufficient.

Plasmapheresis, or therapeutic plasma exchange, is an adjunctive therapy used in patients with severe thyrotoxicosis or thyroid storm who remain critically ill despite standard therapy.[52–55] Treatment has been reported to reduce free thyroid hormone levels and result in clinical improvement. Plasmapheresis has been employed in the preoperative period to improve manifestations of thyrotoxicosis and enable patients to undergo surgery more safely.[56]

The proposed mechanism of plasmapheresis therapy in thyroid storm is removal of circulating thyroid hormone, which has a long serum half-life and is largely protein bound. In this procedure, patient plasma is extracted from other blood components and replaced with a colloid solution, such as fresh frozen plasma and albumin. Thyroid-binding globulin with bound thyroid hormone is removed, and colloid replacement provides new binding sites for circulating free thyroid hormone. Estimated adverse event rates of 5% include transfusion reaction, citrate-related nausea, vasovagal or hypotensive reactions, respiratory distress, and tetany or seizure.

The use of plasmapheresis can be considered in patients refractory to conventional therapy, particularly when ATD are contraindicated, as a stabilizing measure or bridge to safer definitive surgery, or for destructive etiologies of thyroid storm (e.g., thyroiditis, AIT) that are less responsive to ATD. The usual plasmapheresis protocols reported in patients with thyroid storm used a 2.5- to 3-L volume of combined fresh-frozen plasma and 5% albumin.[53,55,57–59]

Additionally, use of albumin-based dialysis when initial plasmapheresis was unsuccessful has been reported.[60,61] Thyroid hormone is ineffectively cleared by usual hemodialysis, but rapid hormone clearance may be achieved with continuous renal replacement therapy or other equivalent forms of continuous hemodialysis with albumin supplementation to dialysate in hemodynamically unstable patients. Techniques extrapolated from those used in liver failure and hepatorenal syndrome have been reported for thyroid storm, including 4% human serum albumin with blood flow at 150 mL/minute, dialysate flow at 1.5 L/hour, and durations lasting 12 hours.[61] Furthermore, because of the continuous nature of these therapies, which are not dose limited by the exchange transfusion risks of plasmapheresis, more cumulative thyroxine may be removed.[60,61]

L-carnitine has been suggested as a therapy for hyperthyroidism and thyroid storm, usually in cases refractory to conventional therapy or where ATD are contraindicated. The proposed mechanism of action is inhibition of thyroid hormone (T3) uptake into cell nuclei by amine L-carnitine. Several case reports of L-carnitine in thyroid storm claim clinical improvement in mental status, but results are confounded by concurrent administration of other treatments.[62–64] The current data are insufficient to suggest use of L-carnitine in thyroid storm patients.

Thyroidectomy provides definitive therapy for thyrotoxicosis caused by thyroidal production or release of hormone. Thyroid surgery may be considered particularly in cases with hyperthyroidism due to more persistent and recalcitrant causes, such as refractory AIT or Graves' disease. In thyroid storm, the benefit of thyroidectomy is often weighed against the risk of anesthesia and surgery. Retrospective reports of total or subtotal thyroidectomy in thyrotoxic patients demonstrate decreased serum thyroid hormone levels and clinical improvement over 2 to 10 days postoperatively. Kaderli et al.[65] described a cohort of 11 patients with AIT who failed medical therapy and were treated with total thyroidectomy under general anesthesia. In this series there were no major intraoperative complications, no incident thyroid storm, and all patients survived. Similar results were seen in earlier series of AIT, including in patients with significant heart failure.[66–68] In patients with thyrotoxicosis due to Graves' disease, a recent retrospective case series compared surgical outcomes in 247 patients undergoing elective thyroidectomy after complete medical control of Graves' disease versus 19 patients undergoing urgent thyroidectomy after rapid optimization for 1 to 2 weeks, at a single center.[69] This study found no differences between populations with regard to the incidence of thyroid storm, vocal cord palsy, postoperative bleeding, or hypoparathyroidism. Although prospective, randomized data is lacking, these studies suggest that, in patients intolerant of standard medical management, with an experienced multidisciplinary team, surgery may be considered as an alternative definitive therapy.

TREATMENT OF COMPENSATED THYROTOXICOSIS

Patients without thyroid storm who are nonetheless thyrotoxic may benefit from disease-specific treatment while hospitalized. Adequate fluid resuscitation should be provided to adequately correct hypovolemia. The application of beta-blockers for the amelioration of adrenergic symptoms is generally appropriate regardless of the etiology of thyrotoxicosis, with initial doses of propranolol of 10 to 40 mg every 8 hours, or an equivalent, depending on the degree of symptoms, blood pressure and heart rate tolerability, the presence of CHF, and any contraindications. The use of beta-blockers, diuretics for management of volume excess, or sedative-hypnotics for treating insomnia or anxiety must be monitored closely, as blood pressure reductions and hypoperfusion can precipitate thyroid storm.

Socioeconomic Factors

Compared with compensated thyrotoxicosis, thyroid storm portends a higher hospital mortality, greater incidence of ICU admission and intubation, and overall longer hospital and ICU length of stay.[8,9] Additionally, within patients diagnosed with thyroid storm, patients who were male, older than 65 years, Black, and who had multiple other comorbid conditions had longer hospitalizations and greater healthcare costs.[9] Sherman et al.[70] previously reported that poor socioeconomic conditions were a risk factor for complicated thyrotoxicosis and thyroid storm. These findings were recently corroborated by a retrospective study of thyrotoxic patients from 2011–2017 by Rivas et al.,[19] with an increased risk of thyroid storm associated with lack of health insurance, lower education, and residing in areas with lower median income. These factors likely underlie, in part, the higher frequency of thyroid storm reported among patients with thyrotoxicosis in studies based at medical centers serving large underserved populations[8,19] compared with nationwide, database studies.[9] Given the higher morbidity, mortality, and healthcare costs associated with thyroid storm, improving access to medical care and addressing societal factors leading to medication noncompliance or late diagnosis of thyrotoxicosis may be steps to improve outcomes for thyroid storm.

Follow-up After Discharge

Discharge plan should include a timely follow-up visit with an endocrinologist for continued treatment. Interruption of prescribed doses of beta-blockers, antithyroid drugs, or steroids can result in recurrence of clinical symptoms. Strong consideration should be given to definitive treatment of persistent causes of thyrotoxicosis, such as Graves' disease, given the possibility of further morbidity or thyroid storm if there is recurrent thyrotoxicosis.

Conclusions

Thyroid storm is a rare but life-threatening endocrine emergency that must be considered in the presentation of a patient with thyrotoxicosis. When diagnosed, prompt treatment should be initiated to correct hemodynamic instability and attenuate the presence and effects of excess thyroid hormones. Application of current critical care medicine and multimodality treatment of thyrotoxicosis has been successful in substantially lowering the mortality of thyroid storm.

References

1. Mazzaferri EL, Skillman TG. Thyroid storm. A review of 22 episodes with special emphasis on the use of guanethidine. *Arch Intern Med.* 1969;124(6):684–690.
2. Pimentel L, Hansen KN. Thyroid disease in the emergency department. A clinical and laboratory review. *Clin Lab Em Med.* 2005;28(2):201–209.
3. Tietgens ST, Leinung MC. Thyroid storm. *Med Clin North Am.* 1995;79(1):169–184.
4. Nicoloff JT. Thyroid storm and myxedema coma. *Med Clin North Am.* 1985;69(5):1005–1017.
5. Maddock WG, Pedersen S, Coller FA. Studies of the blood chemistry in thyroid crisis. *JAMA.* 1937; 109(26):2130–2135.

6. Roizen M, Becker CE. Thyroid storm. A review of cases at University of California, San Francisco. *Calif Med.* 1971;115(4):5–9.
7. Dillon PT, Babe J, Meloni CR, Canary JJ. Reserpine in thyrotoxic crisis. *N Engl J Med.* 1970;283(19):1020–1023.
8. Angell TE, Lechner MG, Nguyen CT, Salvato VL, Nicoloff JT, LoPresti JS. Clinical features and hospital outcomes in thyroid storm: a retrospective cohort study. *J Clin Endocrinol Metab.* 2015;100(2):451–459.
9. Galindo RJ, Hurtado CR, Pasquel FJ, García Tome R, Peng L, Umpierrez GE. National trends in incidence, mortality, and clinical outcomes of patients hospitalized for thyrotoxicosis with and without thyroid storm in the United States, 2004-2013. *Thyroid.* 2019;29(1):36–43.
10. Klein I, Danzi S. Thyroid disease and the heart. *Curr Probl Cardiol.* 2016;41(2):65–92.
11. Klein I, Danzi S. Thyroid disease and the heart. *Circulation.* 2007;116(15):1725–1735.
12. Kahaly GJ, Kampmann C, Mohr-Kahaly S. Cardiovascular hemodynamics and exercise tolerance in thyroid disease. *Thyroid.* 2002;12(6):473–481.
13. Ingbar SH. Management of emergencies. IX. Thyrotoxic storm. *N Engl J Med.* 1966;274(22):1252–1254.
14. Mohananey D, Smilowitz N, Villablanca PA, et al. Trends in the incidence and in-hospital outcomes of cardiogenic shock complicating thyroid storm. *Am J Med Sci.* 2017;354(2):159–164.
15. Braverman LE, Cooper DS. Introduction to thyrotoxicosis. In: Braverman LE, Cooper D, eds. *Werner & Ingbar's The Thyroid: A Fundamental and Clinical Text.* 10th ed. Philadelphia: Lippincott Williams and Wilkins; 2013.
16. Burch HB. Drug effects on the thyroid. *N Engl J Med.* 2019;381:749–761.
17. Yonezaki K, Kobayashi T, Imachi H, et al. Combination therapy of ipilimumab and nivolumab induced thyroid storm in a patient with Hashimoto's disease and diabetes mellitus: a case report. *J Med Case Rep.* 2018;12(1):171.
18. Ma C, Hodi FS, Giobbie-Hurder A, et al. the impact of high-dose glucocorticoids on the outcome of immune-checkpoint inhibitor-related thyroid disorders. *Cancer Immunol Res.* 2019;7(7):1214–1220.
19. Rivas AM, Larumbe E, Thavaraputta S, Juarez E, Adiga A, Lado-Abeal J. Unfavorable socioeconomic factors underlie high rates of hospitalization for complicated thyrotoxicosis in some regions of the United States. *Thyroid.* 2019;29(1):27–35.
20. Ross DS, Burch HB, Cooper DS, et al. American Thyroid Association guidelines for diagnosis and management of hyperthyroidism and other causes of thyrotoxicosis *Thyroid.*. 2016;26(10):1343–1421.
21. Ramírez JI, Petrone P, Kuncir EJ, Asensio JA. Thyroid storm induced by strangulation. *South Med J.* 2004;97(6):608–610.
22. Noh KW, Seon CS, Choi JW, Cho YB, Park JY, Kim HJ. Thyroid storm and reversible thyrotoxic cardiomyopathy after ingestion of seafood stew thought to contain marine neurotoxin. *Thyroid.* 2011;21(6):679–682.
23. Delikoukos S, Mantzos F. Thyroid storm induced by trauma due to spear fishing-gun trident impaction in the neck. *Emerg Med J.* 2007;24(5):355–356.
24. Brooks MH, Waldstein SS, Bronsky D, Sterling K. Serum triiodothyronine concentration in thyroid storm. *J Clin Endocrinol Metab.* 1975;40(2):339–341.
25. Brooks MH, Waldstein SS. Free thyroxine concentrations in thyroid storm. *Ann Intern Med.* 1980;93(5):694–697.
26. Klubo-Gwiezdzinska J, Wartofsky L. Thyroid emergencies. *Med Clin North Am.* 2012;96(2):385–403.
27. Choudhary AM, Roberts I. Thyroid storm presenting with liver failure. *J Clin Gastroenterol.* 1999;29(4):318–321.
28. McArthur JW, Rawson RW, Means JH, Cope O. Thyrotoxic crisis; an analysis of the thirty-six cases at the Massachusetts General Hospital during the past twenty-five years. *J Am Med Assoc.* 1947;134(10):868–874.
29. Weldstein SS, Slodki SJ, Kagantec GI, Bronsky D. A clinical study of thyroid storm. *Ann Intern Med.* 1960;52(3):626–642.
30. Burch HB, Wartofsky L. Life-threatening thyrotoxicosis. Thyroid storm. *Endocrinol Metab Clin North Am.* 1993;22(2):263–277.
31. Akamizu T, Satoh T, et al. Diagnostic criteria, clinical features, and incidence of thyroid storm based on nationwide surveys *Thyroid.*. 2012;22(7):661–679.
32. Swee du S, Chng CL, Lim A. Clinical characteristics and outcome of thyroid storm: a case series and review of neuropsychiatric derangements in thyrotoxicosis. *Endocr Pract.* 2015;21(2):182–189.

33. Larsen PR. Salicylate-induced increases in free triiodothyronine in human serum. Evidence of inhibition of triiodothyronine binding to thyroxine-binding globulin and thyroxine-binding prealbumin. *J Clin Invest*. 1972;51(5):1125–1134.
34. Knighton JD, Crosse MM. Anaesthetic management of childhood thyrotoxicosis and the use of esmolol. *Anaesthesia*. 1997;52(1):67–70.
35. Duggal J, Singh S, Kuchinic P, Butler P, Arora R. Utility of esmolol in thyroid crisis. *Can J Clin Pharmacol*. 2006;13(3):e292–e295.
36. Dalan R, Leow MK. Cardiovascular collapse associated with beta blockade in thyroid storm. *Exp Clin Endocrinol Diabetes*. 2007;115(6):392–396.
37. Ashikaga H, Abreu R, Schneider R. Propranolol administration in a patient with thyroid storm. *Ann Intern Med*. 2000;132(8):681–682.
38. Boccalandro C, Boccalandro F, Orlander P, Wei CP. Severe reversible dilated cardiomyopathy and hyperthyroidism: case report and review of literature. *Endocr Pract*. 2003;9(2):140–146.
39. Fraser T, Green D. Weathering the storm: beta-blockade and the potential for disaster in severe hyperthyroidism. *Emerg Med (Fremantle)*. 2001;13(3):376–380.
40. Vijayakumar H, Thomas W, Ferrara J. Perioperative management of severe thyrotoxicosis with esmolol. *Anaesthesia*. 1989;44(5):406–408.
41. Nayak B, Burman K. Thyrotoxicosis and thyroid storm. *Endocrinol Metab Clin North Am*. 2006;35(4):663–686, vii.
42. Cooper DS, Saxe VC, Meskell M, Maloof F, Ridgway EC. Acute effects of propylthiouracil (PTU) on thyroidal iodide organification and peripheral iodothyronine deiodination: correlation with serum PTU levels measured by radioimmunoassay. *J Clin Endocrinol Metab*. 1982;54(1):101–107.
43. Abuid J, Larsen PR. Triiodothyronine and thyroxine in hyperthyroidism. Comparison of the acute changes during therapy with antithyroid agents. *J Clin Invest*. 1974;54(1):201–208.
44. Roti E, Robuschi G, Gardini E, et al. Comparison of methimazole, methimazole and sodium ipodate, and methimazole and saturated solution of potassium iodide in the early treatment of hyperthyroid Graves' disease. *Clin Endocrinol (Oxf)*. 1988;28(3):305–314.
45. Alfadhli E, Gianoukakis AG. Management of severe thyrotoxicosis when the gastrointestinal tract is compromised. *Thyroid*. 2011;21(3):215–220.
46. Hodak SP, Huang C, Clarke D, Burman KD, Jonklaas J, Janicic-Kharic N. Intravenous methimazole in the treatment of refractory hyperthyroidism. *Thyroid*. 2006;16(7):691–695.
47. Thomas DJ, Hardy J, Sarwar R, et al. Thyroid storm treated with intravenous methimazole in patients with gastrointestinal dysfunction. *Br J Hosp Med (Lond)*. 2006;67(9):492–493.
48. Wartofsky L, Ransil BJ, Ingbar SH. Inhibition by iodine of the release of thyroxine from the thyroid glands of patients with thyrotoxicosis. *J Clin Invest*. 1970;94:174–183.
49. Boehm TM, Burman KD, Barnes S, Wartofsky L. Lithium and iodine combination therapy for thyrotoxicosis. *Acta Endocrinol (Copenh)*. 1980;94(2):174–183.
50. Sholter DE, Armstrong PW. Adverse effects of corticosteroids on the cardiovascular system. *Can J Cardiol*. 2000;16(4):505–511.
51. Giugliano GR, Giugliano RP, Gibson CM, Kuntz RE. Meta-analysis of corticosteroid treatment in acute myocardial infarction. *Am J Cardiol*. 2003;91(9):1055–1059.
52. Muller C, Perrin P, Faller B, Richter S, Chantrel F. Role of plasma exchange in the thyroid storm. *Ther Apher Dial*. 2011;15(6):522–531.
53. Ashkar FS, Katims RB, Smoak 3rd WM, Gilson AJ. Thyroid storm treatment with blood exchange and plasmapheresis. *JAMA*. 1970;214(7):1275–1279.
54. Vyas AA, Vyas P, Fillipon NL, Vijayakrishnan R, Trivedi N. Successful treatment of thyroid storm with plasmapheresis in a patient with methimazole-induced agranulocytosis. *Endocr Pract*. 2010;16(4):673–676.
55. Carhill A, Gutierrez A, Lakhia R, Nalini R. Surviving the storm: two cases of thyroid storm successfully treated with plasmapheresis. *BMJ Case Rep*. 2012;2012. pii: bcr2012006696.
56. Ezer A, Caliskan K, Parlakgumus A, Belli S, Kozanoglu I, Yildirim S. Preoperative therapeutic plasma exchange in patients with thyrotoxicosis. *J Clin Apher*. 2009;24(3):111–114.
57. Zhu L, Zainudin SB, Kaushik M, Khor LY, Chng CL. Plasma exchange in the treatment of thyroid storm secondary to type II amiodarone-induced thyrotoxicosis. *Endocrinol Diabetes Metab Case Rep*. 2016;2016:160039.

58. Samaras K, Marel GM. Failure of plasmapheresis, corticosteroids and thionamides to ameliorate a case of protracted amiodarone-induced thyroiditis. *Clin Endocrinol (Oxf)*. 1996;45(3):365–368.
59. Shah KK, Mbughuni MM, Burgstaler EA, Block DR, Winters JL. Iatrogenic thyrotoxicosis and the role of therapeutic plasma exchange. *J Clin Apher*. 2017;32(6):579–583.
60. Park HS, Kwon SK, Kim YN. Successful treatment of thyroid storm presenting as recurrent cardiac arrest and subsequent multiorgan failure by continuous renal replacement therapy. *Endocrinol Diabetes Metab Case Rep*. 2017;2017. pii:16-0115.
61. Koball S, Hickstein H, Gloger M, et al. Treatment of thyrotoxic crisis with plasmapheresis and single pass albumin dialysis: a case report. *Artif Organs*. 2010;34(2):E55–E58.
62. Benvenga S, Lapa D, Cannavò S, Trimarchi F. Successive thyroid storms treated with L-carnitine and low doses of methimazole. *Am J Med*. 2003;115(5):417–418.
63. Chee R, Agah R, Vita R, Benvenga S. L-carnitine treatment in a seriously ill cancer patient with severe hyperthyroidism. *Hormones (Athens)*. 2014;13(3):407–412.
64. Kimmoun A, Munagamage G, Dessalles N, Gerard A, Feillet F, Levy B. Unexpected awakening from comatose thyroid storm after a single intravenous injection of L-carnitine. *Intensive Care Med*. 2011;37(10):1716–1717.
65. Kaderli RM, Fahrner R, Christ ER, et al. Total thyroidectomy for amiodarone-induced thyrotoxicosis in the hyperthyroid state. *Exp Clin Endocrinol Diabetes*. 2016;124(1):45–48.
66. Hamoir E, Meurisse M, Defechereux T, Joris J, Vivario J, Hennen G. Surgical management of amiodarone-associated thyrotoxicosis: too risky or too effective? *World J Surg*. 1998;22(6):537–542; discussion 542-543.
67. Gough J, Gough IR. Total thyroidectomy for amiodarone-associated thyrotoxicosis in patients with severe cardiac disease. *World J Surg*. 2006;30(11):1957–1961.
68. Tomisti L, Materazzi G, Bartalena L, et al. Total thyroidectomy in patients with amiodarone-induced thyrotoxicosis and severe left ventricular systolic dysfunction. *J Clin Endocrinol Metab*. 2012;97(10):3515–3521.
69. Ali A, Debono M, Balasubramanian SP. Outcomes after urgent thyroidectomy following rapid control of thyrotoxicosis in Graves' disease are similar to those after elective surgery in well-controlled disease. *World J Surg*. 2019;43(12):3051–3058.
70. Sherman SI, Simonson L, Ladenson PW. Clinical and socioeconomic predispositions to complicated thyrotoxicosis: a predictable and preventable syndrome? *Am J Med*. 1996;101(2):192–198.

CHAPTER 2

Amiodarone-Induced Thyrotoxicosis

Anupam Kotwal ■ Marius N. Stan

CHAPTER OUTLINE

Introduction

Amiodarone is a benzofuranic acid with potent antiarrhythmic properties that contains iodine amounting to 37% of its weight. Thus a 200-mg tablet (typical maintenance daily dose) provides approximately 70 mg of iodine of which 50% is bioavailable. This should be considered in the context of daily recommended iodine intake of 150 mcg per person.[1] Consequently, amiodarone causes thyroid dysfunction in 15% to 20% of cases,[2–4] with the incidence of thyrotoxicosis being approximately 3% to 9%.[4–7] Amiodarone-induced hypothyroidism is more common in iodine-replete regions[7] but fortunately easier to manage than the less commonly encountered entity of amiodarone-induced thyrotoxicosis (AIT). The approach to AIT has subtype, diagnostic, and management challenges, and at times this condition leads to life-threatening complications. This is due to multiple factors, including the use of this drug in patients with preexisting cardiovascular conditions, the lack of a consistently effective therapy, the prolonged half-life of amiodarone (2 to 3 months),[8] and the fact that its discontinuation is not always feasible in the setting of life-threatening arrhythmias refractory to conventional antiarrhythmic medications.

AIT is particularly associated with increased mortality in older individuals and in those with impaired ventricular function, possibly due to a combination of preexisting cardiac dysfunction and a superimposed high-output thyrotoxic state, precipitating heart failure in these patients.[9–12] Yiu et al. demonstrated that AIT predicted an adverse cardiovascular outcome in up to 31.6% and cardiovascular mortality in 12.6% of these patients.[11] Similarly, O'Sullivan et al. demonstrated that AIT was associated with a mortality rate of 10% overall, but up to 50% in those with systolic heart failure (left ventricular ejection fraction less than 45%).[12] These observations are consistent with the recent findings in France where AIT was shown to be the most common cause of thyroid storm in patients admitted to an intensive care unit (ICU).[13] From a general viewpoint, any patient with AIT is at increased risk of deterioration because thyrotoxicosis can precipitate cardiac dysfunction even in asymptomatic patients, especially in those with cardiac conditions like systolic heart failure, ventricular arrhythmias, and congenital heart disease. The general approach to AIT and the role of specific therapeutic modalities in its management are discussed in the sections below.

Pathogenesis and Subtypes

Amiodarone causes thyroid dysfunction by one or a combination of the following mechanisms: (1) intrinsic drug factors that exhibit a dose-dependent direct toxic effect on thyroid follicular cells; and (2) iodine effects that include inhibition of deiodination of thyroxine (T4) to triiodothyronine (T3) but are further nuanced by the presence or absence of autoimmune thyroid disease or thyroid nodules.[14–16] Classically, AIT has been categorized as type 1 or type 2, but many times the cases are mixed, especially at initial presentation,[14] as shown in Table 2.1. Type 1 AIT is characterized by iodine-induced hyperthyroidism due to excess hormone synthesis, usually occurring in patients with underlying thyroid disease such as nodular goiter or latent Graves' disease.[2,14,17] On the other hand, type 2 AIT is characterized by destructive thyroiditis causing excessive thyroid hormone release and is reported to occur in patients with normal thyroid or small goiter.[2,14,17] Type 1 AIT has been more commonly reported in iodine-deficient areas, whereas type 2 AIT is more prevalent in iodine replete areas,[2,14,17,18] and is the most frequent form of AIT overall,[6] accounting for 79% of cases in one large series.[19] However, this clean separation is not evident in many cases that seem to have a mixed presentation with a combination of diagnostic features and probably mixed pathogenesis of both type 1 and type 2 AIT.[14,18,20,21]

Diagnostic Evaluation and Classification

Given the high incidence of thyroid dysfunction, patients treated with amiodarone should be screened for thyroid dysfunction by monitoring thyroid function tests (TFTs). The 2016 American

TABLE 2.1 ■ **Comparison of Types of Amiodarone-Induced Thyrotoxicosis**

Features of AIT	Type 1 AIT	Type 2 AIT	Mixed AIT
Mechanism	Excess thyroid hormone synthesis (iodine induced)	Excess release of thyroid hormone (destructive thyroiditis)	Features of both
Preexistent thyroid structure and function	Abnormal (nodules or latent Graves' disease)	Apparently normal or small goiter	Features of both
Iodine-123 thyroid uptake	Most commonly low or low-normal, but sometimes normal or increased	Usually very low or absent	Features of both
Thyroid ultrasound with CFDS	Hypervascularity	Absent or decreased vascularity	Features of both
Initial treatment	Thionamides	Antiinflammatory therapy like prednisone	Combination of both
	Rare need to add potassium perchlorate (not FDA approved)		

AIT, Amiodarone-induced thyrotoxicosis; *CFDS*, color-flow Doppler sonography; *FDA*, Food and Drug Administration.

Thyroid Association (ATA) Guidelines for Diagnosis and Management of Hyperthyroidism and Other Causes of Thyrotoxicosis[22] suggest monitoring TFTs before commencing treatment and after the first 3 months following initiation of amiodarone, and at 3- and 6-month intervals thereafter. It is important to avoid making a diagnosis of thyroid dysfunction when testing early after amiodarone initiation, as it causes transient changes in TFTs in many patients. It causes these changes by inhibiting type 1 5′-deiodinase enzyme activity, thereby decreasing the peripheral conversion of T4 to T3 and reducing the clearance of both T4 and reverse T3 (rT3). Consequently, the serum levels of T4 and rT3 increase and the serum levels of T3 decrease by 20% to 25%. Subsequently, the feedback mechanism leads to thyroid-stimulating hormone (TSH) elevation that will increase thyroid hormone production in an otherwise healthy thyroid and the equilibrium is restored with normalization of TSH. These changes typically resolve within the first 3 to 6 months. Hence, the diagnosis of hypothyroidism should be made based on TFTs obtained after 3 to 6 months of amiodarone treatment. However, the diagnosis of AIT can be made earlier if the biochemical changes of thyrotoxicosis are present and they are overt, such as undetectable TSH and elevated T4/T3. Although patients may present with clinical features similar to any other form of thyrotoxicosis, there are clinical features that may be unique to AIT. The effect of amiodarone may prevent the occurrence of symptomatic tachycardia. Also, there is a higher chance of apathetic thyrotoxicosis where the typical sympathetic features of thyrotoxicosis are absent but the patient develops weight loss, muscle weakness, and worsening of cardiac function, a concern especially in elderly patients. Some patients may only present with worsening of fluid retention, congestive heart failure, recurrence of the underlying arrhythmia after a period of quiescence, or may develop a new arrhythmia, which should raise the concern for AIT.

LABORATORY EVALUATION

AIT presents with the typical laboratory features of thyrotoxicosis of suppressed TSH and elevated thyroid hormones T4 and/or T3. Subclinical thyrotoxicosis can also be present in mild cases where T3/T4 remain normal in association with suppressed TSH. As amiodarone has no effect on the serum concentration of thyroid hormone-binding globulin (TBG), changes in the levels of free T4 and free T3 mirror those for total T4 and total T3. It is important to rule out nonthyroidal illness or drugs (heparin, dopamine, glucocorticoids, and biotin) as the only cause of the thyroid laboratory abnormalities before making a diagnosis of AIT. Patients with AIT, especially those who are hospitalized, may also have concomitant nonthyroidal illness, which decreases T3 levels; hence those may be normal when there is a combination of AIT and nonthyroidal illness.[23] The T3/T4 ratio, which tends to be higher in patients with autonomous hyperthyroidism as compared with destructive thyroiditis, is not very helpful in diagnosing AIT because of amiodarone-associated inhibition of T4 monodeiodination.[24] Testing for autoimmune etiology should be performed because presence of TSH receptor antibodies suggests latent Graves' disease, thus categorizing AIT as type 1; thyroid peroxidase (TPO) antibodies are often positive in type 1 AIT,[2] but are not pathognomonic or necessary for this diagnosis[25] (Table 2.1). Interleukin-6 (IL-6) level has been deemed in the past to help with AIT diagnosis[26] but the test is not routinely performed these days as many cases overlap in IL-6 values and the discrimination does not appear to be sensitive and specific enough.

RADIOLOGIC INVESTIGATIONS

Thyroid ultrasonography by itself has low diagnostic value in AIT, but when combined with color-flow Doppler sonography (CFDS), it provides a noninvasive real-time assessment of thyroid vascularity that can be very helpful in separating the AIT types.[13] CFDS scores from 0 (absent vascularity) to 3 (very intense vascularity) are thus employed.[27] Usually, type 2 AIT is characterized by absent thyroid gland vascularity (CFDS score 0) due to destructive thyroiditis, whereas type 1 AIT has normal to increased vascularity (CFDS score 1, 2, or 3)[17,27–29] (Table 2.1). Even though CFDS is the best option in terms of diagnostic tests to classify AIT, it is not always helpful.[30,31] It has been reported that as many as 42% of patients classified as type 2 (absent vascularity) and 64% classified as type 1 based on CFDS may not respond to the respective therapy.[31] The accuracy of thyroid ultrasonography with CFDS is also highly dependent on the operator skills and expertise. Thus whether the variability of interpreting CFDS has to do with the acquisition of the ultrasound images or to the presence of mixed AIT type remains to be determined. Twenty-four-hour iodine-123 or iodine-131 uptake of the thyroid has also been studied as a modality to classify the type of AIT. This will theoretically be very low or absent in type 2 AIT, whereas it can be low, normal, or high in type 1 AIT.[2] However, in iodine-replete areas, especially with the iodine load from amiodarone, most cases of AIT have very low or absent uptake irrespective of the type; hence this diagnostic modality is not usually a useful distinguishing investigation.[2] Other nuclear isotopes have been employed for their predictive nature in separating AIT types. The predictive nature of technetium-99m (99mTc)-sestamibi scintigraphy for AIT is low, and the numbers of patients reported as studied with these isotopes are small.[17,32,33] Hence these methods have limited clinical validation in the diagnostic evaluation of AIT and should be reserved mainly for research studies.

SUMMARIZING CLASSIFICATION OF AMIODARONE-INDUCED THYROTOXICOSIS

An effort should be made to subtype AIT based on laboratory and radiologic investigations (usually CFDS); however, many cases demonstrated features of both (Table 2.1) or may not respond to the respective therapies instituted based on the initial subtype. Hence no single investigation can accurately define the best treatment strategy, which is at least partially due to the presence of mixed forms of the disease. At the Mayo Clinic, we incorporated previously reported criteria[2,18,34] as well as our clinical experience, in addition to information obtained from thyroidectomy surgical pathology, to classify AIT subtypes as below. We used the lower limit of normal for 24-hour radioactive iodine uptake in our population, as we have reported in previous publications.[35–37]

1. Type 1 AIT: nodular thyroid or diffuse goiter greater than 15 g or positive TSH receptor antibody titer; with normal/increased thyroid vascularity on CFDS or 24-hour radioactive iodine uptake greater than 8%.
2. Type 2 AIT: normal thyroid or small diffuse goiter less than 15 g; with negative TSH receptor antibody titer and low thyroid vascularity on ultrasound CFDS.
3. Mixed: nodular thyroid or diffuse goiter greater than 15 g or positive antithyroid antibodies; with low thyroid vascularity on ultrasound CFDS.

From the clinical standpoint, AIT can develop at any time during or even after the discontinuation of amiodarone because of the large deposits of this lipophilic medication in the adipose tissues, which explains its long half-life.[8] Following prospectively 200 AIT patients, Tomisti et al showed that type 1 AIT cases demonstrated significantly higher thyroid hormone levels and an earlier average onset of disease after amiodarone initiation as compared with type 2 (average of 3.5 months versus 30 months);[19] hence higher severity and earlier onset of thyrotoxicosis may be used as additional criteria to subtype AIT as type 1.

Approach to Management

There is a degree of divergence between the experts regarding the importance of identifying the type of AIT (Table 2.1) in order to guide its management. This is because the data on this issue are mixed, with some studies clearly supporting its role and others demonstrating that initial therapy choice and the subsequent response to it are not altered by the type of AIT. The 2016

ATA Guidelines for Diagnosis and Management of Hyperthyroidism and Other Causes of Thyrotoxicosis[22] argue that as the pathogenesis of AIT is not fully understood, the classic division of AIT into two subtypes likely represents an oversimplification. They argue that many patients have mixed AIT forms, patients classified as type 1 or 2 often fail to respond to the subtype directed therapy, and, lastly, that some cases of type 2 AIT respond to measures not typically useful in destructive thyroiditis, such as perchlorate and oral cholecystographic agents. It is probably for this reason that several recent series did not attempt to classify the AIT subtypes.[12,38,39] On the other hand, the European Thyroid Association (ETA) Guidelines for the Management of Amiodarone-Associated Thyroid Dysfunction[18] propose that investigations should be performed to distinguish the subtype of AIT as best as possible so as to guide initial therapy. We consider it useful to utilize the clinical data and diagnostic tests for the purpose of AIT subclassification and subsequent therapy selection. Additionally, we emphasize the need for considering the preexistent cardiovascular comorbidities along with the severity of thyrotoxicosis in choosing the appropriate therapy for the patient. This therapy is then modified based on initial response (Fig. 2.1). Thus, in our practice, we recommend that patients who are stable from a cardiovascular standpoint, and have definitive evidence supporting a distinct subtype of overt AIT, may be tried on appropriate monotherapy, either antithyroid drug (thionamide) or glucocorticoid[22] (Fig. 2.1). Because AIT, especially mixed and type 1, may present with severe thyrotoxicosis or thyroid storm, special consideration should be given to the intensity of antithyroid therapy and the necessary systemic support measures (discussed in Chapter 1, "Thyroid Storm: Acute Thyrotoxicosis"). However, the management of thyroid storm associated with AIT as compared with other causes of thyrotoxicosis is slightly different due to the lack of efficacy of iodine-based therapies.

Type 1 AIT is best treated initially with thionamides[2,18,22] when medical therapy is advisable, due to its presumed pathogenic mechanism of iodine-induced increased thyroid hormone production. Thionamides work by inhibiting the enzyme thyroid peroxidase, inhibiting iodine organification and thus reducing synthesis of T3 and T4.[40] Because the iodine-loaded thyroid gland is less responsive to the inhibitory action of these medications, higher dosages (40 to 60 mg/day of methimazole or equivalent doses of propylthiouracil) and longer periods of therapy (generally 3 to 6 months) may be required before euthyroidism is restored.[2,18,22] Potassium perchlorate (250 mg four times daily) can be added to thionamides,[14] though this is not routinely available in the United States. At high doses, this can cause agranulocytosis and aplastic anemia; hence therapy should be limited to 1 g per day and up to 4 weeks only. Amiodarone discontinuation in this situation should be considered based on the factors discussed later. There is no consistent data on the time required to restore euthyroidism in type 1 AIT; however, if thyrotoxicosis does not respond to thionamides after 4 to 6 weeks of therapy, then the case should be considered as mixed AIT, and glucocorticoids should be added. Where perchlorate is available, it can also be added before or after glucocorticoids, with the caveats discussed previously, particularly considering the risk of agranulocytosis in combination with thionamides. In the case of unresponsiveness to combined therapy with both thionamides and glucocorticoids or worsening of cardiovascular status, emergency total thyroidectomy should be offered[2,18,22] (Fig. 2.1). If euthyroidism is achieved with medical therapy, then definitive ablative therapy should be performed, especially if amiodarone is continued or will be resumed. This is usually in the form of total thyroidectomy, but radioactive iodine ablation could also be offered provided that amiodarone has been discontinued for at least 6 months, along with normalized urinary iodine excretion and 24-hour thyroid radioactive iodine uptake greater than 8% to 10%.[2,18,22]

Type 2 AIT tends to be mild and is usually self-resolving[41,42]; however, it can exacerbate the underlying cardiac dysfunction, and should be treated appropriately.[41,42] Glucocorticoids are the treatment of choice, based on studies demonstrating poor response with methimazole,[43] iopanoic acid, and perchlorate[44] as compared with glucocorticoids in type 2 AIT, and supported by its pathophysiology of destructive thyroiditis. In addition to controlling the inflammatory destruction

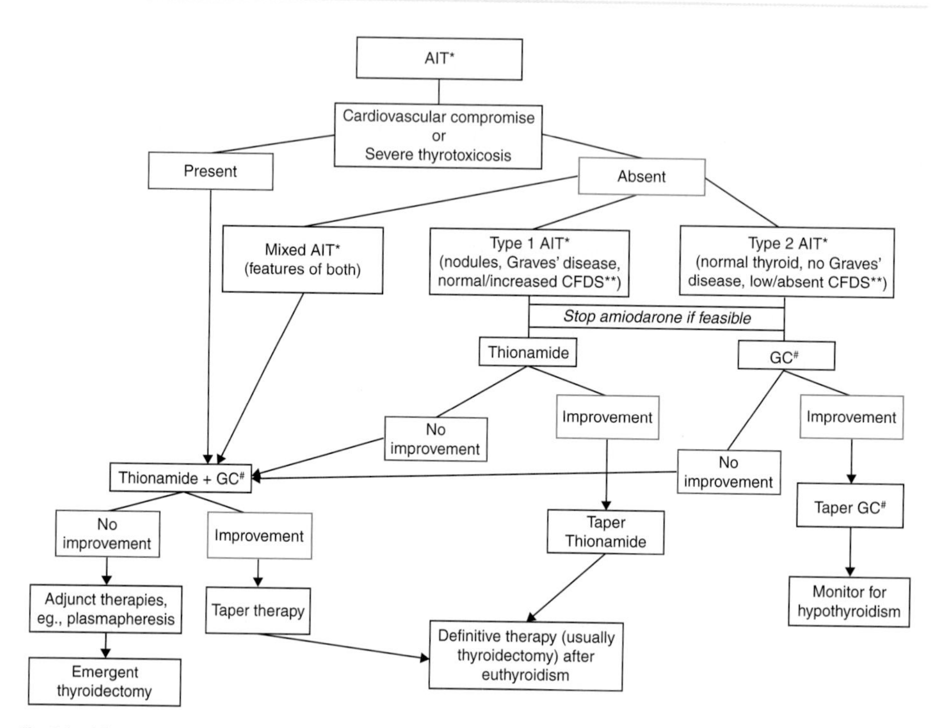

Fig. 2.1 Management algorithm for amiodarone-induced thyrotoxicosis. Red box signifies worse prognosis of AIT. Green box signifies fair or improving prognosis of AIT. *AIT**, Amiodarone-induced thyrotoxicosis; *CFDS***, color-flow Doppler sonography; *GC#*, glucocorticoid. (Adapted from Ross DS, Burch HB, Cooper DS, et al. 2016 American Thyroid Association guidelines for diagnosis and management of hyperthyroidism and other causes of thyrotoxicosis. *Thyroid.* 2016;26(10):1343–1421; Bartalena L, Bogazzi F, Chiovato L, Hubalewska-Dydejczyk A, Links TP, Vanderpump M. 2018 European Thyroid Association (ETA) guidelines for the management of amiodarone-associated thyroid dysfunction. *Eur Thyroid J.* 2018;7(2):55–66.)

of the thyroid, glucocorticoids also inhibit peripheral conversion of T4 to T3, thus limiting the manifestations of thyrotoxicosis. The usual initial dose is 0.5 to 0.7 mg/kg per day or 30 to 40 mg/day of prednisone for approximately 4 weeks, then tapered over 2 to 3 months based on the patient's clinical and biochemical response.[2,18,22] Exacerbation of thyrotoxicosis during the glucocorticoid taper should be managed by temporarily increasing the dose and then trying to taper more slowly. Due to its destructive nature, resolution of type 2 AIT can be followed by long-term hypothyroidism, in which case thyroid hormone replacement should be instituted. If there is no response to glucocorticoids after 4 to 6 weeks or there is worsening of cardiovascular status, then thionamides should be added[22] (Fig. 2.1). If, despite escalating the therapy, clinical deterioration is emerging or impending, then thyroidectomy should be offered.[2,18,22]

The most difficult management challenge is represented by mixed forms of AIT. In these cases, both pathogenic mechanisms (increased thyroid hormone synthesis and thyroid hormone release due to glandular damage) are likely taking place. Thus the best initial treatment is represented by a combination of thionamides (with or without potassium perchlorate) and oral glucocorticoids[2,18,22] (Fig. 2.1). According to the 2016 ATA guidelines,[22] and consistent with our practice,[36,37] combination treatment should also be started in the setting of significant cardiovascular compromise (Fig. 2.1). If there is rapid improvement in the clinical and biochemical features of thyrotoxicosis, and cardiac function does not worsen, it is very likely that the predominant mechanism was destructive thyroiditis, and the thionamide can be tapered. Definitive therapy should be similarly performed after restoration of euthyroidism, as described for cases after euthyroidism in type 1 AIT. However, if the clinical or biochemical status does not improve after 4 to 6 weeks of combination therapy, or if the cardiovascular status worsens, then emergency thyroidectomy should be considered[2,18,22] (Fig. 2.1), with the preoperative management discussed in a separate section.

Adjunct Therapies

Certain adjunct therapies have been tried for poorly controlled AIT but have not demonstrated consistent efficacy. **Potassium perchlorate** inhibits the sodium/iodide symporter and blocks active transport of iodide into the thyroid and helps deplete intrathyroidal iodine stores to improve the therapeutic efficacy of thionamides.[14] Potassium perchlorate (250 mg four times daily) can be added to thionamides in type 1 AIT,[12] but it is not routinely available in the United States. At high doses, this can cause agranulocytosis and aplastic anemia, hence therapy should be limited to 1 g per day and up to 4 weeks only. **Lithium carbonate** increases intrathyroidal iodine content and inhibits both the formation and release of thyroid hormones,[45] but can have prominent side effects like diabetes insipidus and arrhythmias. There is only one study reporting its use in AIT, where the combination of lithium and propylthiouracil was associated with shorter time to euthyroidism as compared with propylthiouracil alone, but all patients did eventually become euthyroid in this study.[46] Hence, the evidence is too limited to support its effectiveness in AIT. **Iopanoic acid**, an iodine-containing radiocontrast medium used in cholecystography, inhibits both thyroid hormone release and peripheral conversion of T4 to T3. It was initially proposed as a medical therapy for AIT patients,[47] but later shown to be less effective than glucocorticoids in type 2 AIT by Bogazzi et al.[48] This could be used in the preparation of AIT patients for thyroidectomy, because it rapidly lowers serum T3 concentrations[49]; however, it is not currently available in the United States. **Bile acid sequestrants** such as colestipol and cholestyramine bind to thyroid hormones in the enterohepatic circulation, thus removing them from circulation.[50] They can be used as adjunct to thionamides or for rapid control of thyrotoxicosis in preparation for thyroidectomy. Bloating and the need for multiple daily doses are their main limiting factors. The treatment should be continued for 7 to 10 days after the surgery to prevent the T3 surge after the drug is withdrawn. **Plasmapheresis** or **therapeutic plasma exchange** works by eliminating large molecular substances, including protein-bound thyroid hormones, from the plasma through extracorporeal blood purification technique. This induces a shift of intracellular thyroid hormones into the circulation, which are bound onto new binding sites provided by the plasma or albumin replacement solution, thereby effectively decreasing the total thyroid hormone concentrations. Plasmapheresis can be employed in cases of severe thyrotoxicosis when rapid correction of thyroid hormone excess is required.[51] The expectation is that a session of plasmapheresis can lower thyroid hormone levels by approximately 30%[21,52,53]; therefore multiple sessions are required to significantly reduce thyroid hormone levels. This therapy has no impact on the mechanism of thyroid hormone generation or release, and its effect is transient. Its main role is to provide a bridge toward definitive therapy by rapidly lowering circulating thyroid hormone levels in preparation for thyroidectomy.[21,52,53] Unfortunately it is not devoid of side effects such as hypotension and arrhythmia,[54] it has limited availability, and is costly, which are all likely to affect its utility in the management of severe AIT.[2] **Potassium iodide,** which acutely lowers thyroid hormone levels by reducing hormone secretion and inhibiting iodide organification, has been used prior to thyroidectomy for Graves' hyperthyroidism,[55] but is not indicated for AIT.

Role of Amiodarone Discontinuation and Resumption

There is currently no strong evidence or consensus to support the discontinuation of amiodarone in patients with AIT. Both the 2018 ETA[18] and the 2016 ATA guidelines[22] recommend that this decision should be individualized with respect to risk stratification, and be taken in a multidisciplinary manner with involvement of the cardiologists and endocrinologists. Amiodarone should be continued if the cardiac indication demands it, for example, uncontrolled arrhythmia[5] refractory to other agents. Amiodarone may also be continued in cases of definite type 2 AIT, which are usually milder and will resolve after the destructive thyroiditis. This is supported by observations from a few studies reporting no impact of amiodarone continuation on resolution of type 2 AIT,[42,44,56] including a randomized clinical trial by Eskes et al.[44] of 36 type 2 AIT patients where all patients became euthyroid after medical treatment of AIT despite ongoing treatment with amiodarone. In a retrospective study by Bogazzi et al., continuation of amiodarone did delay achieving euthyroidism in 83 type 2 AIT patients treated with prednisone, but AIT did resolve in all, irrespective of amiodarone continuation or withdrawal.[57]

This issue becomes complicated in cases of type 1 or mixed AIT, which are usually more severe and likely to have a protracted course as compared with type 2 AIT. Amiodarone can be discontinued if, after discussion with the cardiologist, the cardiac indication for it has either resolved or can be safely managed by other therapies. It should be noted that discontinuing amiodarone may not help at all in the initial control of thyrotoxicosis due its long half-life and lipophilic nature, and thyrotoxicosis may take as long as 8 months to subside after amiodarone is discontinued. The other issue that should be considered in a patient who has discontinued amiodarone is the possibility that amiodarone might need to be restarted at some point after AIT has resolved. Typically, this is an issue in patients who had previous type 1 or mixed AIT that was managed by medical therapy. In a study of 172 AIT patients, resuming amiodarone was associated with AIT recurrence in 30% of cases, the majority being recurrent type 1 AIT.[58] Therefore, when considering resuming amiodarone, the managing team should pay attention to the type and course of the previous AIT episode. If this was protracted, severe, type 1, or mixed AIT, then definitive therapy with total thyroidectomy should be performed. Radioactive iodine ablation could also be offered if amiodarone has been discontinued for at least 6 months, along with normalized urinary iodine excretion and 24-hour thyroid radioactive iodine uptake is greater than 8% to 10%. Often the need for amiodarone resumption comes under urgent circumstances (recurrent severe tachyarrhythmia) and there is no opportunity for definitive thyroid ablation. Therefore, Maqdasy et al. have explored the role of preventive thionamides prior to reintroduction of amiodarone and found the recurrence of type 1 AIT to be reduced by preventive thionamide therapy.[58] However, there is no additional data to strongly support this preventive modality. As of now, total thyroidectomy is preferred as the definitive management to prevent recurrence of type 1 or mixed AIT before amiodarone is resumed.[18,22]

Role of Thyroidectomy in Management

Both the 2018 ETA[18] and the 2016 ATA guidelines[22] recommend total thyroidectomy without delay when urgent control of thyrotoxicosis is required in AIT patients (i.e., deterioration of cardiac function or severe underlying cardiac disease, in patients whose thyrotoxicosis is unresponsive to medical therapies or those with adverse effects of medical therapy). Our practice is consistent with these recommendations[37,59] (Fig. 2.1). The role of emergency thyroidectomy in these situations has been substantiated by cohort studies from a number of institutions.[37,59–61] They demonstrated the effectiveness and relative safety of this intervention for critical AIT cases, especially when associated with cardiac compromise and refractoriness to medical therapy. Cappellani et al.[61] compared medical management to thyroidectomy in a prospective AIT cohort, and found that total thyroidectomy was superior to medical therapy in those with severe systolic dysfunction. Our group at Mayo Clinic reported on the role of thyroidectomy in AIT in 2004[59] and more recently in 2018,[37] showing that the complication rate and mortality rate have decreased over the years (from 9% to 5.4%), and that thyroidectomy remains a valuable option for AIT management, particularly for patients with suboptimal response to medical therapy and high risk for cardiac complications who, inevitably, have high morbidity[12,36] and mortality with uncontrolled thyrotoxicosis.[11,12] In these situations, emergency thyroidectomy not only leads to resolution of thyrotoxicosis but also improves cardiac function in those with preexisting systolic dysfunction.[37,60,61] Thyrotoxicosis should be controlled as much as possible with thionamides with or without glucocorticoids, beta blockers, or temporary use of adjunct therapies (plasmapheresis ± lithium or bile acid sequestrants) prior to thyroidectomy to minimize the surgical risk and decrease the risk of precipitating thyroid storm. Thyroidectomy is also considered a definitive ablative therapy for patients who are at risk for AIT recurrence while they need to continue or resume amiodarone.[2,18,22] For the best surgical outcome, thyroidectomy should be performed by a high-volume thyroid surgeon (one who performs more than 25 thyroid surgeries/year), as this approach significantly reduces the complication rate.[62]

Conclusions

AIT can present a diagnostic and management challenge. It can be classified as type 1 or 2 based on underlying thyroid dysfunction and vascularity of the thyroid, but many cases are mixed. The morbidity from AIT is especially high in the elderly and those with cardiovascular compromise, especially systolic dysfunction. In such cases, combined therapy with thionamides and glucocorticoids should be initiated. Refractoriness to medical therapy and cardiovascular decompensation are indications for emergent total thyroidectomy, which treats the thyrotoxicosis and improves the cardiac function. Adjunct therapies such as plasmapheresis and bile acid sequestrants may be used when available as a bridge to thyroidectomy. Multidisciplinary care by endocrinologists, cardiologists, surgeons, and anesthesiologists is essential for the optimal management of complicated and high-risk AIT cases.

References

1. Trumbo P, Yates AA, Schlicker S, Poos M. Dietary reference intakes: vitamin A, vitamin K, arsenic, boron, chromium, copper, iodine, iron, manganese, molybdenum, nickel, silicon, vanadium, and zinc. *J Am Diet Assoc*. 2001;101(3):294–301.
2. Bogazzi F, Bartalena L, Martino E. Approach to the patient with amiodarone-induced thyrotoxicosis. *J Clin Endocrinol Metab*. 2010;95(6):2529–2535.
3. Batcher EL, Tang XC, Singh BN, et al. Thyroid function abnormalities during amiodarone therapy for persistent atrial fibrillation. *Am J Med*. 2007;120(10):880–885.
4. Farhan H, Albulushi A, Taqi A, et al. Incidence and pattern of thyroid dysfunction in patients on chronic amiodarone therapy: experience at a tertiary care centre in Oman. *Open Cardiovasc Med J*. 2013;7:122–126.
5. Uchida T, Kasai T, Takagi A, et al. Prevalence of amiodarone-induced thyrotoxicosis and associated risk factors in Japanese patients. *Int J Endocrinol*. 2014;2014:534904.
6. Bogazzi F, Bartalena L, Dell'Unto E, et al. Proportion of type 1 and type 2 amiodarone-induced thyrotoxicosis has changed over a 27-year period in Italy. *Clin Endocrinol (Oxf)*. 2007;67(4):533–537.
7. Martino E, Safran M, Aghini-Lombardi F, et al. Environmental iodine intake and thyroid dysfunction during chronic amiodarone therapy. *Ann Intern Med*. 1984;101(1):28–34.
8. Plomp TA, van Rossum JM, Robles de Medina EO, van Lier T, Maes RA. Pharmacokinetics and body distribution of amiodarone in man. *Arzneimittelforschung*. 1984;34(4):513–520.
9. Conen D, Melly L, Kaufmann C, et al. Amiodarone-induced thyrotoxicosis: clinical course and predictors of outcome. *J Am Coll Cardiol*. 2007;49(24):2350–2355.
10. Bogazzi F, Dell'Unto E, Tanda ML, et al. Long-term outcome of thyroid function after amiodarone-induced thyrotoxicosis, as compared to subacute thyroiditis. *J Endocrinol Invest*. 2006;29(8):694–699.
11. Yiu KH, Jim MH, Siu CW, et al. Amiodarone-induced thyrotoxicosis is a predictor of adverse cardiovascular outcome. *J Clin Endocrinol Metab*. 2009;94(1):109–114.
12. O'Sullivan AJ, Lewis M, Diamond T. Amiodarone-induced thyrotoxicosis: left ventricular dysfunction is associated with increased mortality. *Eur J Endocrinol*. 2006;154(4):533–536.

13. Bourcier S, Coutrot M, Kimmoun A, et al. Thyroid storm in the ICU: a retrospective multicenter study. *Crit Care Med.* 2020;48(1):83–90.
14. Martino E, Bartalena L, Bogazzi F, Braverman LE. The effects of amiodarone on the thyroid. *Endocr Rev.* 2001;22(2):240–254.
15. Bogazzi F, Tomisti L, Bartalena L, Aghini-Lombardi F, Martino E. Amiodarone and the thyroid: a 2012 update. *J Endocrinol Invest.* 2012;35(3):340–348.
16. Brennan MD, Erickson DZ, Carney JA, Bahn RS. Nongoitrous (type I) amiodarone-associated thyrotoxicosis: evidence of follicular disruption in vitro and in vivo. *Thyroid.* 1995;5(3):177–183.
17. Theodoraki A, Vanderpump MP. Thyrotoxicosis associated with the use of amiodarone: the utility of ultrasound in patient management. *Clin Endocrinol (Oxf).* 2015.
18. Bartalena L, Bogazzi F, Chiovato L, Hubalewska-Dydejczyk A, Links TP, Vanderpump M. 2018 European Thyroid Association (ETA) guidelines for the management of amiodarone-associated thyroid dysfunction. *Eur Thyroid J.* 2018;7(2):55–66.
19. Tomisti L, Rossi G, Bartalena L, Martino E, Bogazzi F. The onset time of amiodarone-induced thyrotoxicosis (AIT) depends on AIT type. *Eur J Endocrinol.* 2014;171(3):363–368.
20. Bartalena L, Bogazzi F, Martino E. Amiodarone-induced thyrotoxicosis: a difficult diagnostic and therapeutic challenge. *Clin Endocrinol (Oxf).* 2002;56(1):23–24.
21. Kotwal A, Touchan B, Seetharaman KY, Haas RA, Lithgow M, Malkani S. Mixed amiodarone-induced thyrotoxicosis refractory to medical therapy and plasmapheresis. *J Endocrinol Metab.* 2015;5(3):220–223.
22. Ross DS, Burch HB, Cooper DS, et al. 2016 American Thyroid Association guidelines for diagnosis and management of hyperthyroidism and other causes of thyrotoxicosis. *Thyroid.* 2016;26(10):1343–1421.
23. Balzano S, Sau F, Bartalena L, et al. Diagnosis of amiodarone-iodine-induced thyrotoxicosis(AIIT) associated with severe nonthyroidal illness. *J Endocrinol Invest.* 1987;10(6):589–591.
24. Daniels GH. Amiodarone-induced thyrotoxicosis. *J Clin Endocrinol Metab.* 2001;86(1):3–8.
25. Tomisti L, Urbani C, Rossi G, et al. The presence of anti-thyroglobulin (TgAb) and/or anti-thyroperoxidase antibodies (TPOAb) does not exclude the diagnosis of type 2 amiodarone-induced thyrotoxicosis. *J Endocrinol Invest.* 2016;39(5):585–591.
26. Bartalena L, Grasso L, Brogioni S, Aghini-Lombardi F, Braverman LE, Martino E. Serum interleukin-6 in amiodarone-induced thyrotoxicosis. *J Clin Endocrinol Metab.* 1994;78(2):423–427.
27. Bogazzi F, Martino E, Dell'Unto E, et al. Thyroid color flow Doppler sonography and radioiodine uptake in 55 consecutive patients with amiodarone-induced thyrotoxicosis. *J Endocrinol Invest.* 2003;26(7):635–640.
28. Loy M, Perra E, Melis A, et al. Color-flow Doppler sonography in the differential diagnosis and management of amiodarone-induced thyrotoxicosis. *Acta Radiol.* 2007;48(6):628–634.
29. Macedo TA, Chammas MC, Jorge PT, et al. Differentiation between the two types of amiodarone-associated thyrotoxicosis using duplex and amplitude Doppler sonography. *Acta Radiol.* 2007;48(4):412–421.
30. Eaton SE, Euinton HA, Newman CM, Weetman AP, Bennet WM. Clinical experience of amiodarone-induced thyrotoxicosis over a 3-year period: role of colour-flow Doppler sonography. *Clin Endocrinol (Oxf).* 2002;56(1):33–38.
31. Wong R, Cheung W, Stockigt JR, Topliss DJ. Heterogeneity of amiodarone-induced thyrotoxicosis: evaluation of colour-flow Doppler sonography in predicting therapeutic response. *Intern Med J.* 2003;33(9-10):420–426.
32. Pattison DA, Westcott J, Lichtenstein M, et al. Quantitative assessment of thyroid-to-background ratio improves the interobserver reliability of technetium-99m sestamibi thyroid scintigraphy for investigation of amiodarone-induced thyrotoxicosis. *Nucl Med Commun.* 2015;36(4):356–362.
33. Piga M, Cocco MC, Serra A, Boi F, Loy M, Mariotti S. The usefulness of 99mTc-sestaMIBI thyroid scan in the differential diagnosis and management of amiodarone-induced thyrotoxicosis. *Eur J Endocrinol.* 2008;159(4):423–429.
34. Eskes SA, Wiersinga WM. Amiodarone and thyroid. *Best Pract Res Clin Endocrinol Metab.* 2009;23(6):735–751.
35. Stan MN, Ammash NM, Warnes CA, et al. Body mass index and the development of amiodarone-induced thyrotoxicosis in adults with congenital heart disease–a cohort study. *Int J Cardiol.* 2013;167(3):821–826.
36. Stan MN, Sathananthan M, Warnes CA, Brennan MD, Thapa P, Bahn RS. Amiodarone-induced thyrotoxicosis in adults with congenital heart disease–clinical presentation and response to therapy. *Endocr Pract.* 2014;20(1):33–40.

37. Kotwal A. Thyroidectomy for amiodarone-induced thyrotoxicosis: Mayo Clinic experience. *J Endocr Soc.* 2018;2(11):1226–1235.
38. Huang CJ, Chen PJ, Chang JW, et al. Amiodarone-induced thyroid dysfunction in Taiwan: a retrospective cohort study. *Int J Clin Pharm.* 2014;36(2):405–411.
39. Patel N, Inder WJ, Sullivan C, Kaye G. An audit of amiodarone-induced thyrotoxicosis–do anti-thyroid drugs alone provide adequate treatment? *Heart Lung Circ.* 2014;23(6):549–554.
40. Cooper DS. Antithyroid drugs. *N Engl J Med.* 2005;352(9):905–917.
41. Osman F, Franklyn JA, Sheppard MC, Gammage MD. Successful treatment of amiodarone-induced thyrotoxicosis. *Circulation.* 2002;105(11):1275–1277.
42. Uzan L, Guignat L, Meune C, et al. Continuation of amiodarone therapy despite type II amiodarone-induced thyrotoxicosis. *Drug Saf.* 2006;29(3):231–236.
43. Bogazzi F, Tomisti L, Rossi G, et al. Glucocorticoids are preferable to thionamides as first-line treatment for amiodarone-induced thyrotoxicosis due to destructive thyroiditis: a matched retrospective cohort study. *J Clin Endocrinol Metab.* 2009;94(10):3757–3762.
44. Eskes SA, Endert E, Fliers E, et al. Treatment of amiodarone-induced thyrotoxicosis type 2: a randomized clinical trial. *J Clin Endocrinol Metab.* 2012;97(2):499–506.
45. Burrow GN, Burke WR, Himmelhoch JM, Spencer RP, Hershman JM. Effect of lithium on thyroid function. *J Clin Endocrinol Metab.* 1971;32(5):647–652.
46. Dickstein G, Shechner C, Adawi F, Kaplan J, Baron E, Ish-Shalom S. Lithium treatment in amiodarone-induced thyrotoxicosis. *Am J Med.* 1997;102(5):454–458.
47. Chopra IJ, Baber K. Use of oral cholecystographic agents in the treatment of amiodarone-induced hyperthyroidism. *J Clin Endocrinol Metab.* 2001;86(10):4707–4710.
48. Bogazzi F, Bartalena L, Cosci C, et al. Treatment of type II amiodarone-induced thyrotoxicosis by either iopanoic acid or glucocorticoids: a prospective, randomized study. *J Clin Endocrinol Metab.* 2003;88(5):1999–2002.
49. Bogazzi F, Aghini-Lombardi F, Cosci C, et al. Iopanoic acid rapidly controls type I amiodarone-induced thyrotoxicosis prior to thyroidectomy. *J Endocrinol Invest.* 2002;25(2):176–180.
50. Mercado M, Mendoza-Zubieta V, Bautista-Osorio R, Espinoza-de los Monteros AL. Treatment of hyperthyroidism with a combination of methimazole and cholestyramine. *J Clin Endocrinol Metab.* 1996;81(9):3191–3193.
51. Jha S, Waghdhare S, Reddi R, Bhattacharya P. Thyroid storm due to inappropriate administration of a compounded thyroid hormone preparation successfully treated with plasmapheresis. *Thyroid.* 2012;22(12):1283–1286.
52. Zhu L, Zainudin SB, Kaushik M, Khor LY, Chng CL. Plasma exchange in the treatment of thyroid storm secondary to type II amiodarone-induced thyrotoxicosis. *Endocrinol Diabetes Metab Case Rep.* 2016;2016:160039.
53. Tonnelier A, de Filette J, De Becker A, Deweer S, Velkeniers B. Successful pretreatment using plasma exchange before thyroidectomy in a patient with amiodarone-induced thyrotoxicosis. *Eur Thyroid J.* 2017;6(2):108–112.
54. Szczeklik W, Wawrzycka K, Wludarczyk A, et al. Complications in patients treated with plasmapheresis in the intensive care unit. *Anaesthesiol Intensive Ther.* 2013;45(1):7–13.
55. Randle RW, Bates MF, Long KL, Pitt SC, Schneider DF, Sippel RS. Impact of potassium iodide on thyroidectomy for Graves' disease: implications for safety and operative difficulty. *Surgery.* 2018;163(1):68–72.
56. Sato K, Shiga T, Matsuda N, et al. Mild and short recurrence of type II amiodarone-induced thyrotoxicosis in three patients receiving amiodarone continuously for more than 10 years. *Endocr J.* 2006;53(4):531–538.
57. Bogazzi F, Bartalena L, Tomisti L, Rossi G, Brogioni S, Martino E. Continuation of amiodarone delays restoration of euthyroidism in patients with type 2 amiodarone-induced thyrotoxicosis treated with prednisone: a pilot study. *J Clin Endocrinol Metab.* 2011;96(11):3374–3380.
58. Maqdasy S, Batisse-Lignier M, Auclair C, et al. Amiodarone-induced thyrotoxicosis recurrence after amiodarone reintroduction. *Am J Cardiol.* 2016;117(7):1112–1116.
59. Houghton SG, Farley DR, Brennan MD, van Heerden JA, Thompson GB, Grant CS. Surgical management of amiodarone-associated thyrotoxicosis: Mayo Clinic experience. *World J Surg.* 2004;28(11):1083–1087.

60. Tomisti L, Materazzi G, Bartalena L, et al. Total thyroidectomy in patients with amiodarone-induced thyrotoxicosis and severe left ventricular systolic dysfunction. *J Clin Endocrinol Metab*. 2012;97(10):3515–3521.
61. Cappellani D, Papini P, Pingitore A, et al. Comparison between total thyroidectomy and medical therapy for amiodarone-induced thyrotoxicosis. *J Clin Endocrinol Metab*. 2020;105(1).
62. Adam MA, Thomas S, Youngwirth L, et al. Is there a minimum number of thyroidectomies a surgeon should perform to optimize patient outcomes? *Ann Surg*. 2017;265(2):402–407.

CHAPTER 3

Ocular Emergencies in Graves' Ophthalmopathy

Ann Q. Tran ■ Michael Kazim

CHAPTER OUTLINE

Introduction

Thyroid eye disease (TED), also known as thyroid orbitopathy and Graves' ophthalmopathy, is an autoimmune-driven process that results in pathologic changes of the extraocular muscles, orbital fat, and surrounding tissues. Most patients with TED have a self-limited course, not requiring medical or surgical intervention.[1] Mild ophthalmic complaints include ocular surface irritation, excessive tearing, or pressure sensation. More moderate involvement includes diplopia, eyelid retraction, and proptosis. Vision-threatening disease includes compressive optic neuropathy, corneal ulceration and perforation, globe subluxation, and choroidal folds. The diagnosis and management of TED can be particularly challenging. The goal of this chapter is to help providers recognize emergency ophthalmic conditions in TED that warrant referral to ophthalmologists or oculoplastic specialists and their current treatment strategies.

Demographics

Thyroid eye disease more commonly affects women, with a bimodal distribution that peaks in incidence between 50 and 70 years of age.[2] Annually, 16 women and 3 men per 100,000 people are newly diagnosed.[1] Among patients with TED, the majority have Graves' disease (90%), while a small subset are primarily hypothyroid (1%), have Hashimoto's thyroiditis (3%), or are euthyroid (6%).[3] Overall, among patients with Graves' disease, approximately one in four will develop TED.[4] Risk factors for developing TED include smoking, older age, extreme physical or psychological stress, prior treatment with radioactive iodine, and increased titers of antithyroid stimulating hormone receptor antibodies.[5,6]

The exact pathophysiology of TED is incompletely understood. However, it is believed to be an autoimmune inflammatory condition.[7] A combination of genetic, environmental, and epigenetic factors that result in the production of autoreactive T-cells, B-cells, and antibodies stimulates the proliferation of orbital fibroblasts and adipocytes and upregulates a cascade of inflammatory mediators. The cytokine-mediated activation results in tissue remodeling and production of fibrosis and adipogenesis.

The natural course of the disease consists of an initial inflammatory phase followed by a durable quiescent phase.[8] The inflammatory (active) phase typically lasts between 6 to 18 months in a nonsmoker and 24 to 36 months in an active smoker. The quiescent/cicatricial phase follows after the inflammation subsides and features varying degrees of fibrosis and fat expansion in the orbit and eyelid. Differentiating between the active inflammatory phase and the quiescent phase is critical in guiding treatment of TED. The timing of surgical management of TED depends on the patient's overall clinical stability.

Clinical Evaluation

A systematic approach is critical when evaluating a patient with TED, as the clinical presentation may be highly variable. A comprehensive medical history of thyroid condition should be documented including timing and clinical presentation of diagnosis, thyroid status at the time of diagnosis, and prior treatment history (antithyroidal medication, surgical thyroidectomy, radioactive iodine). One must establish the stability of the thyroid status and recent changes in thyroid medications. Family history of thyroid and autoimmune conditions should be noted. If the patient is an active smoker, smoking cessation counseling should be actively pursued.

A careful history and duration of the eye symptoms should be documented to help determine where in the timeline of thyroid eye disease activity the patient resides. The International Thyroid Eye Disease Society's VISA (Vision, Inflammation, Strabismus, Appearance) classification can be a useful framework to help monitor activity and severity. It includes both subjective and objective measures of disease. Subjective assessment of vision loss includes blurriness and decreased color perception. Inflammatory symptoms include retrobulbar ache at rest or with gaze, and lid swelling. Symptoms of diplopia may occur at rest, intermittently, or constantly and may produce a compensatory head tilt. Appearance changes include the presence of lid stare, tearing, irritation, or light sensitivity.

Objective measures of vision and optic nerve function are assessed with tests of visual acuity, color perception, pupillary response, and visual field. Additional pertinent clinical findings include chemosis, conjunctival injection, periocular redness or edema, extraocular motility restriction, upper or lower eyelid retraction, lagophthalmos, proptosis, corneal abnormalities, and elevation of intraocular pressure (Fig. 3.1). An exophthalmometer is used to quantify the distance from the orbital rim to the corneal surface of each eye as a measure of proptosis. Photographs taken prior to the development of TED help determine the magnitude of change in the eyes from baseline.

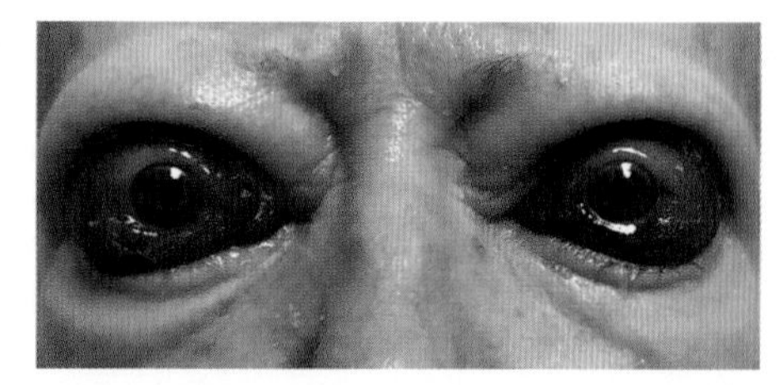

Fig. 3.1 Clinical photograph of a patient with severe active thyroid eye disease demonstrating periorbital edema, proptosis, upper eyelid and lower eyelid retraction, chemosis and injection, corneal keratopathy, ocular motility restriction, and compressive optic neuropathy.

Laboratory investigations should include T3, free T4, thyroid-stimulating hormone (TSH) levels, thyroid peroxidase, TSH receptor antibody, and thyroid stimulating immunoglobulins.[9] Neuroimaging with computed tomography or magnetic resonance imaging aid in determining the degree of orbital fat and extraocular muscle expansion.[10,11] Fusiform enlargement of the extraocular muscles, which spares the tendons helps differentiate TED from other etiologic causes of muscle enlargement, including idiopathic orbital inflammation and lymphoma.

External Pathology

PERIORBITAL EDEMA

Periorbital edema involving the upper and lower eyelids is an early sign of orbital congestion. Over time, the eyelids can become thickened in chronic cases. Severe periorbital congestion may be seen in cases featuring compressive optic neuropathy. However, it should be noted that among octogenarians, compressive optic neuropathy often occurs in the absence of periorbital edema or erythema. High-salt-content foods should be avoided to mitigate the swelling.

UPPER AND LOWER EYELID RETRACTION

The most common ocular manifestation of TED is eyelid retraction, which is seen in 90% of patients. Eyelid retraction may manifest prior to symptoms of hyperthyroidism or serologic evidence of hyperthyroidism by as many as 6 to 12 months. The internist and general ophthalmologist should remain vigilant in a patient who presents with asymptomatic unilateral eyelid retraction and maintain a low threshold for serial serologic thyroid evaluations. Once the patient is within the quiescent phase of TED, upper eyelid retraction can be corrected surgically by procedures including graded blepharotomy.[12,13] Lower eyelid retraction similarly may be corrected by placement of an autologous or xenograft.

PROPTOSIS

Thyroid eye disease is the most common cause of unilateral and bilateral proptosis. In adults, exophthalmos is seen in almost 60% of cases. Proptosis or exophthalmos may produce eyelid malposition, corneal exposure, and ocular dysmotility. The degree of proptosis is quantified using an exophthalmometer and helps differentiate real from pseudoproptosis produced by eyelid retraction. The range of normal exophthalmos is established in the literature; however, normative averages provide little guidance for the individual patient where baseline measurements are unknown. A review of old photos is therefore helpful to understand the magnitude of change consequent to the TED.

After establishing that the TED has been stable for a period of 6 months, decompression may be considered. Depending upon the phenotype of the proptosis (fat or muscle predominant expansion) and the degree of proptosis reduction desired, bony decompression and/or fat decompression can be employed to reverse proptosis. Typically, decompression should be avoided in the active phase of TED, unless medically urgent relief of proptosis is required.

SPONTANEOUS SUBLUXATION OF THE GLOBE

Globe subluxation occurs when the eyelids slip behind the equator of the globe resulting in acute stretch of the optic nerve and exquisite pain. Approximately 0.1% of patients with TED develop globe subluxation.[14] Subluxation is more typically seen when proptosis is severe, and results from expansion of the orbital fat and when there is upper lid retraction or preexisting laxity of the eyelids.

Spontaneous subluxation is a vision-threatening condition that can produce stretch optic neuropathy. Although reversable if the globe can be repositioned, if there is prolonged stretch or repeated insults, optic nerve damage may be irreversible. The severe pain results from both the stretching of the orbital tissues and the frequent association with corneal abrasion. The pain and shock of the unexpected event make home management of subluxation challenging. The globe can be repositioned in the emergency room by first applying topical anesthetic to relieve corneal pain. The patient is asked to maintain a downward gaze. Then, using one hand to pull on the upper eyelid skin and the other hand on the globe to place posterior pressure, the upper lid is returned to its normal position.[15] If this fails, the use of Desmarres retractors or a paper clip bent as a shoehorn can help reposition upper lid over the globe. Intravenous corticosteroids may be used to limit acute inflammatory swelling and potentially provide neuro-protection. A temporary lateral tarsorrhaphy may be used to reduce the acute risk of recurrent subluxation. Definitive treatment options include orbital decompression to reduce proptosis, lid retraction repair, and permanent tarsorrhaphy.

DIPLOPIA

Diplopia is a debilitating symptom of TED and may manifest in the horizontal, vertical, or oblique planes. Up to 42% of adult TED patients will demonstrate progressive extraocular motility changes.[16] Extraocular muscle involvement can be assessed by measuring the amount of ocular rotation of the eye in degrees from 0 to 45 in each field of gaze. Ocular misalignment resulting in symptomatic diplopia is measured with neutralizing prisms and often with the assistance of a certified orthoptist.

Diplopia is the most disabling feature of TED. Treatment varies based on the phase of the orbitopathy.[17] If only present in eccentric gaze, aggressive immunosuppression may be helpful in preventing progression of diplopia into primary gaze. If the diplopia is in primary or reading gaze, temporary relief can be obtained by occluding vision from the nondominant eye with frosted adhesive tape on the lens of eyeglasses. Alternatively, an orthoptist can help provide temporary (Fresnel) prisms applied to either or both distance or reading glasses to eliminate diplopia and maintain binocular depth perception. Orthoptics measurements should be repeated quarterly with adjustments in the prisms as required. When orthoptics measurements remain unchanged for 6 months, TED is considered to have entered the stable phase and rehabilitative surgery may be considered. Strabismus surgery is an effective measure to restore single binocular vision in primary and reading gaze.[18,19]

Anterior Segment Pathology

CORNEAL KERATOPATHY

Assessment of the cornea in patients with TED is critical, as vision loss from corneal keratopathy may be confused with that caused by compressive optic neuropathy. Severe corneal keratopathy can result in permanent vision loss due to scarring or perforation. A slit lamp examination should evaluate for abnormal tear film, superior limbal keratitis, mild punctate epithelial erosions, and signs of chronic exposure with corneal scarring. The pathogenesis of corneal keratopathy is multifactorial including unstable tear film, eyelid retraction, proptosis, reduced motility, and poor Bell's reflex.[20]

Many patients in the active phase of TED complain of ocular irritation, light sensitivity, and tearing. For mild disease, treatment includes topical lubrication with preservative-free artificial tears and lubricating gel at night. Moisture chambers and Saran Wrap occlusion at bedtime should also be considered.[21] If there are signs of corneal keratopathy with progressive corneal thinning, the cornea may be further protected by closure of the eyelids by placement of a temporary tarsorrhaphy or injection of botulinum toxin to induce a ptosis of the upper eyelids. A longer-term solution can be achieved with a permanent tarsorrhaphy.[22] Amniotic membrane grafts to the cornea have been reported, especially if a corneal dellen (focal thinning of the cornea) develops. Emergency corneal gluing or corneal transplantation may be required if perforation occurs.

Corneal ulcers or infectious keratitis develops when the epithelial surface disruption becomes colonized with bacteria. This is a rare complication, as only 1.3% of TED patients develop microbial keratitis. The spectrum of the corneal involvement includes corneal infiltrates, corneal melt, severe corneal thinning, and, in rare cases, corneal perforation. A mixture of gram-negative and gram-positive flora has been isolated from corneal cultures.[23]

The majority of the corneal keratopathy is related to upper and/or lower eyelid retraction and lagophthalmos. Once in the stable phase, eyelid retraction repair reduces the risk of corneal disease.

CONJUNCTIVAL INJECTION AND CHEMOSIS

Conjunctival injection or hyperemia and chemosis are common clinical features of active TED disease. Symptomatic medical management with topical lubrication is recommended. Over-the-counter topical redness-relief medications have active decongestants containing either selective or mixed alpha-1 and alpha-2 adrenergic receptor agonists. These agents include tetrahydrozoline, naphazoline, and brimonidine, which should be avoided due to their association with rebound redness and irritation. Conjunctival injection should be managed with lubricating artificial tear drops.

Posterior Segment Pathology

RETINAL PATHOLOGY—CHOROIDAL FOLDS

Chorioretinal folds are rarely seen in TED.[24] The etiology of chorioretinal folds in TED is variably speculated to be secondary to vascular engorgement from apical crowding, traction on the optic nerve, and posterior pressure on the globe due to enlarged rectus muscles.[25] The visual acuity in these patients can vary; however, many patients will report metamorphopsias. A dilated fundoscopic examination and use of optical coherence tomography can aid in diagnosis. Despite medical therapy or surgical decompression, chorioretinal folds may variably persist indefinitely.[26,27]

COMPRESSIVE OPTIC NEUROPATHY

Compressive optic neuropathy occurs in 4% to 8% of TED patients.[1] Male and older patients are more likely to develop compressive optic neuropathy.[28] The etiology is multifactorial and thought to be secondary to the mass effect of the pathologically enlarged and inflamed extraocular muscles in the orbital apex, producing variable degrees of optic nerve compression, stretch, and inflammation.[29] Optic neuropathy may be challenging to diagnose and relies on changes in visual acuity, pupillary reactions, color vision, and visual fields. Younger patients with compressive optic neuropathy tend to have better visual acuity and color vision, fewer visual field deficits, and greater exophthalmos as compared with older patients.[30] A mathematical formula to aid in the diagnosis of compressive optic neuropathy has been found to have good specificity and sensitivity, when employing multiple clinical parameters.[31]

Oral corticosteroids have been a primary treatment for moderate to severe active TED for the past 50 years.[32] Intravenous corticosteroids may be more effective and have a lower rate of therapeutic morbidity.[33] The most widely utilized treatment protocol, developed by EUGOGO (European Union Graves Ophthalmopathy Group) infuses 500 mg IV methylprednisolone weekly for 6 weeks, followed by 250 mg weekly for 6 weeks to suppress active TED.[34] Although the therapeutic response is favorable, the relapse rate is between 20% and 40% after completion of the infusion protocol.[35] The use of high-dose corticosteroids has been shown to be effective in reversing vision loss from compressive optic neuropathy in active-phase TED, but it does not shorten the overall duration of the active phase.[36] Conversely, compressive optic neuropathy identified in the stable phase is not responsive to medical therapy. In these cases, and those in which active-phase compressive optic neuropathy is unresponsive to corticosteroid therapy, surgical decompression is required to restore optic nerve function.

The first report of surgical decompression performed for severe TED with compressive optic neuropathy in 1911 described removal of the lateral orbital wall to relieve the orbital congestion.[37] Subsequently, surgical innovation has expanded and refined both the decompressive techniques and surgical planning.[38] Surgical decompression in the acute phase of TED should be reserved for patients who do not respond to medical therapy or have contraindications to medical treatment.[39] In the majority of patients surgical decompression should be postponed until the stable phase is achieved and the outcome of surgery can be more reliably predicted.

Complications associated with bony decompressions should not be taken lightly as they include ptosis, worsening strabismus, trigeminal nerve paresthesia, orbital cellulitis, cerebral spinal fluid leak, hypoglobus, change in voice quality, and permanent vision loss. Surgical decompressions during the active phase have increased risk of orbital hemorrhage, enophthalmos, hypoglobus, and diplopia.[40,41]

Orbital radiotherapy was first used to treat TED in 1936. The standard radiotherapy protocol is 2000 cGy delivered in 10 treatments to the orbital tissue over a 2-week course. It is most commonly used in the acute phase to supplement corticosteroid treatment of compressive optic neuropathy, rapidly progressive orbitopathy, and steroid-dependent orbitopathy.[42] In a study of patients with compressive optic neuropathy responsive to corticosteroids who received adjuvant orbital radiation therapy, only 6% of patients required an urgent surgical decompression as a result of persistent optic neuropathy.[43]

Conclusion

Management of TED poses many challenges. The clinical presentation can range from mild to severe ocular. Recognizing the signs and symptoms of TED and making the appropriate referral for treatment is vital to the preservation of both form and function. A multidisciplinary approach including endocrinology and ophthalmology is required to optimize management.

References

1. Bartley GB. The epidemiologic characteristics and clinical course of ophthalmopathy associated with autoimmune thyroid disease in Olmsted County, Minnesota. *Trans Am Ophthalmol Soc.* 1994;92:477–588.
2. Wiersinga WM, Bartalena L. Epidemiology and prevention of Graves' ophthalmopathy. *Thyroid.* 2002;12:855–860.
3. Bartley GB, Fatourechi V, Kadrmas EF, et al. Clinical features of Graves' ophthalmopathy in an incidence cohort. *Am J Ophthalmol.* 1996;121:284–290.
4. Tanda ML, Piantanida E, Liparulo L, et al. Prevalence and natural history of Graves' orbitopathy in a large series of patients with newly diagnosed Graves' hyperthyroidism seen at a single center. *J Clin Endocrinol Metab.* 2013;98:1443–1449.
5. Khong JJ, Finch S, De Silva C, et al. Risk factors for Graves' orbitopathy; the Australian Thyroid-Associated Orbitopathy Research (ATOR) study. *J Clin Endocrinol Metab.* 2016;101:2711–2720.
6. Kung AW, Yau CC, Cheng A. The incidence of ophthalmopathy after radioiodine therapy for Graves' disease: prognostic factors and the role of methimazole. *J Clin Endocrinol Metab.* 1994;79:542–546.
7. Weiler DL. Thyroid eye disease: a review. *Clin Exp Optom.* 2017;100:20–25.
8. Li Z, Cestari DM, Fortin E. Thyroid eye disease: what is new to know? *Curr Opin Ophthalmol.* 2018;29:528–534.

9. Bahn RS. Graves' ophthalmopathy. *N Engl J Med*. 2010;362:726–738.
10. Trokel SL, Hilal SK. Recognition and differential diagnosis of enlarged extraocular muscles in computed tomography. *Am J Ophthalmol*. 1979;87:503–512.
11. Bailey CC, Kabala J, Laitt R, et al. Magnetic resonance imaging in thyroid eye disease. *Eye (Lond)*. 1996;10:617–619.
12. Elner VM, Hassan AS, Frueh BR. Graded full-thickness anterior blepharotomy for upper eyelid retraction. *Arch Ophthalmol*. 2004;122:55–60.
13. Nimitwongsakul A, Zoumalan CI, Kazim M. Modified full-thickness blepharotomy for treatment of thyroid eye disease. *Ophthalmic Plast Reconstr Surg*. 2013;29(1):44–47.
14. Rubin PA, Watkins LM, Rumelt S, et al. Orbital computed tomographic characteristics of globe subluxation in thyroid orbitopathy. *Ophthalmology*. 1998;105:2061–2064.
15. Tse DT. A simple maneuver to reposit a subluxed globe. *Arch Ophthalmol*. 2000;118:410–411.
16. Gruters A. Ocular manifestations in children and adolescents with thyrotoxicosis. *Exp Clin Endocrinol Diabetes*. 1999;107:S172–S174.
17. Schotthoefer EO, Wallace DK. Strabismus associated with thyroid eye disease. *Curr Opin Ophthalmol*. 2007;18:361–365.
18. Zoumalan CI, Lelli Jr GJ, Kazim M. Tenon recession: a novel adjunct to improve outcome in the treatment of large-angle strabismus in thyroid eye disease. *Ophthalmic Plast Reconstr Surg*. 2011;27(4):287–292.
19. Scofield-Kaplan SM, Dunbar K, Stein G, Kazim M. Improvement in both primary and eccentric ocular alignment after thyroid eye disease—strabismus surgery with Tenon's recession. *Ophthalmic Plast Reconstr Surg*. 2018;34(4S Suppl 1):S85–S89.
20. Gilbard JP, Farris RL. Ocular surface drying and tear film osmolarity in thyroid eye disease. *Acta Ophthalmol (Copenh)*. 1983;61:108–116.
21. Scofield-Kaplan S, Dunbar K, Kazim M. Glad Press'n Seal for the treatment of chronic exposure keratopathy. *Ophthalmic Plast Reconstr Surg*. 2017;33:152–153.
22. Heinz C, Eckstein A, Steuhl KP, Meller D. Amniotic membrane transplantation for reconstruction of corneal ulcer in graves ophthalmopathy. *Cornea*. 2004;23:524–526.
23. Naik MN, Vasanthapuram VH, Joseph J, Murthy SI. Microbial keratitis in thyroid eye disease: clinical features, microbiological profile, and treatment outcome. *Ophthalmic Plast Reconstr Surg*. 2019;35:543–548.
24. Kowal L, Georgievski Z. Choroidal folds in Graves' ophthalmopathy. *Aust N Z J Ophthalmol*. 1994;22:216.
25. Bullock JD, Egbert PR. The origin of choroidal folds a clinical, histopathological, and experimental study. *Doc Ophthalmol*. 1974;37:261–293.
26. Kroll AJ, Norton EWD. Regression of choroidal folds. *Trans Am Acad Ophthalmol Otolaryngol*. 1970; 74:515–526.
27. Jorge R, Scott IU, Akaishi PM, Velasco Cruz AA, Flynn HW Jr. Resolution of choroidal folds and improvement in visual acuity after orbital decompression for graves orbitopathy. *Retina*. 2003;23:563–565.
28. Trobe JD, Glaser JS, Laflamme P. Dysthyroid optic neuropathy. Clinical profile and rationale for management. *Arch Ophthalmol*. 1978;96:1199–1209.
29. Neigel JM, Rootman J, Belkin RI, et al. Dysthyroid optic neuropathy. The crowded orbital apex syndrome. *Ophthalmology*. 1988;95:1515–1521.
30. Campbell AA, Nanda T, Oropesa S, Kazim M. Age-related changes in the clinical phenotype of compressive optic neuropathy in thyroid eye disease. *Ophthalmic Plast Reconstr Surg*. 2019;35:238–242.
31. Callahan AB, Campbell AA, Oropesa S, Baraban A, Kazim M. The Columbia thyroid eye disease-compressive optic neuropathy diagnostic formula. *Ophthalmic Plast Reconstr Surg*. 2018;34:S68–S71.
32. Snyder NJ, Green DE, Solomon DH. Glucocorticoid-induced disappearance of long-acting thyroid stimulator in the ophthalmopathy of graves' disease. *J Clin Endocrinol Metab*. 1964;24:1129–1135.
33. Kahaly GJ, Pitz S, Hommel G, Dittmar M. Randomized, single blind trial of intravenous versus oral steroid monotherapy in Graves' orbitopathy. *J Clin Endocrinol Metab*. 2005;90:5234–5240.
34. Bartalena L, Baldeschi L, Boboridis K, et al. The 2016 European Thyroid Association/European Group on Graves' orbitopathy guidelines for the management of Graves' orbitopathy. *Eur Thyroid J*. 2016;5(1): 9–26.
35. Zang S, Ponto KA, Kahaly GJ. Clinical review: intravenous glucocorticoids for Graves' orbitopathy: efficacy and morbidity. *Journal of Clinical Endocrinology and Metabolism*. 2011;96(2):320–332.

36. Brown J, Coburn JW, Wigod RA, Hiss JM Jr, Dowling JT. Adrenal steroid therapy of severe infiltrative ophthalmopathy of Graves' disease. *Am J Med.* 1963;34:786–795.
37. Dollinger J. Die Druckentlastung der Augenhohle durch Entfernung der 1iu/3eren Orbitalwand bei hochgradigem Exophthalmus (Morbus Basedowii) und konsekutiver Hornhauterkrankung. Dtsch. *Med Wochenschr.* 1911;37:1888–1890.
38. Tooley AA, Godfrey KJ, Kazim M. Evolution of thyroid eye disease decompression-dysthyroid optic neuropathy. *Eye (Lond).* 2019;33:206–211.
39. Perumal B, Meyer DR. Treatment of severe thyroid eye disease: a survey of the American Society of Ophthalmic Plastic and Reconstructive Surgery (ASOPRS). *Ophthal Plast Reconstr Surg.* 2015;31:127–131.
40. McNab AA. Orbital decompression for thyroid orbitopathy. *Aust N Z J Ophthalmol.* 1997;25:55–61.
41. Dumont N, Bouletreau P, Guyot L. [Reoperation after orbital decompression for Graves' ophthalmopathy]. *Rev Stomatol Chirm Maxillofac.* 2012;113:81–86.
42. Jones A. Orbital x-ray therapy of progressive exophthalmos. *Br J Radiol.* 1951;24:637–646.
43. Gold KG, Scofield S, Isaacson SR, Stewart MW, Kazim M. Orbital radiotherapy combined with corticosteroid treatment for thyroid eye disease-compressive optic neuropathy. *Ophthalmic Plast Reconstr Surg.* 2018;34(2):172–177.

CHAPTER 4

Myxedema Coma

Dorina Ylli ■ Leonard Wartofsky

CHAPTER OUTLINE

Introduction

Myxedema coma is an important endocrine emergency caused by untreated or prolonged hypothyroidism that culminates in a comatose state. It is seen more commonly in elderly women during the winter months, typically having been triggered by exposure to cold weather, an infectious process, trauma, gastrointestinal (GI) bleeding, or other nonthyroidal illness superimposed on preexisting severe hypothyroidism. The estimated incidence of myxedema coma varies from 0.2 to 1.08 per million people per year,[1,2] and despite the high mortality rate of 29% to 60%, timely diagnosis and immediate treatment will increase the chance for survival.[1,3,4]

Pathophysiology

Myxedema coma always presents in the setting of a patient with a diagnosis of hypothyroidism that either is long-standing and not being treated or is recently established. The hypothyroidism may be due to any cause, for example, post-radioiodine ablation or thyroidectomy, but the most common cause will be underlying Hashimoto's thyroiditis. Patients often have a known history of Hashimoto's disease treated with levothyroxine but for various or uncertain reasons had interrupted or discontinued the treatment. Another relatively less frequent setting for myxedema coma is when it is due to secondary or tertiary hypothyroidism on a pituitary or hypothalamic basis. These patients are encountered in less than 5% of reported cases of myxedema coma.[5]

BOX 4.1 ■ Myxedema Coma: Causes and Precipitating Factors

Causes of Hypothyroidism

- Hashimoto's thyroiditis
- Total thyroidectomy
- Radiation therapy
- Post radioactive Iodine 131 treatment for hyperthyroidism
- Drugs:
  - Lithium carbonate
  - Amiodarone
  - Tyrosine kinase inhibitors
  - Antithyroid drugs

Precipitating Factors to Myxedema Coma

- Infections
- Trauma
- Gastrointestinal bleeding
- Hypothermia
- Congestive heart failure
- Cerebrovascular accidents
- Metabolic disturbances
- Drugs:
  - Anesthetics
  - Sedatives
  - Tranquillizers
  - Narcotics

In almost all instances, the clinical state of an otherwise stable hypothyroid patient is overcome by a precipitating event such as a pulmonary infection, congestive heart failure, or a cerebrovascular accident (Box 4.1). Less frequent causes have included subclinical thyroiditis, diabetic ketoacidosis, and consumption of large amounts of raw bok choy (Box 4.1).[6–8] Why some superimposed nonthyroidal illness or event might lead to coma is unclear, but could be related to inhibition of conversion of thyroxine (T4) to triiodothyronine (T3) as occurs in the "euthyroid sick syndrome," thereby worsening the hypothyroidism. Related to this possible mechanism, particular attention should be paid to the patient's medications, as drugs such as amiodarone, lithium carbonate, or tyrosine kinase inhibitors may affect thyroid function.[9,10] Amiodarone, for example, also causes inhibition of T4 to T3 conversion, and lithium would inhibit any residual thyroid function in an already compromised thyroid gland. Other mechanisms that might underly decompensation are common in hospitalized patients and include the use of drugs such as opioids, anesthetics, and sedatives that suppress respiratory drive, facilitating the deterioration into coma. As is the case with most drugs administered to a hypothyroid subject, blood levels of these agents are higher and more prolonged due to the reduced distribution space and slowed metabolic turnover in these patients.

Clinical Presentation

As noted earlier, the syndrome will typically present in a patient who develops an infection or other systemic disease superimposed upon previously undiagnosed, untreated, or inadequately treated hypothyroidism. Reported cases in the literature and designated as myxedema coma have included patients who were not frankly comatose, but rather presented in a lethargic, disoriented, and obtunded state; such patients, if not properly diagnosed and treated, are highly likely to progress into a comatose state. The physician first examining a lethargic subject may not have the benefit of a history of hypothyroidism, but slow speech and a hoarse voice can be important clues. On physical examination, a scar present in the anterior part of the neck should suggest prior thyroidectomy as the cause of the hypothyroidism. Other clues include dry, scaly skin, non-pitting edema of the face, hands, and feet, macroglossia, delayed deep tendon reflexes, and thinning or sparse body hair. In two series that identified 12 and 14 patients, respectively, with myxedema coma, the findings on presentation included hypoxemia in 36% to 80%, hypotension in 50%, hypercapnia in 36% to 54%, bradycardia in 36%, and hypothermia with a temperature below 94°F (34.4°C) in 50% to 88%.[11,12] The belief that early and aggressive therapeutic intervention is required is supported by the observed mortality of 50% of patients who died despite subsequent treatment with thyroid hormone. Patients with myxedema coma may manifest hypoglycemia, hypercalcemia, hyponatremia, hypercapnia, and hypoxemia as either precipitating factors or secondary consequences of the condition. Hypoventilation with hypercapnia and hypoxemia are particularly dreaded prognostic indicators, as they herald further CO_2 retention and progression into worsening respiratory failure, lethargy, stupor, and coma.

MANIFESTATIONS IN THE RESPIRATORY SYSTEM

An appreciation of the pathologic mechanisms threatening the integrity of the respiratory system in the myxedema coma patient is crucial to understanding both the cause of a patient's deterioration and the intervention necessary to reduce the risk of their demise. In overtly hypothyroid patients, decreases in the respiratory response to hypercapnia are observed in combination with a decrease in respiratory drive. Hypothyroid patients retain fluid and may present with generalized edema, pleural or pericardial effusions, or ascites. The presence of pleural or pericardial effusion may compromise normal respiratory function with further deterioration provided by concomitant bronchopulmonary infection. Edema and swelling of the tongue occur in profound hypothyroidism and, together with the marked edema of the vocal cords, contribute to mechanical narrowing of the upper respiratory airways. After initiation of T4 therapy, the respiratory response to CO_2 has been reported to improve in most but not all cases.[13–16]

CARDIOVASCULAR MANIFESTATIONS

In a patient with myxedema coma, bradycardia is often present, as it often is in uncomplicated hypothyroidism. Other electrocardiogram (ECG) findings may include low voltage, inverted T waves, and a prolonged QT interval, the latter exposing patients to risk of *torsades de pointes* and potentially dangerous arrhythmias.[17] Cardiac ultrasound will reveal an enlarged cardiac silhouette due either to ventricular dilatation or pericardial effusion. When present, pericardial effusions are likely to have slowly accumulated over time, and only rarely cause cardiac tamponade.

Bradycardia with ventricular dilatation and reduced contractility results in reduced stroke volume and cardiac output. Whereas administration of cardioactive drugs may be considered, it requires only the initiation of treatment with T4 to reverse the above-mentioned abnormalities. However, overly aggressive or injudicious T4 replacement may increase the risk of myocardial infarction, especially when T3 is combined with T4 therapy. Hypotension may be present in spite of the increased retention of total body water, as fluids primarily accumulate in the extravascular compartments and intravascular volume is reduced. With initiation of T4 replacement, blood pressure should normalize, but the use of vasopressor agents may be required prior to onset of the vascular effects of T4 in order to avoid progression to severe hypotension or shock (see Management later). In view of the potential for shock, fatal arrhythmia, and mortality, myxedema coma patients should be admitted to, and managed in, an intensive care unit.

GASTROINTESTINAL MANIFESTATIONS

One of the first signs of altered GI physiology in myxedema is often slowed peristalsis, due mainly to impairment of GI innervation and edematous infiltration of the muscularis mucosae. Constipation is common, and the more severe cases can evolve into a paralytic ileus.[18] Given the risks of anesthesia in the profoundly hypothyroid patient, surgical intervention should be temporized for suspected obstruction by conservative management with decompression until the therapeutic response to thyroid hormone might occur. Because absorption may be impaired due to intestinal edema and gastric atony, the initial therapy with T4 or T3 should be administered parenterally in preference to oral administration. Ascites has been documented in 51 cases,[19] and GI bleeding can occur secondary to a coagulopathy.

RENAL AND ELECTROLYTE MANIFESTATIONS

Renal function is impaired in profound hypothyroidism, with decreases in glomerular filtration rate, renal clearance, renal plasma flow, and plasma osmolarity. As a consequence, total body water, urine sodium, and urine osmolarity are increased. Hypoperfusion of the distal nephron[20] will trigger an increase of antidiuretic hormone (ADH) secretion[21] leading to water retention and worsening of hyponatremia. Hyponatremia per se may cause altered mental status and, when severe, may be largely responsible for precipitating the comatose state.

HYPOTHERMIA

One of the cardinal signs of myxedema coma is hypothermia, which occurs in 50% to 75% of patients with myxedema, and its presence should prompt timely diagnosis of the syndrome. In some cases, it may reach dramatic levels (below 80°F [26.7°C]), and temperatures below 90°F (32.2°C) are associated with poorer prognosis.[12] Because the presence of hypothermia may mask an underlying infection, a diagnosis of overt hypothyroidism or myxedema coma should be considered in any patient with a known infection but absent fever. Broad-spectrum empiric antibiotic therapy also should be considered in such patients. Infectious diseases, and pneumonia in particular, often serve as the triggering events to drive a patient with hypothyroidism into myxedema coma. Absent early diagnosis and treatment, the infection can lead to sepsis with vascular collapse and possible death. The presence of underlying hypoglycemia may further compound the observed decrement in body temperature.

NEUROPSYCHIATRIC MANIFESTATIONS

Although coma is the predominant and most dramatic clinical presentation in myxedema coma, an earlier history of disorientation, depression, paranoia, or hallucinations ("myxedema madness") may often be elicited. Other neurologic findings that may have been present either just before entering the comatose state or which appear early during recovery include cerebellar signs, such as poorly coordinated purposeful movements of the hands and feet, ataxia, diadochokinesis, poor memory and recall, or even frank amnesia. Abnormal findings on electroencephalography are few and include low amplitude and a decreased rate of α-wave activity. Status epilepticus has been described,[22] and up to 25% of patients with myxedema coma may experience minor to major seizures, possibly related to hyponatremia, hypoglycemia, and/or hypoxemia (due to reduced cerebrovascular perfusion from low cardiac output and atherosclerotic vessels in elderly patients). T4 treatment will generally lead to demonstrable clinical improvement of the condition.

HEMATOLOGIC MANIFESTATIONS

A microcytic anemia may be seen secondary to GI hemorrhage, or there may be a macrocytic anemia due to vitamin B12 deficiency, which, if present, may also be associated with a worsening of the neurologic state. Granulocytopenia with a decreased cell-mediated immunologic response may contribute to a higher risk of severe infection. In contrast to the tendency to thrombosis seen in mild hypothyroidism, severe hypothyroidism is associated with a higher risk of bleeding due to coagulopathy related to an acquired von Willebrand syndrome (type 1) and decreases in factors V, VII, VIII, IX, and X.[23] The von Willebrand syndrome is reversible with T4 therapy.[24] Another potential cause of bleeding in these patients may be disseminated intravascular coagulation when there is associated sepsis.

Diagnosis

Myxedema coma is fortunately a rare event, and its rarity suggests that physicians will generally have had little prior experience in making a proper and timely diagnosis. Diagnosis is indeed a clinical one and should be based on the concomitant presence of the abovementioned signs and symptoms (see Clinical Presentation) in the setting of a patient with either a history of or suspected hypothyroidism. Because the diagnosis is not achieved on the basis of laboratory tests or imaging results, some authors have proposed a scoring system based on the presence of some of the most crucial aspects of the myxedema presentation (e.g., personal medical history, precipitating event, hypothermia, cardiovascular dysfunction, nervous system manifestations, metabolic disorders, and GI findings). The Popoveniuc et al. scoring system has a sensitivity of 100% and specificity of 80%.[12] According to the score achieved, the diagnosis of myxedema coma in a patient would be classified as either highly suggestive or unlikely (Box 4.2). Another objective screening tool has been proposed based on heart rate, temperature, Glasgow coma scale, TSH, free thyroxine, and history of a precipitating event, and was associated with a sensitivity and specificity of

BOX 4.2 ■ Diagnostic Scoring System for Myxedema Coma

Thermoregulatory Dysfunction (Temperature °C)		**Cardiovascular Dysfunction**	
>35	0	Bradycardia	
32–35	10	Absent	0
<32	20	50–59	10
Central Nervous System Effects		40–49	20
Absent	0	<40	30
Somnolent/lethargic	10	Other ECG changes[a]	10
Obtunded	15	Pericardial/pleural effusions	10
Stupor	20	Pulmonary edema	15
Coma/seizures	30	Cardiomegaly	15
Gastrointestinal Findings		Hypotension	20
Anorexia/abdominal pain/ constipation	5	**Metabolic Disturbances**	
Decreased intestinal motility	15	Hyponatremia	10
Paralytic ileus	20	Hypoglycemia	10
Precipitating Event		Hypoxemia	10
Absent	0	Hypercarbia	10
Present	10	Decrease in GFR	10

A score of 60 or higher is highly suggestive/diagnostic of myxedema coma; a score of 25 to 59 is suggestive of risk for myxedema coma, and a score below 25 is unlikely to indicate myxedema coma.
[a]Other ECG changes: QT prolongation, or low voltage complexes, or bundle branch blocks, or nonspecific ST-T changes, or heart blocks.
ECG, Electrocardiogram; *GFR,* glomerular filtration rate.

Adapted from Popoveniuc G, Chandra T, Sud A, et al. A diagnostic scoring system for myxedema coma. *Endocr Pract.* 2014;20(8):808–817.

approximately 80%.[25] Even though these scoring systems may have some utility for rapid diagnosis of myxedema coma, it should be acknowledged that the scores were proposed based on data obtained from a limited sample of patients, and thus, further external validation may be needed.

In order to confirm the clinical suspicion of hypothyroidism in a comatose patient, blood should be immediately obtained for thyroid function testing. However, in view of the potential for mortality when robust signs and symptoms of myxedema coma are present, treatment could be initiated without awaiting laboratory confirmation. However, the pros and cons of early, aggressive therapy with T4 or T3 should always be properly weighed, especially in the elderly population where the risk of inducing fatal cardiac arrhythmias or a coronary event obtains.

The thyroid function laboratory findings will include a low free thyroxine (FT4) and free triiodothyronine (FT3) together with a high thyroid-stimulating hormone (TSH) in patients with primary hypothyroidism or a low FT4 and FT3 with a low or normal TSH in the rarer circumstance when the hypothyroidism is on the basis of pituitary TSH insufficiency. Other laboratory results may indicate evidence of anemia, hyponatremia, hypercholesterolemia, and increased serum lactate dehydrogenase and creatine kinase levels.[26]

An elevated serum TSH concentration is generally considered to be the most important laboratory evidence for the diagnosis of hypothyroidism. One caveat applies to interpretation of the TSH level in myxedema coma, however, and that is because the presence of severe systemic illness or treatment with drugs such as dopamine, dobutamine, or corticosteroids may serve to reduce the elevation in TSH levels.[27,28] Other than the performance of laboratory tests to confirm a diagnosis of myxedema coma, the performance of ancillary studies critical for the management of these patients is also important, i.e., evaluation for CO_2 retention, hypoxia, hyponatremia, or infection. Rare patients with hypothyroidism may have a polyglandular syndrome with either pituitary or adrenal disease, and until ruled out, corticosteroid therapy is recommended in addition to T4.

Management

The importance of myxedema coma as an endocrine emergency with a high mortality rate cannot be overemphasized. The multisystemic dysfunction usually present renders diagnosis more complex and treatment more challenging. As soon as myxedema coma is suspected, for example, in the Emergency Department, the patient should be transferred to the intensive care unit for close monitoring and prompt treatment. Any delay caused by either inability to diagnose or temporizing while waiting for blood test confirmation is unacceptable and may contribute to an increased risk of mortality.

THYROID HORMONE REPLACEMENT

Thyroid hormone treatment stands at the core of the therapy for myxedema coma. Numerous modalities or regimens have been proposed, varying in regard to doses, frequencies, and routes of administration. Perhaps the most debatable matter is whether to administer only T4, thereby relying on the individual to convert it to the more active T3, or to give T3 itself. However, because myxedema coma is not common and systematic randomized studies with a large cohort of patients are unavailable, the optimum treatment approach remains still uncertain.

Physiologically, the thyroid gland produces both T4 and T3, with only 20% of T3 derived from thyroidal secretion, whereas 80% of circulating T3 comes from the peripheral metabolic activation of T4 mediated by deiodinases I and II. Thus T3 is considered the more active thyroid hormone, with T4 serving as a "prohormone." Nevertheless, as has been reported, administration of only T4 may be sufficient in the treatment of myxedema coma because tissue deiodinases make possible its conversion to T3. However, based on its more rapid onset of action, the administration of T3 directly has been considered preferential in order to achieve a faster beneficial effect on the compromised systems and hence promote earlier transition toward a euthyroid state.[29,30] Nevertheless, some studies suggest that T4 provides a steadier and smoother onset of action with a lower risk of adverse effects. In our view, the choice of therapy with T4 alone or T3 alone, or T4 plus T3 may depend on the clinical severity of the patient's status and the willingness to take on a possible greater risk attendant to T3 therapy factored against estimates of risk benefit. Hence, the importance of personalizing the patient's therapy by balancing the need for quickly attaining physiologically effective thyroid hormone levels against the risk of precipitating a fatal tachyarrhythmia or myocardial infarction.

Routes of Administration

Both T4 and T3 are available for oral and parenteral administration and both routes have been reported to be used with success. However, as there may be gastrointestinal involvement in myxedema with impaired absorption and gastric atony, the intravenous administration could be more effective. The oral route can even be employed in comatose patients by placement of a nasogastric tube.

Doses

A loading dose of 200 to 400 mcg of levothyroxine (T4) may be given intravenously followed by a maintenance dose of 1.6 mcg/kg body weight per day, reduced to 75% if being intravenously administered. Within 24 hours, serum T4 levels may approach the normal reference range and a decrease in TSH levels should be observed. Following improvement in the overall general condition of the patient, we may switch to oral therapy. Larger doses of T4 probably have no advantage and may, in fact, be more dangerous.[31] Due to its conversion from T4, a progressive increase in serum T3 is seen after a dose of 300 to 600 mcg of T4, as has been described by Ridgway et al.[31]

Although the therapeutic approach of administering a bolus followed by maintenance therapy has been more widely accepted as optimal, the initial amount of the dose of T4 is still debated. In a retrospective study analyzing 11 patients with myxedema coma, it was observed that those patients who died had received larger amounts of thyroid hormone and had circulating levels of T3 that were 1.9 times higher than the surviving patients.[3] Together with advanced age, high serum levels of T3 were associated with a fatal outcome. It was on this basis that Hylander et al. suggested that the use of T4 instead of T3 would lead to lower serum levels of T3, which are probably less stressful for the patients.[3]

In a more recent prospective study, 11 patients were randomized to receive either a 500-mcg loading dose of intravenous T4 followed by a 100-mcg daily maintenance dose, or only the maintenance dose. The overall mortality rate was 36.4%, and despite the absence of statistically significant results between the two groups, a lower mortality was noted in the high-dose group (17%) versus the low-dose group (60%).[32] Factors associated with a worse outcome included a decreased level of consciousness, lower Glasgow coma score, and increased severity of illness on entry as determined by an APACHE II score of more than 20.[32]

"Thyroid Sick Syndrome"

As mentioned earlier, whether treatment with T4 alone or a combination of T3 and T4 is more beneficial for the patients is still debatable. Although T3 is the active form of thyroid hormone and its administration will have a faster onset of action, it will also expose the patient to a higher risk for tachyarrhythmias and an ischemic heart event. By its slower and gradual conversion to T3, T4 instead would provide an ostensibly safer source of thyroid hormone. However, although historically the treatment of myxedema coma with T4 alone has been generally successful, there is one important potential drawback to total reliance on T3 generation from T4. The concern is based on the fact that conversion of T4 to T3 is impaired in several nonthyroidal illnesses and critical conditions (euthyroid sick syndrome)[28] and this situation may apply to myxedema coma wherein T4 conversion to T3 may also be impaired by an underling illness.[33] If so, then rates of conversion of T4 to T3 would be reduced and recovery or even survival of the patient may be threatened. Based on this concern, we recommend that when only T4 is to be administered that there be frequent periodic monitoring of blood T4, FT4, FT3, and TSH. If clinical recovery is delayed in parallel with failure of T3 to rise and TSH to fall, we believe it prudent to then administer small supplemental doses of T3 (10–20 mcg twice daily), particularly when an obvious associated illness is present that would be affecting T4 to T3 conversion. One patient has been reported with postpartum hypopituitary insufficiency presenting with cardiogenic shock who did not respond to T4 treatment but improved once T3 was used.[29] According to a (weak) recommendation of the American Thyroid Association (ATA), a loading dose of T3 of 5 to 20 mcg can be given concomitantly with T4, followed by a maintenance dose of 2.5 to 10 mcg every 8 hours.[34] When therapy is approached with T3 alone, it may be given as a 10 to 20 mcg bolus followed by 10 mcg every 4 hours for the first 24 hours, dropping to 10 mcg every 6 hours for days 2 to 3, by which time oral administration should be feasible.[35]

Preferred Regimen

Taking all the aforementioned considerations into account, our preferred regimen reflects a compromise approach with administration of both forms of thyroid hormones. We would initially administer both T4 and T3 simultaneously, with T4 at a dose of 4 mcg/kg lean body weight (approximately 200 to 300 mcg) followed by 100 mcg 24 hours later and then 50 mcg daily either intravenously or orally. Simultaneously with the initial dose of T4, we recommend an initial bolus of T3 (5 to 20 mcg), followed by 2.5 to 10 mcg of T3 intravenously every 8 to 12 hours until the patient is conscious and able to tolerate oral intake (Box 4.3).[34] Clinical improvement has also been reported with a single dose of T3.[30] Recently published ATA guidelines for treatment of hypothyroidism and myxedema coma[34] emphasize individualizing dosage based upon age, weight, and cardiac status, suggesting the initial use of intravenous T4 in a dose of 200 to 400 mcg, with a lower dose given to elderly patients or those with cardiac disease. It is wise to monitor the patient for any untoward effects of therapy before administering each dose of thyroid hormone.[36]

ANTIBIOTIC THERAPY

Although the principal cause of myxedema coma is severe hypothyroidism, treatment with thyroid hormone alone may not be sufficient to address the complex multisystemic decompensation that is often present. As it is quite common that pulmonary or systemic infections serve as triggering events for progression to coma, it has been suggested that initiation of empiric broad spectrum antibiotic therapy may be beneficial even in the absence of fever or leukocytosis.

VENTILATOR SUPPORT

The high mortality rate is often related to inexorable respiratory failure, and hence maintenance of an adequate airway and prevention of hypoxemia is one of the most important supportive measures required to avoid a disastrous outcome. Presence of hypoventilation and increased retention of CO_2 will contribute to aggravation of the comatose state by worsening the hypoxemia and causing respiratory acidosis. Given the presence of frank coma, in almost all cases intubation and respiratory assistance are necessary for the first days, especially if drugs have contributed to respiratory depression. Even when consciousness is regained, noninvasive respiratory ventilation may be necessary for 2 to 3 weeks for some patients.

Initial intubation leads to improvement of the respiratory state by reducing hypercapnia and improving the respiratory acidosis, although hypoxia may be noted to persist longer, a phenomenon

BOX 4.3 ■ Management of Myxedema Coma

Thyroid Hormone Treatment

- T4 bolus 4 mcg/kg lean body weight (approximately 200–400 mcg) followed by 100 mcg 24 h later and then 50 mcg daily either intravenously or orally
- T3 bolus (5–20 mcg), followed by 2.5–10 mcg T3 intravenously every 8–12 h until the patient is conscious and able to tolerate oral intake.

lower dose should be given to older patients or those with cardiac disease

Ventilation

- If hypoxia and/or hypercapnia present
- Extubate only when patient is fully conscious
- If necessary, keep noninvasive assisted ventilation for 2–3 weeks

Empiric Antibiotic Therapy

Hyponatremia

If Na plasma levels <120 mEq/L:

- Slow administration of hypertonic saline infusion 50–100 mL 3% sodium chloride
- Furosemide intravenous bolus dose of 40–80 mg

(limit sodium correction to less than 10–12 mmol/L in 24 h and less than 18 mmol/L in 48 h)

- Vaptans
  - Conivaptan: 20 mg loading dose infused in 30 min followed by 20 mg/day continuous infusion for up to 4 days
  - Tolvaptan: starting dose of 15 mg the first day followed by titration up to 30 mg and 60 mg at 24-hours if necessary.

If Na plasma levels are 120–130 mEq/L

- Water restriction

Hypothermia

Blankets
Warm room temperature

Hypotension

Fluids 5%–10% glucose in 0.5 N NaCl initially or as isotonic normal saline if hyponatremia is present.

Glucocorticoids

Hydrocortisone 50–100 mg IV every 6–8 h during the first 7–10 days with tapering of the dosage thereafter based upon clinical response and further diagnostic evaluation.

thought due to shunting in nonaerated areas.[37] Given the gravity of the situation and the compromised respiratory state usually present, arterial blood gases should be monitored regularly until the full recovery of the patient. Moreover, extubation should be approached cautiously, as patients may relapse, especially if extubation is attempted before the patient is fully conscious.

HYPONATREMIA

Renal function is impaired in profound hypothyroidism, resulting in fluid retention, electrolyte dilution, and hyponatremia. Sodium levels must be closely monitored and properly corrected. Although the comatose state results from multiple factors, hyponatremia per se can cause disorientation, altered consciousness, lethargy, and coma. With marked hyponatremia (serum sodium concentration less than 120 mEq/L), the slow administration of hypertonic saline (50 to 100 mL 3% sodium chloride) is justified and should suffice to increase the sodium concentration by 2 mmol/L early in the course of treatment.[33] Too rapid correction can result in worsening central nervous system function due to central pontine myelinolysis. In patients with chronic hyponatremia this complication is avoided by limiting the sodium correction to less than 10 to 12 mmol/L in 24 hours and to less than 18 mmol/L in 48 hours.

Otherwise, only normal saline or mixed saline/glucose should be employed and will also address the volume depletion present. The water diuresis can be enhanced by administering an intravenous bolus dose of 40 to 80 mg furosemide after the saline infusion.[33] Even slight improvement of hyponatremia (2 to 4 mmol/L) may contribute to a reduction in brain edema.[38] After achieving a sodium level of more than 120 mmol/L, no further hypertonic saline infusion should be required, and restriction of fluids may be all that is necessary to correct any persistent hyponatremia, especially if it is mild (120 to 130 mmol/L).

The high ADH levels reported in myxedema coma play a key role in water retention and worsening of hyponatremia. For this reason, the use of ADH antagonists may contribute to correction of the plasma sodium. The Food and Drug Administration has approved use of vasopressin antagonists called vaptans (conivaptan and tolvaptan) for the treatment of hypervolemic hyponatremia.[39] Conivaptan current dosing recommendations are 20 mg loading dose to be infused over 30 minutes followed by 20 mg/day continuous infusion for up to 4 days. Tolvaptan is administered orally in a starting dose of 15 mg the first day, followed by titration up to 30 mg and 60 mg at 24 hours if necessary. In order to avoid overcorrection, fluid restriction is not recommended during the active-phase treatment with tolvaptan. Because of the low incidence of myxedema coma, there are as yet no studies indicating that treatment with vaptans alone would be sufficient in these patients with severe hyponatremia.[38]

HYPOTHERMIA

It should be anticipated that initiation of T4 and/or T3 treatment will promote an increase in body temperature to normal. In the interim, blankets or increased room temperature can be used to keep the patient warm. Rapidly increasing body temperature with electric warming blankets is strongly discouraged in order to avoid peripheral vasodilatation that would worsen hypotension and increase the risk of shock.

HYPOTENSION

Maintenance of an effective blood pressure is essential to guarantee organ perfusion and avoid multiorgan failure. With the initiation of thyroid hormone treatment, blood pressure should slowly improve. Persistent hypotension can be addressed by cautious infusion of 5% to 10% glucose in 0.5 N sodium chloride initially, or as isotonic normal saline if hyponatremia is present. Hydrocortisone treatment (100 mg IV every 8 hours) may be administered concomitant with fluids until the blood pressure is corrected. Additional treatment with vasopressors is usually not required and must be carefully weighed in view of the added risk of cardiovascular events.[1] However, if pressors are required, dopamine use could assure improved coronary blood flow. In any event, cardiac function must be carefully monitored for ischemia and administration of vasopressors suspended as soon as possible.[1]

CORTICOSTEROIDS

As indicated above, it could be of crucial importance to rule out the possible concomitant presence of adrenal or pituitary insufficiency in these patients. In the majority of cases, the pituitary adrenal axis is not compromised sufficiently in overt hypothyroidism to prevent sufficient production of cortisol in case of necessity. However, decreased adrenal reserve has been found in 5% to 10% of patients on the basis of either hypopituitarism or primary adrenal failure, accompanying

Hashimoto's disease (Schmidt's syndrome). Thus, a rising urea nitrogen, hypotension, hypothermia, hypoglycemia, hyponatremia, and hyperkalemia may signal the coexistence of adrenal insufficiency. The typical dosage of hydrocortisone is 50 to 100 mg every 6 to 8 hours during the first 7 to 10 days, with tapering of the dosage thereafter based upon clinical response. After a basal blood plasma cortisol level is drawn, there should be no reluctance to administer short-term corticosteroids until the patient is stable and the integrity of the pituitary–adrenal axis can be determined. Even though adrenal insufficiency is present in only a minority of patients, we recommend that corticosteroids always be administered together with thyroid hormone treatment.

Initiating T4 therapy in a setting of adrenal insufficiency without concomitant corticosteroid coverage would risk precipitation of acute adrenal crisis due to the increased cellular metabolism of corticosteroids by the T4.[35]

Myxedema Coma and Surgery

If the factor precipitating the myxedema coma is a condition requiring surgical intervention, surgery must be deferred if possible until the patient's condition is improved. However, if emergency surgery is required, it can proceed with initiation of the indicated therapeutic interventions described previously as feasible, albeit at significant risk of a poor outcome depending on the degree of multisystem dysfunction present. Careful coordination between the treatment team of surgeon, intensivist, endocrinologist, and anesthesiologist will be required.

Although the literature on emergent perioperative management of myxedema coma is scant, it has been advocated that combination T4 and T3 therapy could provide better outcome for the patient, as it would allow a rapid onset of thyroid replacement in the acute perioperative period. However, caution should be exercised in elderly patients with close monitoring of cardiac function.

General Supportive Measures

In addition to the specific therapies outlined, other treatments will be indicated as in the management of any other elderly patient with multisystemic involvement. This might include the treatment of underlying problems such as infection, congestive heart failure, uncontrolled diabetes, or hypertension. The dosage of specific medications (e.g., digoxin for congestive heart failure) may need to be modified based on their altered distribution and slowed metabolism of drugs in myxedema.

Prognosis

Even though myxedema coma has a high mortality, a recent trend of reduction in fatal events has been noted. Mortality has decreased from 60% to 70% to 20% to 25% as a result of more timely diagnosis and improved treatment protocols in intensive care units. However, the prognosis for myxedema coma still remains grim, and elderly patients with severe hypothermia, hypotension, lower degree of consciousness by Glasgow coma scale, and multiorgan impairment can be expected to do worst.[3,32,40–42] The most common causes of death are respiratory failure, sepsis, and GI bleeding. Early diagnosis and prompt treatment, with meticulous attention to the details of management during the first 48 hours, remain critical for the avoidance of a fatal outcome.

References

1. Ono Y, Ono S, Yasunaga H, Matsui H, Fushimi K, Tanaka Y. Clinical characteristics and outcomes of myxedema coma: analysis of a national inpatient database in Japan. *J Epidemiol.* 2017;27(3):117–122.
2. Galofré JC, García-Mayor RV. Densidad de incidencia del coma mixedematoso. *Endocrinologia.* 1997; 44:103–104.

3. Hylander B, Rosenqvist U. Treatment of myxoedema coma: factors associated with fatal outcome. *Acta Endocrinol (Copenh).* 1985;108:65–71.
4. Blignault EJ. Advanced pregnancy in severely myxedematous patient. A case report and review of the literature. *S Afr Med J.* 1980;57:1050–1051.
5. Mathew V, Misgar RA, Ghosh S, et al. Myxedema coma: a new look into an old crisis. *J Thyroid Res.* 2011;2011:493462.
6. Kim JJ, Kim EY. Myxedema coma precipitated by diabetic ketoacidosis after total thyroidectomy: a case report. *J Med Case Rep.* 2019;13(1):50. doi:10.1186/s13256-019-1992-0.
7. Mallipedhi A, Vali H, Okosieme O. Myxedema coma in a patient with subclinical hypothyroidism. *Thyroid.* 2011;21(1):87–89.
8. Chu M, Seltzer TF. Myxedema coma induced by ingestion of raw bok choy. *N Engl J Med.* 2010; 362(20):1945–1946.
9. Lele AV, Clutter S, Price E, De Ruyter ML. Severe hypothyroidism presenting as myxedema coma in the postoperative period in a patient taking sunitinib: case report and review of literature. *J Clin Anesth.* 2013;25(1):47–51.
10. Chen SY, Kao PC, Lin ZZ, Chiang WC, Fang CC. Sunitinib-induced myxedema coma. *Am J Emerg Med.* 2009;27(3):370.e1–370.e3.
11. Reinhardt W, Mann K. Incidence, clinical picture and treatment of hypothyroid coma. Results of a survey. *Med Klin.* 1997;92:521–524.
12. Popoveniuc G, Chandra T, Sud A, et al. A diagnostic scoring system for myxedema coma. *Endocr Pract.* 2014;20(8):808–817.
13. Massumi RA, Winnacker JL. Severe depression of the respiratory center in myxedema. *Am J Med.* 1964;36:876–882.
14. Domm BB, Vassallo CL. Myxedema coma with respiratory failure. *Am Rev Respir Dis.* 1973;107:842–845.
15. Wilson WR, Bedell GN. The pulmonary abnormalities in myxedema. *J Clin Invest.* 1960;39:42–55.
16. Zwillich CW, Pierson DJ, Hofeldt FD, Lufkin EG, Weil JV. Ventilatory control in myxedema and hypothyroidism. *N Engl J Med.* 1975;292:662–665.
17. Schenck JB, Rizvi AA, Lin T. Severe primary hypothyroidism manifesting with torsades de pointes. *Am J Med Sci.* 2006;331:154–156.
18. Garrahy A, Agha A. Dementia, cardiomyopathy and pseudo-obstruction in a 63-year-old female. *Eur J Intern Med.* 2018 Mar 1. pii: S0953-6205(18)30088-8.
19. Ji JS, Chae HS, Cho YS, et al. Myxedema ascites: case report and literature review. *J Korean Med Sci.* 2006;21:761–764.
20. DeRubertis Jr FR, Michelis MF, Bloom ME, Mintz DH, Field JB, Davis BB. Impaired water excretion in myxedema. *Am J Med.* 1971;51:41–53.
21. Skowsky WR, Kikuchi TA. The role of vasopressin in the impaired water excretion of myxedema. *Am J Med.* 1978;64:613–621.
22. Jansen HJ, Doebé SR, Louwerse ES, van der Linden JC, Netten PM. Status epilepticus caused by a myxoedema coma. *Neth J Med.* 2006;64:202–205.
23. Manfredi E, van Zaane B, Gerdes VE, Brandjes DP, Squizzato A. Hypothyroidism and acquired von Willebrand's syndrome: a systematic review. *Haemophilia.* 2008;14:423–433.
24. Michiels JJ, Schroyens W, Berneman Z, van der Planken M. Acquired von Willebrand syndrome type 1 in hypothyroidism: reversal after treatment with thyroxine. *Clin Appl Thromb Hemost.* 2001;7:113–115.
25. Chiong YV, Bammerlin E, Mariash CN. Development of an objective tool for the diagnosis of myxedema coma. *Transl Res.* 2015;166(3):233–243.
26. Benvenga S, Squadrito S, Saporito F, Cimino A, Arrigo F, Trimarchi F. Myxedema coma of both primary and secondary origin, with non-classic presentation and extremely elevated creatine kinase. *Horm Metab Res.* 2000;32(9):364–366.
27. Hooper MJ. Diminished TSH secretion during acute non-thyroidal illness in untreated primary hypothyroidism. *Lancet.* 1976;i:48–49.
28. Wartofsky L, Burman KD. Alterations in thyroid function in patients with systemic illness: the 'euthyroid sick syndrome. *Endocr Rev.* 1982;3:164–217.
29. McKerrow SD, Osborn LA, Levy H, Eaton RP, Economou P. Myxedema-associated cardiogenic shock treated with triiodothyronine. *Ann Intern Med.* 1992;117:1014–1015.

30. McCulloch W, Price P, Hinds CJ, Wass JA. Effects of low dose oral triiodothyronine in myxoedema coma. *Intensive Care Med.* 1985;11:259–262.
31. Ridgway EC, McCammon JA, Benotti J, Maloof F. Acute metabolic responses in myxedema to large doses of intravenous l-thyroxine. *Ann Intern Med.* 1972;77:549–555.
32. Rodríguez I, Fluiters E, Pérez-Méndez LF, Luna R, Páramo C, García-Mayor RV. Factors associated with mortality of patients with myxoedema coma: prospective study in 11 cases treated in a single institution. *J Endocrinol.* 2004;180:347–350.
33. Pereira VG, Haron ES, Lima-Neto N, Medeiros-Neto GA. Management of myxedema coma: report on three successfully treated cases with nasogastric or intravenous administration of triiodothyronine. *J Endocrinol Invest.* 1982;5:331–334.
34. Jonklaas J, Bianco AC, Bauer AJ, et al. Guidelines for the treatment of hypothyroidism: prepared by the American Thyroid Association task force on thyroid hormone replacement. American Thyroid Association Task Force on Thyroid Hormone Replacement. *Thyroid.* 2014;24(12):1670–1751.
35. Klubo-Gwiezdzinska J, Wartofsky L. Myxedema coma. *Oxford Textbook of Endocrinology and Diabetes.* 2nd ed. Oxford: Oxford University Press; 2011:537–543.
36. Ylli D, Klubo-Gwiezdzinska J, Wartofsky L. Thyroid emergencies. *Pol Arch Intern Med.* 2019;129(7-8): 526–534. doi:10.20452/pamw.14876. Epub 2019 Jun 25.
37. Nicoloff JT. Thyroid storm and myxedema coma. *Med Clin North Am.* 1985;69:1005–1017.
38. Verbalis JG, Goldsmith SR, Greenberg A, et al. Diagnosis, evaluation, and treatment of hyponatremia: expert panel recommendations. *Am J Med.* 2013;126(10 Suppl 1):S1–S42.
39. Hline SS, Pham PT, Pham PT, Aung MH, Pham PM, Pham PC. Conivaptan: a step forward in the treatment of hyponatremia. *Ther Clin Risk Manag.* 2008;4:315–326.
40. Yamamoto T, Fukuyama J, Fujiyoshi A. Factors associated with mortality of myxedema coma: report of eight cases and literature survey. *Thyroid.* 1999;9:1167–1174.
41. Jordan RM. Myxedema coma. Pathophysiology, therapy, and factors affecting prognosis. *Med Clin North Am.* 1995;79:185–194.
42. Dutta P, Bhansali A, Masoodi SR, Bhadada S, Sharma N, Rajput R. Predictors of outcome in myxoedema coma: a study from a tertiary care centre. *Crit Care.* 2008;12:1–8.

CHAPTER 5

Acute Suppurative Thyroiditis

Sara Ahmadi ■ Erik K. Alexander

CHAPTER OUTLINE

Background

Acute suppurative thyroiditis (AST) is a rare condition with an incidence of 0.1% to 0.7 % among all thyroid disease.[1] As the thyroid gland is resistant to infection due to protective factors, including high iodine content, high vascularity, extensive lymphatic drainage, and encapsulation, AST is extremely rare.[2] Case reports therefore dominate the published literature, and there are no established guidelines or clinical trials regarding the diagnosis and management of patients with AST.

AST is a potentially life-threatening endocrine emergency that also can be associated with a high mortality rate in certain patients. Potential complications can occur pending abscess extension or rupture in patients with AST, leading to esophageal or tracheal fistula, jugular vein thrombophlebitis, descending necrotizing mediastinitis, or septicemia. A defining dogma is that early diagnosis and appropriate treatment are key factors toward achieving success in the management of patients with AST.

In many cases a predisposing factor to suppurative thyroiditis is identified, including having an immunocompromised state, pyriform sinus fistula (PSF), neck trauma, lymphatic or hemorrhagic spread (e.g., septic emboli), direct inoculation of thyroid gland (e.g., via fine needle aspiration [FNA] or central line placement), ruptured esophagus, or retropharyngeal abscess.[1,3–7] A wide spectrum of microbial pathogens has been reported in patients who suffer from suppurative thyroiditis, including both gram-positive and gram-negative bacteria, as well as fungus, *Nocardia*, and even mycobacteria.

Bacterial Infection

Most patients with acute suppurative thyroiditis are found to have a bacterial etiology, and present with signs and symptoms of infection including neck swelling, redness, warmth, tenderness, and fever.[1] The most common bacterial pathogen of suppurative thyroiditis are gram-positive bacteria such as *Staphylococcus* and *Streptococcus* species.[8–10] However, suppurative thyroiditis due to gram-negative organisms has been also reported. Separately, there are reports of suppurative thyroiditis due to *Brucella* infection,[11,12] as well as *Escherichia coli* infection due to hematogenous spread from urinary tract infection.[13] Finally, *Salmonella* as a causative pathogen as well as[14] and *Porphyromonas* bacteria have been implicated.[13]

Fungal Infection

Infection of the thyroid gland via a fungal pathogen is uncommon, but ranks as the second most common cause of infectious thyroiditis.[15] Fungal AST has been mainly reported in immunosuppressed patients. Specifically, fungal thyroiditis has been described due to *Aspergillus*,[16,17] *Candida*,[18] *Cryptococus*,[19] and *Coccidioides immitis*.[20,21]

Aspergillus is the most common reported fungal thyroiditis.[22-24] It is most often seen in immunosuppressed patients with widespread disseminated *Aspergillus* infection. A thyroid function test can be variable in patients with *Aspergillus* suppurative thyroiditis.[24] The most common presentation in this setting is acute neck pain and swelling accompanied by signs and symptoms of thyrotoxicosis. This can make such a diagnosis difficult to distinguish from subacute granulomatous thyroiditis, which is also painful.[23,25] A clinical presentation of *Aspergillus* thyroiditis presenting as an enlarging mass due to an abscess has been also reported.[26,27]

Granulomatous Infections

Granulomatous infectious thyroiditis is very rare, especially in the developed world. The two most common infectious pathogens causing granulomatous thyroid disease are *Mycobacterium tuberculosis* and *Nocardia*. Patients with tuberculous involvement of the thyroid gland usually present with an enlarging neck mass as part of widespread disseminated disease, though patients are usually euthyroid. Less common presentations of tuberculous thyroid involvement are an acute mycobacterial abscess[28] and new onset hyperthyroidism,[29] as well as hypothyroidism due to gland destruction.[30] Patients with tuberculous thyroid involvement usually have subacute presentations similar to that of acute granulomatous thyroiditis (De Quervain's thyroiditis). For this illness, the diagnosis must be made by histopathologic examination, acid-fast bacilli (AFB) staining, and microbiologic culture, usually in a patient with known disseminated *M. tuberculous* disease.[31,32]

Nocardiosis most commonly presents with pulmonary disease. However, extrapulmonary sites of *Nocardia* infection include the central nervous system and soft tissue. Thyroid involvement by *Nocardia* infection is extremely rare. The majority of patients with nocardiosis are immunosuppressed, often due to HIV infection or organ transplantation. The diagnosis is typically made based on the clinical picture in high-risk patients in whom *Nocardia* has already been identified, as *Nocardia* is an extremely difficult pathogen to grow in culture.[33-36]

Laboratory Testing and Diagnostic Imaging for Acute Suppurative Thyroiditis

When suspected, the initial laboratory evaluation in patients with possible AST should include measurement of a complete blood count (CBC) with differential, a comprehensive metabolic panel (CMP), serial thyroid function testing, an erythrocyte sedimentation rate (ESR) and a C-reactive protein (CRP), urine analysis, and urine culture, as well as blood and fungal cultures with antibiotic sensitivity.[1] Serial thyroid function test is recommended because suppurative thyroiditis could be associated with acute thyrotoxicosis secondary to the release of preformed thyroxine and triiodothyronine given the acute destruction of thyroid follicles.[7,9,13,29] Additional laboratory testing may be appropriate based on clinical and physical examination findings.

It is important to differentiate acute suppurative thyroiditis from other causes of acute neck swelling and pain (e.g., sternocleidomastoid abscess, parathyroid hemorrhage or abscess, lymph node suppuration, thyroglossal duct cyst infection, retropharyngeal abscess, subacute thyroiditis, aggressive thyroid cancer, thyroid nodule/cyst hemorrhage).[1]

Ultrasonography (US) and computed tomography (CT) are two of the imaging modalities that can be used to facilitate the diagnosis of acute suppurative thyroiditis. However, a CT scan may be of limited utility in the early stages of thyroid inflammation, as the imaging findings on CT scan in early stages of AST are low-density areas and slight lobular swellings, both of which are nonspecific. Ultrasound is generally preferred as an imaging modality, and is more capable of diagnosing acute suppurative thyroiditis in the early stages. Ultrasound imaging findings at this stage include identification of hypoechoic areas within the thyroid gland, a finding of perithyroidal hypoechoic spaces, and effacement of the planes between perithyroid tissue and the thyroid gland.[37]

Differentiating acute suppurative thyroiditis from subacute painful thyroiditis (De Quervain's thyroiditis) in the early stage can be challenging and, given this, can result in the prescription of prednisone, which can effectively treat De Quervain's thyroiditis but have an adverse impact and worsen clinical symptoms of acute suppurative disease. Subacute painful thyroiditis is relatively common, and it is associated with anterior neck discomfort overlying the gland, as well as an elevated white blood cell count, ESR, and CRP similar to acute suppurative thyroiditis. An iodine scintigraphy scan will not prove helpful to differentiate these two subtypes of thyroiditis in the setting of thyrotoxicosis, as both demonstrate low radioactive iodine uptake, typically less than 1%. Ultrasound and FNA of any mass or fluid collection is the most helpful method to differentiate between these two subtypes of thyroiditis. Thyroid US usually shows diffuse heterogenicity with low-intensity vascular flow in subacute painful thyroiditis.[1,2]

CT scan and US imaging findings during the acute, symptomatic stages of suppurative thyroiditis are more specific. In a study of 60 patients, CT scans performed during the acute stages demonstrated abscess formation, edema of the ipsilateral hypopharynx, and low density to the thyroid gland in 97%, 83%, and 76% of the patients, respectively. Swelling of the thyroid gland and thyroid shifting/deformity due to abscess formation were less common findings, being seen in 38% and 41% of patients, respectively.[37] This study also examined the role of thyroid US during acute stages of disease. Abscess formation, hypoechoic areas in the thyroid gland, and perithyroidal hypoechoic spaces with effacement of the plane between the perithyroid tissue and thyroid gland were seen in 81%, 94%, and 88% of the patients, respectively.[37]

Given the lack of sensitivity and specificity with other modalities, ultrasound-guided FNA and subsequent cytology/culture remains the best diagnostic method to clarify disease in patients with suspected AST.

Radionuclide imaging of the thyroid with I^{123} or TC^{99} are not helpful in diagnosing AST, as acute infection and thyroid cancer are both associated with focal decreased uptake in euthyroid patients, and diffuse decreased uptake in patients with hyperthyroidism due to destruction of the gland. The diagnostic utility of magnetic resonance imaging (MRI) in patients with AST is unknown due to limited data.[1]

A PSF is a third and fourth pharyngeal pouch anomaly, usually occurring on the left side. PSF should be suspected in pediatric patients with recurrent AST or anterior neck abscess especially when on the left side. CT scan, US, direct laryngoscopy, and barium swallow are imaging modalities that can be used to help diagnose PSF, with barium swallow being the most sensitive method. The ability of imaging studies to detect PSF can vary with the stage of inflammation. One study by Masuoka et al. showed that a barium swallow can detect fistulas in 89% and 97% of cases during the acute and late inflammatory stages. The same study, however, showed that CT scans only detected fistulas in 20% and 54% of cases during these stages.[10,37,38]

Treatment of AST and Recommended Follow-up

AST is a life-threatening endocrine emergency with potential for high mortality. Patients with clinical suspicious of AST should be admitted to an inpatient hospital facility and a monitored setting. Stabilization of respiratory and cardiac function is necessary while the patient is undergoing diagnostic evaluation.

Most patients with bacterial AST are acutely ill and require empiric broad-spectrum antibiotic treatment while diagnostic evaluations, including blood culture, abscess culture, and tissue sampling, are being completed. Most patients with bacterial suppurative thyroiditis require an open surgical procedure including excision or drainage, in addition to antibiotic treatment. There are case reports of successful conservative treatments following only ultrasound-guided drainage of abscesses.[39] But as abscesses are most often complex and loculated, needle drainage is often not a definitive treatment in most cases, and surgical drainage is necessary. Although exceedingly rare, patients with comprised airways require urgent transcutaneous or open-surgical drainage, and conservative diagnostic and therapeutic US-FNA is not appropriate in these patients.

As noted earlier, the rapid initiation of broad-spectrum antibacterial therapy should be initiated promptly with the goals of covering opportunistic infections. Such coverage should be empirically broadened further when treating an immunocompromised host.

The treatment of fungal suppurative thyroiditis includes systemic antifungal therapy, along with aggressive surgical debridement when indicated.[27] In patients with *M. tuberculosis* thyroid involvement, treatment with quadruple antituberculous therapy (e.g., rifampicin, isoniazid, pyrazinamide, and ethambutol) is usually sufficient and has been shown to lead to full resolution involving nonresistant strains. However, occasionally surgery or drainage of an abscess must occur in addition to antituberculous treatment.[29,40]

Surgical thyroidectomy (near-total or hemithyroidectomy) should be considered only when there is evidence of persistent or progressive (nonresponsive to treatment) thyroidal infection despite abscess drainage and medical therapy.[1,21] Patients with multiple, poorly defined, less discrete abscesses with evidence of persistent or progression of disease despite appropriate antibiotic treatment should also undergo thyroidectomy. However, clinicians should consider the higher risks and rates of potential complications following thyroidectomy in these settings given the presence of inflammation which complicates the identification of the recurrent laryngeal nerves and parathyroid glands. In such settings, abscess drainage and medical therapy followed by elective thyroidectomy after the acute inflammatory process has been resolved could be considered.[1]

Unique to AST due to pyriform sinus suppurative thyroiditis is abscess incision and drainage, antimicrobial treatment, and surgical removal of the PSF with or without partial thyroidectomy.[38,41] Endoscopic electrocauterization of the tract is an acceptable alternative to surgery. However, this is a new procedure with limited data regarding long-term outcomes.[42,43]

Rarely, acute suppurative thyroiditis can be associated with thyroid malignancy. Otani et al. reported a case of an adult female who presented with signs and symptoms of AST and responded to antimicrobial agents. Initial FNA did not show any overt evidence of papillary thyroid carcinoma (PTC); however, her thyroid inflammatory area decreased from 47 mm to 27 mm following antimicrobial treatment. At that point a more recognizable thyroid nodule was identified in the tissue and the patient underwent repeat FNA due to worrisome ultrasound features. At this point, FNA cytology was positive for PTC, and confirmed with surgical pathology.[44] Puthanpurayil et al. also reported a case of 17-year-old patient with AST who responded to antibiotic therapy, and where a thyroid inflammatory area reduced from 3 cm to 1.5 cm, and was confirmed as a discrete nodule. The patient underwent repeat FNA outside of the setting of acute inflammation. FNA cytology of the second biopsy was suspicious for PTC and malignancy was confirmed with histopathology.[45]

In summary, acute suppurative thyroiditis is a very rare yet dangerous condition. Host factors that predispose to this entity include pyriform sinus tract formation or other manipulation or exposure of the sterile thyroid to the outside environment, such as skin or oral mucosa. Although bacterial pathogens are most commonly causative, many other infectious agents have been described including *M. tuberculosis*. Prompt treatment is mandated given the risk of systemic infection, and the proximity of any abscess or mass to the vital neck structures. Most often when abscess formation is confirmed, drainage or surgical treatment is required. When detected early, AST can be effective treated, but in other more advanced settings, AST can be deadly.

References

1. Paes JE, Burman KD, Cohen J, et al. Acute bacterial suppurative thyroiditis: a clinical review and expert opinion. *Thyroid: Official Journal of the American Thyroid Association*. 2010;20(3):247–255.
2. Pearce EN, Farwell AP, Braverman LE. Thyroiditis. *The New England Journal of Medicine*. 2003;348(26): 2646–2655.
3. Chen HW, Tseng FY, Su DH, Chang YL, Chang TC. Secondary infection and ischemic necrosis after fine needle aspiration for a painful papillary thyroid carcinoma: a case report. *Acta Cytol*. 2006;50(2): 217–220.
4. Chrobok V, Celakovsky P, Nunez-Fernandez D, Simakova E. Acute purulent thyroiditis with retropharyngeal and retrotracheal abscesses. *J Laryngol Otol*. 2000;114(2):151–153.
5. Lu WH, Feng L, Sang JZ, et al. Various presentations of fourth branchial pouch sinus tract during surgery. *Acta Otolaryngol*. 2012;132(5):540–545.
6. Mollar-Puchades MA, Camara-Gomez R, Perez-Guillen V, Benavides-Gabernet M, Gomez-Vela J, Pinon-Selles F. Thyroid hematoma and infectious thyroiditis after a neck injury. *Thyroid: Official Journal of the American Thyroid Association*. 2006;16(4):421–422.
7. Yildar M, Demirpolat G, Aydin M. Acute suppurative thyroiditis accompanied by thyrotoxicosis after fine-needle aspiration: treatment with catheter drainage. *J Clin Diagn Res*. 2014;8(11):ND12–ND14.
8. Bravo E, Grayev A. Thyroid abscess as a complication of bacterial throat infection. *J Radiol Case Rep*. 2011;5(3):1–7.
9. Yan S, Patti L. Methicillin-sensitive *Staphylococcus aureus* suppurative thyroiditis with thyrotoxicosis. *Case Rep Emerg Med*. 2017;2017:4018193.
10. Wu C, Zhang Y, Gong Y, et al. Two cases of bacterial suppurative thyroiditis caused by *Streptococcus anginosus*. *Endocr Pathol*. 2013;24(1):49–53.
11. Akdemir Z, Karaman E, Akdeniz H, Alptekin C, Arslan H. Giant thyroid abscess related to postpartum Brucella infection. *Case Rep Infect Dis*. 2015;2015:646209.
12. Mousa AR, al-Mudallal DS, Marafie A. Brucella thyroiditis. *J Infect*. 1989;19(3):287–288.
13. Spitzer M, Alexanian S, Farwell AP. Thyrotoxicosis with post-treatment hypothyroidism in a patient with acute suppurative thyroiditis due to porphyromonas. *Thyroid: Official Journal of the American Thyroid Association*. 2012;22(1):97–100.
14. Kazi S, Liu H, Jiang N, et al. Salmonella thyroid abscess in human immunodeficiency virus-positive man: a diagnostic pitfall in fine-needle aspiration biopsy of thyroid lesions. *Diagn Cytopathol*. 2015;43(1):36–39.
15. King C, Clement S, Katugaha S, Brown AW. Fungal thyroiditis in a lung transplant recipient. *BMJ Case Rep*. 2018:2018.
16. Ataca P, Atilla E, Saracoglu P, et al. Aspergillus thyroiditis after allogeneic hematopoietic stem cell transplantation. *Case Rep Hematol*. 2015;2015:537187.
17. Badawy SM, Becktell KD, Muller WJ, Schneiderman J. Aspergillus thyroiditis: first antemortem case diagnosed by fine-needle aspiration culture in a pediatric stem cell transplant patient. *Transpl Infect Dis*. 2015;17(6):868–871.
18. Massolt ET, Rijneveld AW, Vernooij MW, Kevenaar ME, van Kemenade FJ, Peeters RP. Acute Candida thyroiditis complicated by abscess formation in a severely immunocompromised patient. *The Journal of Clinical Endocrinology and Metabolism*. 2014;99(11):3952–3953.
19. Avram AM, Sturm CA, Michael CW, Sisson JC, Jaffe CA. Cryptococcal thyroiditis and hyperthyroidism. *Thyroid: Official Journal of the American Thyroid Association*. 2004;14(6):471–474.
20. Moore JB, Hoang TD, Valentine JC, Maves RC. Coccidioidal thyroiditis. *Endocr Pract*. 2016;22(6):766.

21. McAninch EA, Xu C, Lagari VS, Kim BW. Coccidiomycosis thyroiditis in an immunocompromised host post-transplant: case report and literature review. *The Journal of Clinical Endocrinology and Metabolism*. 2014;99(5):1537–1542.
22. Goldani LZ, Zavascki AP, Maia AL. Fungal thyroiditis: an overview. *Mycopathologia*. 2006;161(3):129–139.
23. Alvi MM, Meyer DS, Hardin NJ, Dekay JG, Marney AM, Gilbert MP. Aspergillus thyroiditis: a complication of respiratory tract infection in an immunocompromised patient. *Case Rep Endocrinol*. 2013;2013:741041.
24. Nguyen J, Manera R, Minutti C. Aspergillus thyroiditis: a review of the literature to highlight clinical challenges. *Eur J Clin Microbiol Infect Dis*. 2012;31(12):3259–3264.
25. Hornef MW, Schopohl J, Zietz C, et al. Thyrotoxicosis induced by thyroid involvement of disseminated *Aspergillus fumigatus* infection. *J Clin Microbiol*. 2000;38(2):886–887.
26. Santiago M, Martinez JH, Palermo C, et al. Rapidly growing thyroid mass in an immunocompromised young male adult. *Case Rep Endocrinol*. 2013;2013:290843.
27. Thada ND, Prasad SC, Alva B, Pokharel M, Prasad KC. A rare case of suppurative aspergillosis of the thyroid. *Case Rep Otolaryngol*. 2013;2013:956236.
28. Parmar H, Hashmi M, Rajput A, Patankar T, Castillo M. Acute tuberculous abscess of the thyroid gland. *Australas Radiol*. 2002;46(2):186–188.
29. Raman L, Murray J, Banka R. Primary tuberculosis of the thyroid gland: an unexpected cause of thyrotoxicosis. *BMJ Case Rep*. 2014:2014.
30. Chaudhary A, Nayak B, Guleria S, Arora R, Gupta R, Sharma MC. Tuberculosis of the thyroid presenting as multinodular goiter with hypothyroidism: a rare presentation. *Indian J Pathol Microbiol*. 2010;53(3):579–581.
31. Ozekinci S, Mizrak B, Saruhan G, Senturk S. Histopathologic diagnosis of thyroid tuberculosis. *Thyroid: Official Journal of the American Thyroid Association*. 2009;19(9):983–986.
32. Majid U, Islam N. Thyroid tuberculosis: a case series and a review of the literature. *Journal of Thyroid Research*. 2011;2011:359864.
33. Trivedi DP, Bhagat R, Nakanishi Y, Wang A, Moroz K, Falk NK. Granulomatous thyroiditis: a case report and literature review. *Ann Clin Lab Sci*. 2017;47(5):620–624.
34. Carriere C, Marchandin H, Andrieu JM, Vandome A, Perez C. Nocardia thyroiditis: unusual location of infection. *J Clin Microbiol*. 1999;37(7):2323–2325.
35. Teckie G, Bhana SA, Tsitsi JM, Shires R. Thyrotoxicosis followed by hypothyroidism due to suppurative thyroiditis caused by *Nocardia brasiliensis* in a patient with advanced acquired immunodeficiency syndrome. *Eur Thyroid J*. 2014;3(1):65–68.
36. Osborn JD, Cariello PF, Pena E, Lee CJ. Nocardia thyroiditis after allogeneic hematopoietic cell transplantation. *Leuk Lymphoma*. 2019:1–4.
37. Masuoka H, Miyauchi A, Tomoda C, et al. Imaging studies in sixty patients with acute suppurative thyroiditis. *Thyroid: Official Journal of the American Thyroid Association*. 2011;21(10):1075–1080.
38. Nicoucar K, Giger R, Pope Jr HG, Jaecklin T, Dulguerov P. Management of congenital fourth branchial arch anomalies: a review and analysis of published cases. *J Pediatr Surg*. 2009;44(7):1432–1439.
39. Ilyin A, Zhelonkina N, Severskaya N, Romanko S. Nonsurgical management of thyroid abscess with sonographically guided fine needle aspiration. *J Clin Ultrasound*. 2007;35(6):333–337.
40. uz-Zaman M, Hussain R, Mirza MK, Khan KA, Khan GM, Ahmad MN. Isolated tuberculous thyroiditis as solitary thyroid nodule. *J Coll Physicians Surg Pak*. 2008;18(2):121–122.
41. Kondo T. Acute suppurative thyroiditis secondary to pyriform sinus fistula. *Lancet Infect Dis*. 2019;19(4):447.
42. Lammers D, Campbell R, Davila J, MacCormick J. Bilateral piriform sinus fistulas: a case study and review of management options. *J Otolaryngol Head Neck Surg*. 2018;47(1):16.
43. Ishinaga H, Kobayashi M, Qtsu K, et al. Endoscopic electrocauterization of pyriform sinus fistula. *Eur Arch Otorhinolaryngol*. 2017;274(11):3927–3931.
44. Otani H, Notsu M, Koike S, et al. Acute suppurative thyroiditis caused by thyroid papillary carcinoma in the right thyroid lobe of a healthy woman. *Thyroid Res*. 2018;11:4.
45. Kalladi Puthanpurayil S, Francis GL, Kraft AO, Prasad U, Petersson RS. Papillary thyroid carcinoma presenting as acute suppurative thyroiditis: a case report and review of the literature. *Int J Pediatr Otorhinolaryngol*. 2018;105:12–15.

CHAPTER 6

Thyrotoxic Periodic Paralysis: A Review and Suggestions for Treatment

Svetlana L. Krasnova ■ Arthur Topilow ■ Jan Calissendorff ■ Henrik Falhammar

CHAPTER OUTLINE

Introduction

Thyrotoxic periodic paralysis (TPP) is considered a neurologic and endocrine emergency. It is a rare, potentially fatal complication of thyrotoxicosis, and is characterized by a variable degree of hypokalemia and muscle paralysis due to a massive shift of potassium into the intracellular space.[1] TPP patients usually seek medical care in the emergency department (ED), but the diagnosis is often missed. The disease has mainly been reported in the male, East Asian population living within East Asian countries. However, published cases from other countries and ethnic groups have increased in the last decade, probably as a result of expanded migration and improved awareness of the condition. A New Zealand study found that Maori Polynesians and Pacific Islanders were also at higher risk for TPP compared to Europeans and European descendants living in New Zealand.[2] Although thyrotoxicosis is more often seen in females than in males, the incidence of TPP is 22 to 76 times more frequent in males compared with females.[3–5] This chapter will focus on the different features and treatments of TPP, in addition to the novel findings on the molecular mechanisms which underly the disorder.

Clinical Presentation

TPP has been described in the literature since the late 1900s. In 1957, Okinaka et al. published that the incidence of TPP was 1.9% in the thyrotoxic Japanese patient population,[3] and a decade later it was described that 1.8% of Chinese patients with thyrotoxicosis had a history suggestive of TPP.[4] The disorder has also been identified in Asian populations of Thais, Vietnamese, Filipinos,

Koreans, Taiwanese,[6] and Malaysians.[7–9] Cases have been reported in many different populations, including Europeans,[10–17] Afro-Americans,[11,18] Native Americans,[11,19] Afro-Caribbeans,[20] Polynesians,[21,22] Hispanics,[23,24] Brazilians,[25] Nepalese,[9] Lebanese,[26] Turks,[27,28] Indians,[9,29–31] and Saudis.[32] The incidence of TPP among thyrotoxic patients in the United States has been estimated to be 0.1% to 0.2%.[10,11]

The typical patient is a 20- to 40-year-old East Asian male. The few reported female cases have had a similar age distribution.[3,4,20,21,33–35] Although it is rare in children and adolescence, some cases of TPP in adolescence have been reported from China, Korea, and in other ethnic groups.[36] Until recently, reported cases of TPP have been attributed to Graves' disease, although autoimmune thyroiditis has been seen to be a very rare cause of TPP in children and adolescences.[37] The hallmark of TPP is recurrent muscle weakness. The attacks tend to be more commonly seen during the hot summer months, likely due to outdoor activities, loss of potassium through perspiration, and the drinking of cold and sweet drinks.[4,9,38] It has been reported[9,21,39] occasionally even on cold winter days.[15] Manoukian et al. reported that the paralysis started between 0100 and 0600 hours in 84% of his patients.[39] The attacks frequently occurred at night or early in the morning upon waking.[39] Others have reported that the attacks tended to occur during weekends, and were often preceded by a heavy meal, high alcohol intake, or strenuous exercise.[9] Other triggering factors that have been described included infections (mainly upper respiratory tract), emotional stress, menstruation, trauma, high-salt diet, beta 2 adrenergic bronchodilators,[40] and glucocorticoid administration.[24,28,41–44] Excessive alcohol intake can result in increased catecholamine secretion and hyperinsulinemia and that, along with hyperthyroidism and the hyperadrenergic state, may lead to a low serum potassium.[45] Affram et al. highlighted a case of TPP after an epidural steroid injection for traumatic low back pain in a patient with severe hypokalemia, hyperthyroidism, and Graves' disease.[46] Corticosteroids have been well-known precipitating factors. The side effect profile of corticosteroids, ranging from the common to the rare, should be kept in mind.[47]

Initial symptoms typically seen on presentation include muscle aches, cramps, and stiffness. Minor muscle aches and weakness accompanied by sore joints can precede the inability to move the legs altogether by approximately 2 weeks.[48] As a rule, the proximal muscles of the lower extremities are initially affected, but in approximately 80%, all four extremities are eventually involved.[35] Symptoms can range in intensity from mild weakness to total paralysis. Asymmetrical weakness has also been noted.[49] Attacks involving all four extremities are frequently linked to urinary retention, oliguria (occasionally polyuria if there is prolonged hypokalemia), and constipation. However, the acute onset of lower motor neuron quadriparesis, without bladder or bowel involvement, has also been described occurring with concomitant hypokalemia and compensated respiratory alkalosis. Improvement in quadriparesis has been achieved with intravenous (IV) potassium, magnesium sulphate, and cautious monitoring.[31]

It is hypothesized that the size of the quadriceps femoris muscle may contribute to TPP. A study by Tang et al. found that the muscle thickness of TPP patients was larger than in nonparalytic hyperthyroid patients. For a hyperthyroid patient, the increase in the quadriceps thickness may indicate a close correlation with TPP, independent of age and body mass index (BMI). Thus, the study concluded that the size of the quadriceps femoris may be, in some way, causally related to the TPP.[50]

Achilles tendon reflexes are absent in about two-thirds of patients, but mental status and sensory functions have been seen to be intact.[9] Ocular, bulbar, and respiratory involvement, although rare, has been documented in a few very severe and occasionally fatal attacks.[29,51–55] Affected muscle groups recover in the reverse order from the paralysis, usually within 36 hours[11] and all within 72 hours.[42] The time from the start of symptoms until the IV potassium treatment is around 3.5 hours in hospitals that have seen many cases of TPP.[56]

In 76% of patients, the thyrotoxicosis had not been diagnosed before the attack, and 79% had no family history of hyperthyroidism.[34] Signs and symptoms of hyperthyroidism were often elusive[1] and were totally absent in 55% of patients.[57] TPP may remain undiagnosed if thyroid function tests are not taken and reviewed in the ED. Occasionally, patients have been subjected to extensive and expensive neurologic investigations and prolonged hospitalization prior to the discovery of TPP.[15,58] A key feature to note is that the attacks may recur, but there is always a complete recovery between the episodes of muscle weakness. About half of the patients had suffered at least one attack before the correct diagnosis was made in one hospital where TPP was seen.[9] The delay in diagnosis is, on average, 14 months.[59] Concurrence of potentially treatable TPP and encephalopathy associated with autoimmune thyroid disease (EAATD) as an initial neurologic manifestation of Graves' disease has been reported. EAATD is a heterogeneous and extremely rare clinical entity that may occur in patients with clinical or subclinical autoimmune thyroid disease.[60] A high level of antithyroid antibodies, increased cerebrospinal fluid protein concentration, nonspecific neurologic symptoms, and psychiatric symptoms with nonspecific electroencephalogram abnormalities are the hallmark of EAATD. High doses of corticosteroids often lead to dramatic improvement in the patients.[60]

Diagnosis

TPP usually occurs when the patient is in a hyperthyroid state, and thyroid function tests, when performed, will lead the clinician to the correct diagnosis. However, attacks after the resolution of hyperthyroidism have been reported.[61] The severity of the attack does not always correspond with the degree of hyperthyroidism,[62] and the thyroid hormone levels are usually lower than in unaffected thyrotoxic patients.[63] This observation suggests that TPP typically occurs in the early stages of thyrotoxicosis and accounts for why the patients display so few thyrotoxic symptoms.[63]

Different etiologies of hyperthyroidism can result in TPP. The majority of patients have Graves' disease, but a small number of cases have been associated with toxic nodular goiter,[34,64,65] thyroiditis,[34,59,66,67] solitary toxic thyroid adenoma,[65,68,69] thyrotropin-secreting pituitary adenoma,[70–72] iodine-induced thyrotoxicosis,[13] excessive thyroxine replacement,[73] misuse of thyroxine/triiodothyronine[59,74,75] or triiodothyroacetic acid (tiratricol),[76] and amiodarone-induced thyrotoxicosis.[77,78] Soonthornpun et al. reported that 90% of TPP individuals were overweight and 40% had an increased waist circumference that was significantly larger than in unaffected thyrotoxic controls.[8] This increase of BMI in TPP has also been confirmed by others.[56,63]

A correlation between the degree of hypokalemia and severity of the paralysis was found in one study[62] but was absent in another.[79] Serum potassium levels ranged from 1.1 to 3.4 mmol/L and was most often less than 3.0 mmol/L.[9,39,59] Sporadic cases of lethal and severe ventricular arrhythmias together with hypokalemia have been described.[67,80,81] In extremely rare cases of TPP, patients with both normokalemia and hyperkalemia have been reported.[29,82,83] In our experience, however, delayed blood sampling can explain why serum potassium levels in many cases were normal, as the patients had already recovered in the interim.

Due to the intracellular shift of potassium, the urinary potassium excretion rate is low in TPP.[84] A study by Abbas et al. describes a case where all TPP patients demonstrated urinary potassium less than 20 mmol/L.[9] However, long-standing hypokalemia can impair the renal ability to concentrate urine, resulting in polyuria, and make a spot urine collection of potassium unreliable. In these cases, the urinary potassium/creatinine ratio may be used. In TPP the ratio is typically less than 2.0 potassium/mmol creatinine.[7] One case report described an atypical presentation of TPP. The findings included hypokalemia with hyperthyroidism and renal potassium wasting in a 36-year-old Chinese man with no previous history of renal disease. TPP was not initially recognized due to the renal potassium wasting, which does not occur normally in patients with TPP. However, his serum potassium level rebounded rapidly within several hours after potassium supplementation, indicating that the intracellular shifting of potassium ions was the main etiology of his hypokalemia.[85]

Bone turnover is stimulated by thyroid hormones, which increase the glomerular filtration rate and decrease the tubular resorption of calcium, leading to a higher urinary calcium concentration in hyperthyroidism. Calcium is often elevated in Graves' disease due to high thyroid hormone levels.

An intracellular shift is the probable reason for the transient hypophosphatemia and hypomagnesemia seen in TPP. In the study conducted by Manoukian et al., 80% of the attacks were associated with mild to moderate serum hypophosphatemia (0.36 to 0.77 mmol/L [1.1 to 3.0 mg/dL]; reference range 0.81–1.55 mmol/L) and all demonstrated low or low-normal serum magnesium levels (0.60 to 0.80 mmol/L [1.5 to 1.9 mg/dL]; reference range 0.7–1.2 mmol/L).[39]

TPP patients usually present with a marked decline in urinary phosphate excretion, although there has been considerable overlap with that of normal. However, a spot urine calcium/phosphate ratio of greater than 1.4 mmol/mmol (1.7 mg/mg) indicated TPP with a sensitivity of 100% and a specificity of 96%.[34] A spot urine calcium/phosphate ratio has therefore been suggested as a useful tool when diagnosing TPP in the ED.

Serum alkaline phosphatase levels were mildly elevated in 75% of patients (118 to 268 U/L; reference range 39–117 U/L).[39] Serum creatine phosphate has been found to be elevated in almost 70% of attacks, especially in those precipitated by exercise. The elevation was predominantly mild but in a few cases it was severe.

The acid-base status is generally normal in TPP,[56] although fear, anxiety, and stress can uncommonly give rise to a mild respiratory alkalosis as a result of hyperventilation. A study performed by Sonkar et al. describes a case of acute onset of lower motor neuron quadriparesis with concomitant hypokalemia and compensated respiratory alkalosis.[31] Occasionally a mild respiratory acidosis is seen as an effect of respiratory muscle weakness attributable to severe hypokalemia.[7]

Hypokalemia increases membrane excitability in the Perkinje fibers of the cardiac conducting system.[86] Severe hypokalemia can induce ventricular arrhythmias and delays ventricular repolarization by inhibiting potassium channel activity.[87] While awaiting thyroid function results, electrocardiographic (ECG) changes in patients with TPP can offer supportive clues to the diagnosis and strengthen the clinical suspicion of TPP in the ED.

Pathological ECG is found in 83% to 100% of patients with TPP.[9,21] The mechanism of TPP includes increases in Na^+/K^+ ATPase activity stimulated by thyroid hormone and/or hyperadrenergic activity along with hyperinsulinemia.[88] Elevated levels of thyroid hormones usually affect the electrophysiologic system in the heart in addition to the typical ECG changes of hypokalemia (U waves, T wave flattening, ST depression, QT prolongation, widened QRS complexes, and high QRS voltage). Sinus tachycardia is commonly seen. Sinus arrest and second-degree atrioventricular block (AVB) have been noted.[89] Dangerous electrocardiographic abnormalities include AVB, atrial fibrillation, ventricular fibrillation, and asystole.[86] The cause of these conduction disturbances was unknown. Atrial fibrillation and other supraventricular arrhythmias and, more rarely, ventricular arrhythmias have also been reported.[4,11,67,80] Almost 75% of TPP patients demonstrate increased QRS voltage,[57] which is also common in ordinary hyperthyroidism.[90] Other cardiogenic effects that have been reported on the electrocardiogram include sinus tachycardia and marked ST segment depression in leads II, III, aVF, and V4–V6, and QT interval prolongation.[17] Acquired long QT interval often results from hypokalemia, hypomagnesemia, or from medications.[48]

Myopathic changes with reduced amplitude of compound muscle action potentials are generally seen when an electromyogram (EMG) is done during an attack.

Nerve conduction studies have been normal. A prolonged exercise test can reproduce EMG changes seen during paralysis and were shown to be very sensitive and specific for TPP (90% and 70%, respectively).[91] Jiaoting et al. described a long exercise test performed during the interphase time between attacks of paralysis in the absence of muscle weakness. The right hand was chosen for the long exercise test. The compound muscle action potential (CMAP) was recorded from the abductor digit minimi muscle. Results showed a significant difference in the CMAP amplitude decrease rate (CMAPADR) between healthy control subjects (non-TPP patients) and TPP patients, with TPP patients showing a decreased CMAPADR rate significantly greater than a healthy control subject.[92] In the euthyroid state, these abnormalities may not completely improve, indicating a permanent latent abnormal excitability of the muscle membrane.[91]

Differential Diagnosis

Periodic paralysis is classified into primary and secondary, depending on the etiology. Primary periodic paralysis is most often familial. Primary causes include hyperkalemic or hypokalemic periodic paralysis and Andersen syndrome, while TPP remains a secondary cause.[93] TPP is seldom associated with a positive family history and has a late onset of paralytic attack, whereas in Andersen syndrome, primary hyperkalemia and hypokalemia are autosomal dominant and manifest within the first two decades of life.[93] In more than half of cases the cause is a shift of potassium from the extracellular to the intracellular space due to TPP or familial hypokalemic periodic paralysis (FHPP). The two can often be distinguished by the case history and the patient's hereditary background. The muscle weakness is similar in the two conditions, but thyroid function tests are normal in FHPP. FHPP is an autosomal dominant condition in which a family history of hypokalemic paralysis and the genetic mutations are often well characterized. White people are generally affected with equal sex distribution, and it usually presents before the age of 20 years.[94] In FHPP, acetazolamide and thyroxin usually lessen the frequency of attacks, in contrast to the situation in TPP, where the attacks may become worse.[42] As the treatment is quite different for the different hypokalemic paralyses, accurate diagnosis is essential. In addition to TPP, the differential diagnosis of lower limb paralysis includes: Guillain-Barre syndrome, polymyositis, myasthenia gravis, acute intermittent porphyria, sagittal sinus thrombosis, severe hypokalemia, familial periodic paralysis, and transverse myelitis.[32]

Pathophysiology

Skeletal muscles contain the largest pool of potassium and have an important role in extracellular potassium homeostasis. Exercise will increase the extracellular potassium pool, whereas rest will restore it to normal. The cell membrane sodium/potassium (Na^+/K^+) ATPase pump actively transports potassium from the extracellular to the intracellular compartment in muscles and the outward flow is controlled by inward rectifying K^+ (Kir) channels and delayed rectifying K^+ channels. Activation of Na^+/K^+-ATPase exists in many conditions, including thyrotoxicosis. Thyroid hormones increase the activity of the cell membrane Na^+/K^+-ATPase pump, and thyroid hormone excess can cause hyperstimulation.[95] The Na^+/K^+-ATPase pump activity in TPP patients is increased by 80% compared to other thyrotoxic patients.[96] However, this is not the cause of hypokalemia in the majority of hyperthyroid patients because the increased activity will in most cases be compensated by an increased outward potassium flow. Only if the outward flux is hampered as well will hypokalemia and subsequent paralysis occur. Gragg et al. described a case of a 26-year-old Black male with normokalemic TPP who developed the syndrome post strenuous exercise. On admission to the ED, he presented with limb paralysis but remained normokalemic on serial testing. This suggests that a single test or even multiple tests showing normokalemia should not rule out TPP.[97]

The Na^+/K^+-ATPase pump activity in skeletal muscle is intensified by catecholamines and as the β-adrenergic responsiveness is increased in hyperthyroidism, the catecholamines will further enhance the activity.[98] This could potentially be one explanation for the effectiveness of nonselective beta-blockers such as propranolol in TPP. The Na^+/K^+-ATPase pump is also stimulated by insulin, explaining why many attacks are preceded by meals overloaded with carbohydrates and sweet snacks.[99] Similarly, drugs that impair the insulin sensitivity, i.e., glucocorticoids, can precipitate an attack.[41] Insulin sensitivity has been indicated to be decreased in TPP compared with other hyperthyroid patients.[8,63] Glucose infusions should therefore be avoided in TPP, as it would increase insulin secretion, exacerbating the intracellular shift and aggravating the hypokalemia.[100] Propranolol decreases insulin secretion, which could be another reason for its therapeutic effect in TPP.[101] Insulin and catecholamines not only stimulate Na^+/K^+-ATPase activity but can also inhibit Kir channels.[102]

In animal models, testosterone increases Na^+/K^+-ATPase pump activity, whereas estrogen and progesterone decrease Na^+/K^+ pump activity.[11,103] This might partly explain why TPP almost exclusively affects males. Male TPP patients have higher testosterone levels than thyrotoxic male patients without paralysis.[63] In two TPP males, unilateral adrenal adenomas and hyperandrogenemia were found.[104] TPP has also been associated with testosterone supplementation in a patient with female to male gender reassignment.[105] Studies in animal models of influenza virus–infected lungs have demonstrated that the release of several cytokines stimulates the hypothalamic-pituitary-adrenal axis, leading to increased cortisol and adrenalin production, which activates the Na^+/K^+-ATPase pump.[95,99]

Genetic Aspects

To date, six mutations of the *KCNJ18* gene encoding an inwardly rectifying potassium channel named Kir2.6 have been described in TPP patients.[17] The loss of Kir2.6 ion channel function leads to a decreased outflow of potassium from the intracellular compartments, and the massive influx of potassium in the skeletal muscle cells due to the increased Na^+/K^+ ATPase activity leads to extracellular hypokalemia and episodic weakness.[106,107] These changes occur during thyrotoxicosis but not during the euthyroid state.[108] Zhao et al. reported a series of 537 patients with TPP in the Chinese Han population. The authors genotyped over 100 TPP-specific single nucleotide polymorphisms (SNPs) and found three loci that were unequivocally associated with TTP.[109]

Jin et al. published a study that included 127 mainland Chinese patients with TPP, in which 3.1% (4/127) of TPP cases harbored the *KCNJ18* gene mutation. No mutations were identified in the *KCNJ2* gene.[92] Mutations in the *KCNJ18* gene may be an important cause of TPP in some patients; however, not all TPP patients have *KCNJ18* gene mutations. *KCNJ18* gene mutations were found in 33% patients from Brazil, USA, and France, and in 26% patients from Singapore, whereas it was seen only in 1.2% of patients from Hong Kong, and none from Thailand.[108] In addition, whereas *KCNJ18* gene mutations were detected in 1.6% of Taiwanese patients with TTP, it was detected in 3.3% of patients with sporadic periodic paralysis.[5] Other gene mutations and channelopathies may also be responsible for the development of TPP. A genetic variant, 75 kb downstream of the *KCNJ2* gene, was associated with TPP in Thai patients with hyperthyroidism[110]; however, no mutations in the actual the *KCNJ2* gene were found. In the Korean population, the genotype and allelic frequency of a single nucleotide polymorphism (SNP;r312691) has shown a significant association with TPP.[111]

Although TPP and FHPP have a similar clinical presentation, there is no common genetic background besides the fact that FHPP is an autosomal dominant disease. The main difference appears to be racial: FHPP usually affects White people,[94] whereas TPP mainly affects East Asian males.[42] FHPP is caused by mutations in the gene encoding the L-type α1 calcium channel subunit ($Ca_v1.1$; *CACN1AS*) in skeletal muscle, leading to ionic channel defects. These mutations could not be routinely demonstrated in Brazilian or Chinese patients with TPP,[5,112,113] with only two cases being reported. The mutation in the $K_v3.4$ gene (*KCNE3*), which encodes for a voltage-gated potassium channel, was found in a Brazilian patient with TPP.[114] Another mutation in the voltage-gated sodium channel, $Na_v1.4$ (*SCN4A*), was reported in a White family with TPP.[115] Whether these cases represent a true genetic overlap or a random genetic variation is unclear, as in four studies of a total of 251 Asian people affected by TPP, similar mutations were not found.[5,113,116,117] It has been shown, however, that both in FHPP and in TPP, insulin is able to reduce Kir conductance, suggesting similarities in insulin regulation.[102]

Thus our present knowledge indicates that TPP is caused by a mixture of genetic predispositions, the presence of thyrotoxicosis, dietary excesses of various types, and other, yet unknown stimulants. The diagnosis of TPP is still primarily based on the clinical presentation, the presence of hypokalemia, and the demonstration of hyperthyroidism with elevated serum T4, free T3, and suppression of TSH.[17]

Acute Treatment

Guidelines for the management of thyrotoxic hypokalemic periodic paralysis have been updated by Correa et al., who encourage early beta-blockade, with potassium replacement "taking the backseat," as beta-blockers treat the underlying disease process driving the periodic paralysis.[118] Propranolol, a nonselective beta-blocker, is used for blocking the hyperadrenergic activity seen in the pathogenesis of TPP.[119] The rationale for choosing a nonselective beta-blocker is that a beta-1 selective agent is less likely to inhibit the beta-2 receptor mediated hypokalemic effect of epinephrine.[120] Propranolol should be started as a solitary treatment at a rate of 3.0 mg/kg orally. If the oral route is not tolerated, an intravenous infusion of 1.0 mg every 10 minutes up to a total of three doses can be given. The goal of the currently recommended therapy focuses on the importance of preventing rebound hyperkalemia. If potassium is given, it should be administered as a 5-mEq (1.95 g) oral dose every 2 hours, with a maximum of 90 mEq (3.52 g).[121] The patient's serum electrolytes should be obtained within 3 hours of potassium administration and frequently thereafter, to minimize the development of hyperkalemia.[122] It has been demonstrated that propranolol IV (1.0 mg IV every 10 minutes for a total of 3 doses) was successful in treating attacks of TPP when potassium chloride (KCl) supplementation was shown to be ineffective.[52,123] Falhammar et al. have summarized the need for vigilant monitoring.[1] Fatal arrhythmias have been reported when high doses of potassium have been given (hyperkalemia of greater than 10 mmol/L).[124] With an IV KCl infusion at a rate of 10 mmol/hour, 59% to 70% of patients treated had rebound hyperkalemia of greater than 5.0 mmol/L.[56,125] Among those receiving in total 50 mmol or less of KCl IV, few developed hyperkalemia.[125] Most likely this lower dose of KCl is sufficient in the majority of TPP patients, and severe hyperkalemia could thus be avoided.[125] A fatal outcome has been reported with simultaneous administration of IV KCl and IV glucose.[126] As a glucose infusion can further aggravate the hypokalemia, saline is the preferred solution.

Paradoxical hypokalemia, defined as a paradoxical drop in serum potassium level when potassium is given for severe hypokalemia, has been mentioned in the literature as it was reported initially in the TPP patient population. These patients had higher serum free thyroxin concentrations, higher heart rate, and higher systolic blood pressure compared to TPP patients without paradoxical hypokalemia but with similar lead time, age, BMI, and initial potassium concentration. It is postulated that it affects one-quarter of patients. It is quantified as a fall in serum potassium of 0.1 mmol/L or greater during IV KCl. These patients needed more than double the recovery time, and their potassium infusions resulted in more severe hyperkalemia.[56] Potassium supplementation as prophylaxis against further attacks was ineffective, and it was recommended that it should be avoided.[42] Nevertheless, rebound hyperkalemia with cardiac arrhythmias developed, although paralytic symptoms were rapidly reversed.[52,123]

Oral propranolol (40 mg four times a day) also prevented recurrent attacks by inhibiting the Na^+/K^+-ATPase pump activity.[119] Propranolol, however, must be used with precaution, especially if given IV and/or in cases of heart block, to prevent adverse effects such as severe bradycardia, complete heart block, and cardiac failure. Cardiovascular collapse has been associated with both oral and IV administration of propranolol in thyroid storm. A safer alternative in the emergency situation may be the use of ultra-short-acting beta-blockers, for example, IV esmolol.[127] If thyroid storm is present, methimazole or propylthiouricil should also be administered along with steroids at least 1 hour prior to administration of iodine.[118]

Although some authors advocate propranolol as the first-line treatment in the ED for TPP,[43,128] others consider that further studies are needed before this is the definitive treatment strategy.[7,42,125] The use of propranolol, with its beneficial effects of nonselective beta-blockade, includes the beneficial effects of lysis of the physiologic response to catecholamines and beta-2 mediated insulin release. This places a brake on the Na/K pump and rapidly normalizes potassium levels. It also reduces conversion of T4 to T3 and mitigates associated symptoms.[118] Whether propranolol should be combined with a low dose of KCl is also an unsettled issue.

Definitive Treatment

Curative therapy of the underlying hyperthyroidism is the main treatment option, as TPP, with very few exceptions, does not recur in the euthyroid state. In Graves' disease, toxic nodular goiter, and solitary toxic thyroid adenoma, antithyroid drugs are usually used until definitive treatment with radioactive iodine or surgery can be done. If radioactive iodine is given, an ablative dose should be used to minimize the risk of relapse. Patients should avoid known precipitating factors of TPP, which include heavy carbohydrate intake, a high-salt diet, alcohol ingestion, and undue exertion, until the thyrotoxicosis condition is under control.[88] It should also be suggested that they continue to use propranolol until a euthyroid status has been achieved.[7,42] Treating Graves' disease with only antithyroid drugs for 12 to 18 months is not a preferred option considering the high risk of relapse of Graves' after cessation of these drugs.[129] In one study, 56% of patients diagnosed with TPP treated with only antithyroid drugs and beta-blockade had a new attack within 7 months, most probably as a result of an insufficient dose of the drug and/or non-compliance.[9] Based on the American Thyroid Association guidelines, both fixed dose and thyroid weight-adjusted dose calculation can be used in treating hyperthyroidism with radioactive iodine, with the goal of reaching a hypothyroid status.[130,131] In China, only the thyroid weight-adjusted radioactive iodine dose is recommended to achieve euthyroid status.[132,133]

Anesthesia Considerations

If possible, surgery should be postponed until the patient reaches a euthyroid state. In case of surgery in emergency situations, the thyrotoxic patient with TPP should be given propranolol pre- and intraoperatively, and if hypokalemic, KCl should be administered. At the present time it is understood that both regional and general anesthesia may be performed safely with no specific induction method. Glucose-containing IV solutions should be avoided, as these can precipitate or worsen an attack due to insulin release stimulating Na^+/K^+-ATPase activity.[134]

Summary

A decline in the incidence of TPP has been reported from Japan. However, it has become increasingly common in the Western countries not only due to population migration but also because of improved awareness of the condition. Many patients are not correctly diagnosed in the ED, as thyroid function tests may not be readily available and there can be delays in controlling serum potassium levels. Rapid recognition and management of TPP is essential to reduce morbidity and prevent mortality. Emergency treatment includes KCl and/or propranolol; however, the definitive treatment is control and cure of the hyperthyroidism. At the present time we can say novel insights of the pathophysiology and molecular aspects of TPP have been achieved. The present concept is that TPP is a result of a combination of genetic predisposition, thyrotoxicosis, dietary, and other miscellaneous factors. In addition to the known factors, the underlying mechanisms still remain incompletely understood and further investigations are required.

References

1. Okinaka S, Shizume K, Iino S, et al. The association of periodic paralysis and hyperthyroidism in Japan. *J Clin Endocrinol Metab*. 1957;17(12):1454–1459.
2. McFadzean AJ, Yeung R. Periodic paralysis complicating thyrotoxicosis in Chinese. *Br Med J1*. 1967(5538):451–455.
3. Cheng CJ, Lin SH, Lo YF, et al. Identification and functional characterization of Kir2.6 mutations associated with non-familial hypokalemic periodic paralysis. *J Biol Chem*. 2011;286(31):27425–27435. doi:10.1074/jbc.M111.249656 M111.249656 [pii].
4. Cheema MA, Zain MA, Cheema K, Ullah W. Thyroxine-induced periodic paralysis: a rare complication of nutritional supplements. *BMJ Case Rep*. 2018;11(1):e227946. doi:10.1136/bcr-2018-227946 pii.
5. Lin SH. Thyrotoxic periodic paralysis. *Mayo Clin Proc*. 2005;80(1):99–105. doi:10.1016/S0025-6196(11)62965-0.
6. Soonthornpun S, Setasuban W, Thamprasit A. Insulin resistance in subjects with a history of thyrotoxic periodic paralysis (TPP). *Clin Endocrinol (Oxf)*. 2009;70(5):794–797. doi:10.1111/j.1365-2265.2008.03395.x.
7. Abbas MT, Khan FY, Errayes M, Baidaa AD, Haleem AH. Thyrotoxic periodic paralysis admitted to the medical department in Qatar. *Neth J Med*. 2008;66(9):384–388.
8. Kelley DE, Gharib H, Kennedy FP, Duda Jr RJ, McManis PG. Thyrotoxic periodic paralysis. Report of 10 cases and review of electromyographic findings. *Arch Intern Med*. 1989;149(11):2597–2600.
9. Ober KP. Thyrotoxic periodic paralysis in the United States. Report of 7 cases and review of the literature. *Medicine (Baltimore)*. 1992;71(3):109–120.
10. Schalin-Jantti C, Laine T, Valli-Jaakola K, Lonnqvist T, Kontula K, Valimaki MJ. Manifestation, management and molecular analysis of candidate genes in two rare cases of thyrotoxic hypokalemic periodic paralysis. *Horm Res*. 2005;63(3):139–144. doi:10.1159/000084689.
11. Kane MP, Busch RS. Drug-induced thyrotoxic periodic paralysis. *Ann Pharmacother*. 2006;40(4):778–781. doi:10.1345/aph.1G543.
12. Vendrame F, Verrienti A, Parlapiano C, Filetti S, Dotta F, Morano S. Thyrotoxic periodic paralysis in an Italian man: clinical manifestation and genetic analysis. *Ann Clin Biochem*. 2008;45(Pt 2):218–220. doi:10.1258/acb.2007.007117.
13. Korno MR, Hagen C. Hypokalemic thyrotoxic periodic paralysis—a rare differential diagnosis in patients presenting acute tetraparesis. *Ugeskr Laeger*. 2008;170(39):3070.
14. Guilloton L, De Carvalho A, Quesnel L, Pasquet F, Mounier C, Drouet A. Thyrotoxic hypokaliemic periodic paralysis revealing Graves' disease in a male Caucasian. *Rev Neurol (Paris)*. 2012;168(2):170–172.
15. Sayiner ZA, Eraydın A, Akarsu E. Steroid-induced thyrotoxic periodic paralysis during Graves' ophthalmopathy treatment. *Postgrad Med J*. 2016;92(1093):682–683. doi:10.1136/postgradmedj-2016-134292.
16. Magsino Jr CH, Ryan Jr AJ. Thyrotoxic periodic paralysis. *South Med J*. 2000;93(10):996–1003.
17. Dietrich C, Miles C, Barth R, Nelson D. Hypokalemic thyrotoxic periodic paralysis: a case report and review. *S D J Med*. 2002;55(3):101–103.
18. Iheonunekwu NC, Ibrahim TM, Davies D, Pickering K. Thyrotoxic hypokalaemic paralysis in a pregnant Afro-Caribbean woman. A case report and review of the literature. *West Indian Med J*. 2004;53(1):47–49.
19. Elston MS, Orr-Walker BJ, Dissanayake AM, Conaglen JV. Thyrotoxic, hypokalaemic periodic paralysis: Polynesians, an ethnic group at risk. *Intern Med J*. 2007;37(5):303–307. doi:10.1111/j.1445-5994.2007.01313.x.
20. Brown JD, Kangwanprasert M, Tice A, Melish J. Thyrotoxic periodic paralysis in a Polynesian male following highly active antiretroviral therapy for HIV infection. *Hawaii Med J*. 2007;66(3):62–63 60.
21. El-Hennawy AS, Nesa M, Mahmood AK. Thyrotoxic hypokalemic periodic paralysis triggered by high carbohydrate diet. *Am J Ther*. 2007;14(5):499–501. doi:10.1097/MJT.0b013e31814daf53.
22. Liu Z, Braverman LE, Malabanan A. Thyrotoxic periodic paralysis in a Hispanic man after the administration of prednisone. *Endocr Pract*. 2006;12(4):427–431.
23. Thornton MD. Lower-extremity weakness in a teenager due to thyrotoxic periodic paralysis. *J Emerg Med*. 2017;52(4):e133–e137. doi:10.1016/j.jemermed.2016.11.006.
24. Atallah P, Dib ER, Khoury M. Thyrotoxic periodic paralysis. A case report. *J Med Liban*. 2007;55(3):167–169.
25. Cesur M, Bayram F, Temel MA, et al. Thyrotoxic hypokalaemic periodic paralysis in a Turkish population: three new case reports and analysis of the case series. *Clin Endocrinol (Oxf)*. 2008;68(1):143–152. doi:10.1111/j.1365-2265.2007.03014.x.

26. Hagel S, Elznerova T, Dietrich W, Schrauzer T, John S. Chest pain and paralysis after pulse prednisolone therapy an unusual case presentation of thyrotoxic periodic paralysis: a case report. *Cases J.* 2009;2:7501. doi:10.4076/1757-1626-2-7501.
27. Satam N, More V, Shanbag P, Kalgutkar A. Fatal thyrotoxic periodic paralysis with normokalemia. *Indian J Pediatr.* 2007;74(11):1041–1043.
28. Rao N, John M, Thomas N, Rajaratnam S, Seshadri MS. Aetiological, clinical and metabolic profile of hypokalaemic periodic paralysis in adults: a single-centre experience. *Natl Med J India.* 2006;19(5):246–249.
29. Jin J, Hu F, Li M, et al. Long exercise test in the interattack period of periodic paralysis: a useful and sensitive diagnostic tool. *Journal of clinical Neurophysiology.* 2017;34(6):497–501. doi:10.1097/WNP.0000000000000405.
30. Affram KO, Reddy TL, Osei KM. A rare case of thyrotoxic periodic paralysis after epidural steroid injection: a case report and literature review. *Am J Case Rep.* 2018;19:1453–1458. doi:10.12659/AJCR.911270.
31. Shizume K, Shishiba Y, Kuma K, et al. Comparison of the incidence of association of periodic paralysis and hyperthyroidism in Japan in 1957 and 1991. *Endocrinol Jpn.* 1992;39(3):315–318.
32. Hsieh MJ, Lyu RK, Chang WN, et al. Hypokalemic thyrotoxic periodic paralysis: clinical characteristics and predictors of recurrent paralytic attacks. *Eur J Neurol.* 2008;15(6):559–564. doi:10.1111/j.1468-1331.2008.02132.x ENE2132 [pii].
33. Wong GW, Leung TF, Lo AF, Ahuja AT, Cheng PS. Thyrotoxic periodic paralysis in a 14-year-old boy. *Eur J Pediatr.* 2000;159(12):934.
34. Vijayakumar A, Ashwath G, Thimmappa D. Thyrotoxic periodic paralysis challenges. *Journal Thyroid Res.* 2014;2014:649502.
35. Tsai IH, Su YJ. Thyrotoxic periodic paralysis with ventricular tachycardia. *J Electrocardiol.* 2019;54:93–95. doi:10.1016/j.jelectrocard.2019.04.001.
36. Birkhahn RH, Gaeta TJ, Melniker L. Thyrotoxic periodic paralysis and intravenous propranolol in the emergency setting. *J Emerg Med.* 2000;18(2):199–202 doi: S0736-4679(99)00194-8 [pii].
37. Wongraoprasert S, Buranasupkajorn P, Sridama V, Snabboon T. Thyrotoxic periodic paralysis induced by pulse methylprednisolone. *Intern Med.* 2007;46(17):1431–1433 doi: JST.JSTAGE/internalmedicine/46.0044 [pii].
38. Sardar Z, Waheed KAF, Javed MA, Akhtar F, Bokhari SRA. Clinical and etiological spectrum of hypokalemic periodic paralysis in a tertiary care hospital in Pakistan. *Cureus.* 2019;11(1):e3921. doi:10.7759/cureus.3921.
39. Diedrich DA, Wedel DJ. Thyrotoxic periodic paralysis and anesthesia report of a case and literature review. *J Clin Anesth.* 2006;18(4):286–292. doi:10.1016/j.jclinane.2005.08.016 S0952-8180(05)00364-8 [pii].
40. Tessier JJ, Neu SK, Horning KK. Thyrotoxic periodic paralysis (TPP) in a 28-year-old Sudanese man started on prednisone. *J Am Board Fam Med.* 2010;23(4):551–554. doi:10.3122/jabfm.2010.04.090220 23/4/551 [pii].
41. Ko GT, Chow CC, Yeung VT, Chan HH, Li JK, Cockram CS. Thyrotoxic periodic paralysis in a Chinese population. *QJM.* 1996;89(6):463–468.
42. Crane MG. Periodic paralysis associated with hyperthyroidism. *Calif Med.* 1960;92(4):285–288.
43. Gragg JI, Federico M, Mellick LB. Normokalemic thyrotoxic periodic paralysis with acute resolution in the emergency department. *Clin Pract Cases Emerg Med.* 2017;1(2):129-131. doi: 10.5811/cpcem.2017.1.33211.
44. Tella SH, Kommalapati A. Thyrotoxic periodic paralysis: an underdiagnosed and under-recognized condition. *Cureus.* 2015;7(10):e342. doi:10.7759/cureus.342.
45. Harrogate SR, Mills E, Qureshi A, de Wolff JF. An unusual case of acute muscle weakness. *Acute Med.* 2016;15(4):209–211.
46. Jung SY, Song KC, Shin JI, Chae HW, Kim HS, Kwon AR. A case of thyrotoxic periodic paralysis as initial manifestation of Graves' disease in a 16-year-old Korean adolescent. *Ann Pediatr Endocrinol Metab.* 2014;19(3):169–173. doi:10.6065/apem.2014.19.3.169.
47. Falhammar H, Thorén M, Calissendorff J. Thyrotoxic periodic paralysis: clinical and molecular aspects. *Endocrine.* 2013;43(2):274–284. doi:10.1007/s12020-012-9777-x.
48. Tassone H, Moulin A, Henderson SO. The pitfalls of potassium replacement in thyrotoxic periodic paralysis: a case report and review of the literature. *J Emerg Med.* 2004;26(2):157–161.
49. Liu YC, Tsai WS, Chau T, Lin SH. Acute hypercapnic respiratory failure due to thyrotoxic periodic paralysis. *Am J Med Sci.* 2004;327(5):264–267 doi: 00000441-200405000-00025 [pii].

50. Thompson MP, Pinckard JK. A rare case of thyrotoxic periodic paralysis presenting to the medical examiner. *Am J Forensic Med Pathol.* 2011;32(3):232–235.
51. Abbasi B, Sharif Z, Sprabery LR. Hypokalemic thyrotoxic periodic paralysis with thyrotoxic psychosis and hypercapnic respiratory failure. *Am J Med Sci.* 2010;340(2):147–153. doi:10.1097/MAJ.0b013e3181cbf567.
52. Shiang JC, Cheng CJ, Tsai MK, et al. Therapeutic analysis in Chinese patients with thyrotoxic periodic paralysis over 6 years. *Eur J Endocrinol.* 2009;161(6):911–916. doi:10.1530/EJE-09-0553 EJE-09-0553 [pii].
53. Hsu YJ, Lin YF, Chau T, Liou JT, Kuo SW, Lin SH. Electrocardiographic manifestations in patients with thyrotoxic periodic paralysis. *Am J Med Sci.* 2003;326(3):128–132.
54. Tran HA, Kay SE, Kende M, Doery JC, Colman PG, Read A. Thyrotoxic, hypokalaemic periodic paralysis in Australasian men. *Intern Med J.* 2003;33(3):91–94 doi: 347 [pii].
55. Maciel RM, Lindsey SC, Dias da Silva MR. Novel etiopathophysiological aspects of thyrotoxic periodic paralysis. *Nat Rev Endocrinol.* 2011;7(11):657–667. doi:10.1038/nrendo.2011.58 nrendo.2011.58 [pii].
56. Rone JK, Brietzke SA. Euthyroid thyrotoxic periodic paralysis. *Mil Med.* 1991;156(8):434–436.
57. Nellen H, Mercado M, Mendoza V, et al. Thyrotoxic periodic paralysis in Mexican mestizo patients: a clinical, biochemical and HLA-serological study. *Arch Med Res.* 1999;30(1):74–76 doi: S0188-0128(98)00014-1 [pii].
58. Tachamo N, Lohani S, Nazir S, Juliano N. Paralysis that easily reverses: a case of thyrotoxic periodic paralysis. *BMJ Case Rep.* 2017:2017. doi:10.1136/bcr-2016-218951 bcr2016218951.
59. Li W, Changsheng C, Jiangfang F, et al. Effects of sex steroid hormones, thyroid hormone levels, and insulin regulation on thyrotoxic periodic paralysis in Chinese men. *Endocrine.* 2010;38(3):386–390. doi:10.1007/s12020-010-9396-3.
60. Norris Jr FH, Clark EC, Biglieri EG. Studies in thyrotoxic periodic paralysis. *J Neurol Sci.* 1971;13(4):431–442.
61. King AD, Chow FC, Ahuja AT, Richards PS. Thyrotoxic periodic paralysis: sonographic appearances of the thyroid. *J Clin Ultrasound.* 2002;30(9):544–547. doi:10.1002/jcu.10119.
62. Ozaki H, Mori K, Nakagawa Y, Hoshikawa S, Ito S, Yoshida K. Autonomously functioning thyroid nodule associated with thyrotoxic periodic paralysis. *Endocr J.* 2008;55(1):113–119 doi: JST.JSTAGE/endocrj/K07E-017 [pii].
63. Tagami T, Usui T, Shimatsu A, Naruse M. Toxic thyroid adenoma presenting as hypokalemic periodic paralysis. *Endocr J.* 2007;54(5):797–803 JST.JSTAGE/endocrj/K07-126 [pii].
64. Hannon MJ, Behan LA, Agha A. Thyrotoxic periodic paralysis due to excessive L-thyroxine replacement in a Caucasian man. *Ann Clin Biochem.* 2009;46(Pt 5):423–425. doi:10.1258/acb.2009.009012 acb.2009.009012 [pii].
65. Chen YC, Fang JT, Chang CT, Chou HH. Thyrotoxic periodic paralysis in a patient abusing thyroxine for weight reduction. *Ren Fail.* 2001;23(1):139–142.
66. Alings AM, Fliers E, de Herder WW, et al. A thyrotropin-secreting pituitary adenoma as a cause of thyrotoxic periodic paralysis. *J Endocrinol Invest.* 1998;21(10):703–706.
67. Hsu FS, Tsai WS, Chau T, Chen HH, Chen YC, Lin SH. Thyrotropin-secreting pituitary adenoma presenting as hypokalemic periodic paralysis. *Am J Med Sci.* 2003;325(1):48–50.
68. Pappa T, Papanastasiou L, Markou A, et al. Thyrotoxic periodic paralysis as the first manifestation of a thyrotropin-secreting pituitary adenoma. *Hormones (Athens).* 2010;9(1):82–86.
69. Tinker TD, Vannatta JB. Thyrotoxic hypokalemic periodic paralysis: report of four cases and review of the literature (2). *J Okla State Med Assoc.* 1987;80(2):76–83.
70. Lee JI, Sohn TS, Son HS, et al. Thyrotoxic periodic paralysis presenting as polymorphic ventricular tachycardia induced by painless thyroiditis. *Thyroid.* 2009;19(12):1433–1434. doi:10.1089/thy.2009.0253.
71. Akinyemi E, Bercovici S, Niranjan S, Paul N, Hemavathy B. Thyrotoxic hypokalemic periodic paralysis due to dietary weight-loss supplement. *Am J Ther.* 2011;18(3):e81–e83. doi:10.1097/MJT.0b013e3181c960a9.
72. Cohen-Lehman J, Charitou MM, Klein I. Tiratricol-induced periodic paralysis: a review of nutraceuticals affecting thyroid function. *Endocr Pract.* 2011;17(4):610–615. doi:10.4158/EP10137.RA 01302X25164Q8824 [pii].
73. Laroia ST, Zaw KM, Ganti AK, Newman W, Akinwande AO. Amiodarone-induced thyrotoxicosis presenting as hypokalemic periodic paralysis. *South Med J.* 2002;95(11):1326–1328.
74. Atienza Morales MP, Jimenez Garcia JA, Beato Perez JL, Aguilar Campos AJ. Amiodarone as cause of periodic thyrotoxic hypopotasemic paralysis. *Rev Clin Esp.* 2006;206(11):598–599 doi: 13096317 [pii].

75. Li J, Yang XB, Zhao Y. Thyrotoxic periodic paralysis in the Chinese population: clinical features in 45 cases. *Exp Clin Endocrinol Diabetes*. 2010;118(1):22–26.
76. Loh KC, Pinheiro L, Ng KS. Thyrotoxic periodic paralysis complicated by near-fatal ventricular arrhythmias. *Singapore Med J*. 2005;46(2):88–89.
77. Randall BB. Fatal hypokalemic thyrotoxic periodic paralysis presenting as the sudden, unexplained death of a Cambodian refugee. *Am J Forensic Med Pathol*. 1992;13(3):204–206.
78. Mehta SR, Verma A, Malhotra H, Mehta S. Normokalaemic periodic paralysis as the presenting manifestation of hyperthyroidism. *J Assoc Physicians India*. 1990;38(4):296–297.
79. Ghosh D, Trivedi N, Kohli A, Mithal A. Hyperkalemic periodic paralysis associated with thyrotoxicosis. *J Assoc Physicians India*. 1993;41(4):239–240.
80. Lin YF, Wu CC, Pei D, Chu SJ, Lin SH. Diagnosing thyrotoxic periodic paralysis in the ED. *Am J Emerg Med*. 2003;21(4):339–342 doi: S0735675703000378 [pii].
81. Ee B, Cheah JS. Electrocardiographic changes in thyrotoxic periodic paralysis. *J Electrocardiol*. 1979; 12(3):263–279.
82. Slovis C, Jenkins R. ABC of clinical electrocardiography: conditions not primarily affecting the heart. *BMJ*. 2002;324(7349):1320–1323.
83. Tang ZW, He Y, Yao Y, Qiu L, Tian HM. Size of quadriceps femoris may contribute to thyrotoxic periodic paralysis. *Med Hypotheses*. 2015;85(6):749–753. doi:10.1016/j.mehy.2015.10.014.
84. Long W, Lin Y. Thyrotoxic periodic paralysis in Chinese patients: milder thyrotoxicosis yet lower dose of (131)I should be avoided. *Clin Nucl Med*. 2013;38(4):248–251. doi:10.1097/RLU.0b013e3182817c31.
85. Bahn RS, Burch HB, Cooper DS, et al. Hyperthyroidism and other causes of thyrotoxicosis: management guidelines of the American Thyroid Association and American Association of Clinical Endocrinologists. *Endocr Pract*. 2011;17(3):456–520.
86. Kook J, Lee H, Kim E, et al. Etiology of hypokalemic paralysis in Korea: data from a single center. *Electrolyte Blood Press*. 2012;10:18–25. doi:10.5049/EBP.2012.10.1.18 http://dx.doi.org/.
87. Arimura K, Arimura Y, Ng AR, Sakoda S, Higuchi I. Muscle membrane excitability after exercise in thyrotoxic periodic paralysis and thyrotoxicosis without periodic paralysis. *Muscle Nerve*. 2007;36(6):784–788. doi:10.1002/mus.20865.
88. Lapie P, Lory P, Fontaine B. Hypokalemic periodic paralysis: an autosomal dominant muscle disorder caused by mutations in a voltage-gated calcium channel. *Neuromuscul Disord*. 1997;7(4):234–240 doi: S0960-8966(97)00435-5 [pii].
89. Chan A, Shinde R, Chow CC, Cockram CS, Swaminathan R. In vivo and in vitro sodium pump activity in subjects with thyrotoxic periodic paralysis. *BMJ*. 1991;303(6810):1096–1099.
90. Park S, Kim TY, Sim S, et al. Association of KCNJ2 genetic variants with susceptibility to thyrotoxic periodic paralysis in patients with Graves' disease. *Exp Clin Endocrinol Diabetes*. 2017;125(2):75–78. doi: 10.1055/s-0042-119527.
91. Yeh FC, Chiang WF, Wang CC, Lin SH. Thyrotoxic periodic paralysis triggered by β2-adrenergic bronchodilators. *CJEM*. 2014;16(3):247–251.
92. Mulder JE. Thyroid disease in women. *Med Clin North Am*. 1998;82(1):103–125.
93. Layzer RB. Periodic paralysis and the sodium-potassium pump. *Ann Neurol*. 1982;11(6):547–552. doi:10.1002/ana.410110602.
94. Chan A, Shinde R, Chow CC, Cockram CS, Swaminathan R. Hyperinsulinaemia and Na+, K(+)-ATPase activity in thyrotoxic periodic paralysis. *Clin Endocrinol (Oxf)*. 1994;41(2):213–216.
95. Tu ML, Fang YW, Leu JG, Tsai MH. An atypical presentation of high potassium renal secretion rate in a patient with thyrotoxic periodic paralysis: a case report. *BMC Nephrol*. 2018;19(1):160. doi:10.1186/s12882-018-0971-9.
96. Griggs RC, Resnick J, Engel WK. Intravenous treatment of hypokalemic periodic paralysis. *Arch Neurol*. 1983;40(9):539–540.
97. Lacey RJ, Berrow NS, London NJ, et al. Differential effects of beta-adrenergic agonists on insulin secretion from pancreatic islets isolated from rat and man. *J Mol Endocrinol*. 1990;5(1):49–54.
98. Azzarolo AM, Mircheff AK, Kaswan RL, et al. Androgen support of lacrimal gland function. *Endocrine*. 1997;6(1):39–45. doi:10.1007/BF02738800.
99. Biering H, Bauditz J, Pirlich M, Lochs H, Gerl H. Manifestation of thyrotoxic periodic paralysis in two patients with adrenal adenomas and hyperandrogenaemia. *Horm Res*. 2003;59(6):301–304. doi:10.1159/00007063070630 [pii].

100. Lin SH, Huang CL. Mechanism of thyrotoxic periodic paralysis. *J Am Soc Nephrol.* 2012;23(6):985–988. doi:10.1681/ASN.2012010046 ASN.2012010046 [pii].
101. Tran HA, Reeves GE. Hepatitis C infection and thyrotoxic periodic paralysis–a novel use of an old drug. *Am J Med Sci.* 2008;336(6):515–518. doi:10.1097/MAJ.0b013e3181643e3d 00000441-200812000-00014 [pii].
102. Ruff RL. Insulin acts in hypokalemic periodic paralysis by reducing inward rectifier K+ current. *Neurology.* 1999;53(7):1556–1563.
103. Ryan DP, da Silva MR, Soong TW, et al. Mutations in potassium channel Kir2.6 cause susceptibility to thyrotoxic hypokalemic periodic paralysis. *Cell.* 2010;140(1):88–98. doi:10.1016/j.cell.2009.12.024 S0092-8674(09)01571-2 [pii].
104. Dias da Silva MR, Cerutti JM, Tengan CH, et al. Mutations linked to familial hypokalaemic periodic paralysis in the calcium channel alpha1 subunit gene (Cav1.1) are not associated with thyrotoxic hypokalaemic periodic paralysis. *Clin Endocrinol (Oxf).* 2002;56(3):367–375 doi: 1481 [pii].
105. Kung AW, Lau KS, Fong GC, Chan V. Association of novel single nucleotide polymorphisms in the calcium channel alpha 1 subunit gene (Ca(v)1.1) and thyrotoxic periodic paralysis. *J Clin Endocrinol Metab.* 2004;89(3):1340–1345.
106. Jongjaroenprasert W, Phusantisampan T, Mahasirimongkol S, et al. A genome-wide association study identifies novel susceptibility genetic variation for thyrotoxic hypokalemic periodic paralysis. *J Hum Genet.* 2012;57(5):301–304. doi:10.1038/jhg.2012.20.
107. Osadchii OE. Mechanisms of hypokalemia-induced ventricular arrhythmogenicity. *Fundam Clin Pharmacol.* 2010;24(5):547–559.
108. Dias Da Silva MR, Cerutti JM, Arnaldi LA, Maciel RM. A mutation in the KCNE3 potassium channel gene is associated with susceptibility to thyrotoxic hypokalemic periodic paralysis. *J Clin Endocrinol Metab.* 2002;87(11):4881–4884.
109. Roh JG, Park KJ, Lee HS, Hwang JS. Thyrotoxic hypokalemic periodic paralysis due to Graves' disease in 2 adolescents. *Ann Pediatr Endocrinol Metab.* 2019;24(2):133–136. doi:10.6065/apem.2019.24.2.133.
110. Lane AH, Markarian K, Braziunene I. Thyrotoxic periodic paralysis associated with a mutation in the sodium channel gene SCN4A. *J Pediatr Endocrinol Metab.* 2004;17(12):1679–1682.
111. Ng WY, Lui KF, Thai AC, Cheah JS. Absence of ion channels CACN1AS and SCN4A mutations in thyrotoxic hypokalemic periodic paralysis. *Thyroid.* 2004;14(3):187–190. doi:10.1089/105072504773297858.
112. Wang W, Jiang L, Ye L, et al. Mutation screening in Chinese hypokalemic periodic paralysis patients. *Mol Genet Metab.* 2006;87(4):359-363. doi:10.1016/j.ymgme.2005.10.020 S1096-7192(05)00379-3 [pii].
113. Lu KC, Hsu YJ, Chiu JS, Hsu YD, Lin SH. Effects of potassium supplementation on the recovery of thyrotoxic periodic paralysis. *Am J Emerg Med.* 2004;22(7):544–547 doi: S0735675704002542 [pii].
114. Ahmed I, Chilimuri SS. Fatal dysrhythmia following potassium replacement for hypokalemic periodic paralysis. *West J Emerg Med.* 2010;11(1):57–59.
115. Chen DY, Schneider P, Zhang XS, He ZM, Chen TH. Fatality after cardiac arrest in thyrotoxic periodic paralysis due to profound hypokalemia resulting from intravenous glucose administration and inadequate potassium replacement. *Thyroid.* 2012;22(9):969–972. doi:10.1089/thy.2011-0352.
116. Elston MS, Orr-Walker BJ, Dissanayake AM, Conaglen JV. Thyrotoxic, hypokalaemic periodic paralysis: Polynesians, an ethnic group at risk. *Intern Med J.* 2007;37(5):303–307.
117. Dalan R, Leow MK. Cardiovascular collapse associated with beta blockade in thyroid storm. *Experimental and Clinical Endocrinology & Diabetes: Official Journal, German Society of Endocrinology [and] German Diabetes Association.* 2007;115(6):392–396. doi:10.1055/s-2007-971065.
118. Correia M, Darocki M, Hirashima ET. Changing management guidelines in thyrotoxic hypokalemic periodic paralysis. *J Emerg Med.* 2018;55(2):252–256. doi:10.1016/j.jemermed.2018.04.063.
119. Manoukian MA, Foote JA, Crapo LM. Clinical and metabolic features of thyrotoxic periodic paralysis in 24 episodes. *Arch Intern Med.* 1999;159(6):601–606.
120. Brent GA. Clinical practice. Graves' disease. *N Engl J Med.* 2008;358(24):2594–2605. doi:10.1056/NEJMcp0801880 358/24/2594 [pii].
121. Shayne P, Hart A. Thyrotoxic periodic paralysis terminated with intravenous propranolol. *Ann Emerg Med.* 1994;24(4):736–740 doi: A58685 [pii].
122. Yeung RT, Tse TF. Thyrotoxic periodic paralysis. Effect of propranolol. *Am J Med.* 1974;57(4):584–590.
123. Lin SH, Lin YF. Propranolol rapidly reverses paralysis, hypokalemia, and hypophosphatemia in thyrotoxic periodic paralysis. *Am J Kidney Dis.* 2001;37(3):620–623 doi: S0272-6386(01)80021-4 [pii].

124. Sonkar SK, Kumar S, Singh NK. Thyrotoxic hypokalemic periodic paralysis. *Indian J Crit Care Med.* 2018;22(5):378–380.
125. Wang PH. Periodic paralysis with normokalemia in a patient with hyperthyroidism. *Medicine.* 2018;97:46. doi:10.1097/MD.0000000000013256 e13256http//dx.doi.org/.
126. Rasheed E, Seheult J, Gibney J, Boran G. Does thyrotoxic periodic paralysis have a genetic predisposition? A case report. *Ann Clin Biochem.* 2018;55(6):713–716. doi:10.1177/0004563218785395.
127. Munir I, Mehmood T, Islam K, Soni L, McFarlane SI. Thyrotoxic periodic paralysis with sensory deficits in young African American male: a case report and literature review. *Am J Med Case Rep.* 2019;7(7):138–142. doi:10.12691/ajmcr-7-7-5.
128. Tsironis T, Tychalas A, Kiourtidis D, et al. Periodic paralysis and encephalopathy as initial manifestations of Graves' disease: case report and review of the literature. *Neurologist.* 2017;22(4):134–137. doi:10.1097/NRL.0000000000000125.
129. Alqahtani SF, Aleithan MM. Thyrotoxic periodic paralysis as an initial presentation of Graves' disease in a Saudi patient. *BMJ Case Rep.* 2017:2017. doi:10.1136/bcr-2017-220224 piibcr-2017-220224.
130. Lin SH, Chu P, Cheng CJ, Chu SJ, Hung YJ, Lin YF. Early diagnosis of thyrotoxic periodic paralysis: spot urine calcium to phosphate ratio. *Crit Care Med.* 2006;34(12):2984–2989. doi:10.1097/01.CCM.0000242249.10856.49.
131. Kung AW. Clinical review: thyrotoxic periodic paralysis: a diagnostic challenge. *J Clin Endocrinol Metab.* 2006;91(7):2490–2495. doi:10.1210/jc.2006-0356 jc.2006-0356 [pii].
132. Dassau L, Conti LR, Radeke CM, Ptacek LJ, Vandenberg CA. Kir2.6 regulates the surface expression of Kir2.x inward rectifier potassium channels. *J Biol Chem.* 2011;286(11):9526–9541. doi:10.1074/jbc.M110.170597 M110.170597 [pii].
133. Zhao SX, Liu W, Liang J, et al. Assessment of molecular subtypes in thyrotoxic periodic paralysis and Graves' disease among Chinese Han adults: a population-based genome-wide association study. *JAMA Netw Open.* 2019;2(5):e193348. doi:10.1001/jamanetworkopen.2019.3348.
134. Chen DY, Schneider PF, Zhang XS, He ZM, Jing J, Chen TH. Striving for euthyroidism in radioiodine therapy of Graves' disease: a 12-year prospective, randomized, open-label blinded end point study. *Thyroid.* 2011;21(6):647–654. doi:10.1089/thy.2010.0348.

PART 2

Postoperative Thyroid Surgical Emergencies

CHAPTER 7

Recurrent Laryngeal Nerve Paralysis – Management of Recurrent Laryngeal Nerve Injuries

Yasuhiro Ito ■ Akira Miyauchi ■ Hiroo Masuoka

CHAPTER OUTLINE

Introduction

Vocal cord paralysis (VCP) is one of the most important complications of thyroid surgery because hoarseness, shortened phonation time, and aspiration derived from VCP significantly reduce the quality of life (QOL) of patients. VCP occasionally occurs for unknown reasons even when the recurrent laryngeal nerve (RLN) is not at risk anatomically. In such cases, VCP may be transient and recover within several months. By contrast, if the RLN was resected surgically because of carcinoma invasion or an accident, VCP will persist. Two points are important for preventing the deterioration of patient QOL. One is to make an effort to avoid injury to the RLN and the other is to appropriately perform reconstruction after RLN resection.

The RLN cannot be preserved in patients with preoperative VCP due to carcinoma invasion. However, surgeons should make an effort to preserve the RLN as much as possible if patients have functioning vocal cords preoperatively. To perform the appropriate surgical management, the RLN on both the peripheral and central sides of the site of the tumor extension must be accurately identified. When a portion of the RLN is surgically resected, the surgeons should reconstruct the nerve without causing deterioration of patient QOL. In this chapter, we describe the intraoperative management of the RLN with thyroid carcinoma invasion.

Intraoperative Management of the RLN With Thyroid Carcinoma Invasion

SHAVING OFF AND PARTIAL LAYER RESECTION

Even in patients with differentiated thyroid carcinoma who have functioning vocal cords preoperatively, the RLN may be found to be involved during thyroid surgery. In such cases, the RLN could be preserved by shaving off the tumor. Nishida et al. reported that the patients who underwent this procedure to preserve the RLN rarely had local recurrence.[1] Our experience

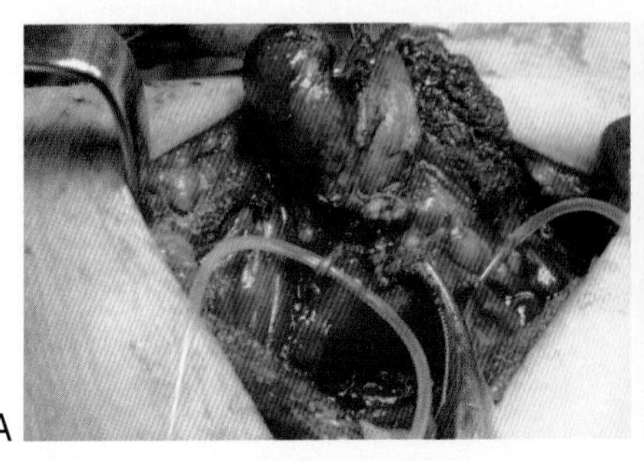

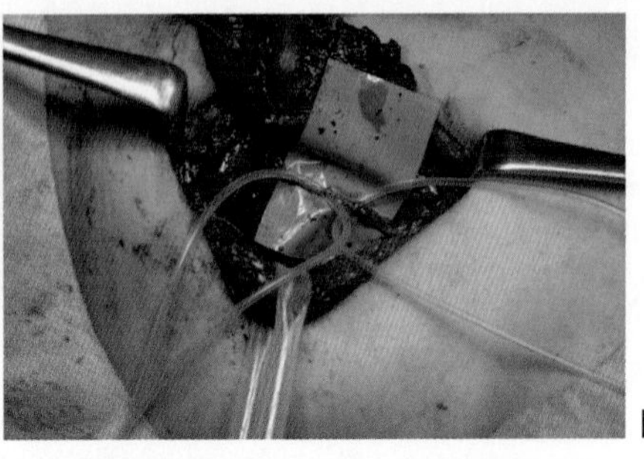

Fig. 7.1 (A) Tumor invading the recurrent laryngeal nerve (RLN). (B) As a result of extensive resection, the RLN became much thinner than its original thickness.

agrees with their report. After extensive dissection, the preserved nerve may become thinner than its original size. We denominated this surgical technique as "partial layer resection" if the thickness of the preserved nerve is less than half of its original size (Fig. 7.1).[2] Kihara et al. reviewed the postoperative vocal cord function of 18 patients who underwent this procedure. Of these patients, 2 had functioning vocal cords, 13 had transient VCP followed by full recovery of vocal cord function, and the remaining 3 had permanent VCP, indicating that 15 (83%) of the 18 patients succeeded in having functioning vocal cords postoperatively.[2] Histologic examination of the normal portion of the resected RLN demonstrated that 78% to 82% of the nerve cross-section was composed of perineural connective tissue.[2] This anatomy explains the excellent outcomes after the partial layer resection of the RLN. Even though the preserved nerve becomes thinner than its original size, partial layer resection is worth trying to preserve the nerve and the vocal cord function of patients who had functioning vocal cords preoperatively.

RECONSTRUCTION AFTER RESECTION OF A PORTION OF THE RLN

Background and Mechanism

When a unilateral RLN is resected, the ipsilateral vocal cord becomes paralytic and atrophic, and is usually fixed at a paramedian position. Symptoms are hoarseness, short phonation and aspiration, and decreasing patient QOL. Aspiration can cause pneumonia, which may be life-threatening, especially in elderly patients.

In the personal series of Akira Miyauchi at Kuma Hospital (Table 7.1), of the 721 patients with thyroid carcinoma who underwent an initial surgery between 1998 and 2008, 31 (4.3%) had

TABLE 7.1 ■ **Number (%) of Patients Who Needed Resection of the Recurrent Laryngeal Nerve in Miyauchi's Personal Series of Primary Thyroid Cancer Cases From 1998 to 2008**

	Preoperative VCP		
	No	Yes	Total
No. of Patients	690 (95.7%)	31 (4.3%)	721 (100.0%)
Patients With RLN Resection	16 (2.2%)	30 (4.2%)	46 (6.4%)

VCP, Vocal cord paralysis.

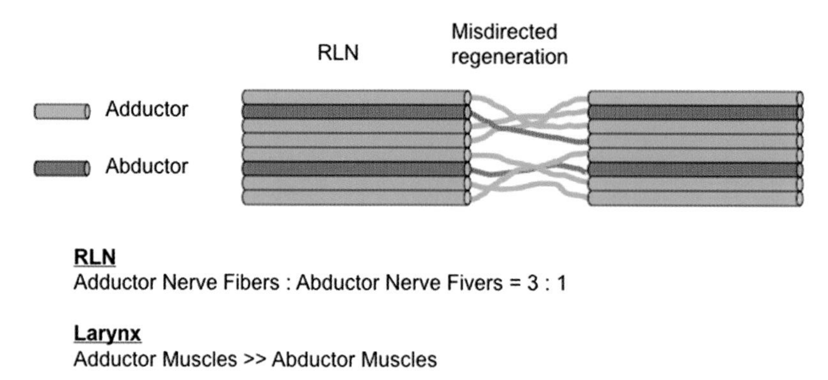

Fig. 7.2 Misdirected regeneration of the recurrent laryngeal nerve (RLN). The RLN contains adductor and abductor nerve fibers without special segregation of the nerve fibers within the RLN. After anastomosis, the nerve fibers regenerate in a mixed fashion.

VCP preoperatively. Thirty of these patients required resection of a portion of the RLN with carcinoma invasion during thyroid surgery. The remaining 690 patients had no VCP on preoperative fiberscopic examination. However, 16 (2.2%) of them required RLN resection due to carcinoma invasion at the time of surgery. In total, 47 patients, accounting for 6.4% of the patients in this series, required RLN resection.

Historically, direct anastomosis of the nerve ends of the transected RLN was performed more than 100 years ago. The first investigators reported that vocal cords on the side of the anastomosis restored their movements after the repair. However, other groups clarified that vocal cord movement was not recovered after anastomosis. Therefore, unfortunately, direct anastomosis of transected RLNs was abandoned for many years. In 1982, Ezaki et al. performed direct end-to-end anastomosis of the transected RLN in seven patients and reported that their voices recovered significantly thereafter, although their vocal cords remained fixed at the median position.[3] According to their explanation of this event, the RLN includes adductor and abductor nerve fibers with no spatial segregation (Fig. 7.2). Even if anastomosis was performed under microscopic surgery, anastomosis of all the fibers precisely is impossible, resulting in a misdirected regeneration among the nerve fibers. Therefore, at the time of inspiration and phonation, the adductor and abductor muscles contract simultaneously. The number of adductor nerve fibers is three times that of the abductor nerve fibers in the RLN, and in the larynx, the adductor muscles are much stronger than the abductor muscles. Therefore, the vocal cord on the side of the nerve anastomosis is fixed in the median position during the inspiration and phonation. This phenomenon is better expressed as synkinesis of the adductor and abductor muscles rather than paralysis. Owing to the reinnervation to its intrinsic muscles, the vocal cord restores tension during phonation, resulting in improvement of phonation.

Several Surgical Procedures for RLN Reconstruction

For reconstruction of the RLN, four surgical procedures can be used, namely direct anastomosis (DA), free nerve grafting (FNG), ansa cervicalis-RLN anastomosis (ARA), and vagus-RLN anastomosis (VRA; Fig. 7.3).

DA simply anastomoses the cut ends of the resected RLN, but its indication is limited. The length of the nerve defect must be short, and realistically, this technique is useful mainly for accidental transection of the RLN. If the defect is long, FNG is necessary to fill the defect to avoid tension on the anastomosis. The graft can be harvested from the supraclavicular cutaneous nerve, transcervical nerve, auricular nerve, or ansa cervicalis, regardless of whether they are motor or

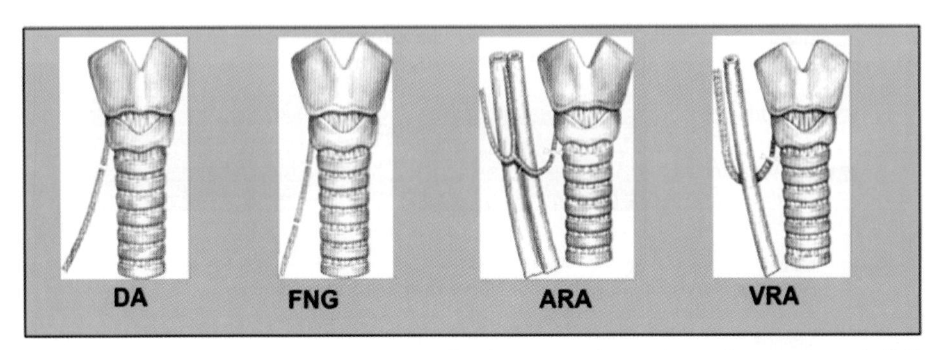

Fig. 7.3 The methods of recurrent laryngeal nerve (RLN) reconstruction used were direct anastomosis (DA), free nerve grafting (FNG), ansa cervicalis-RLN anastomosis (ARA), and vagus-RLN anastomosis (VRA).

sensory nerves. For this method, however, two anastomoses are required, and if the defect extends to the mediastinum, anastomosis on the mediastinal side is technically difficult or even impossible.

VRA was used in several rare cases treated with resection of the RLN and its ipsilateral vagus nerve. The cut end of the central portion of the vagus was anastomosed to the cut end of the peripheral portion of the RLN. These patients showed some recovery in their phonation postoperatively. Some surgeons use a different VRA procedure that involves splitting of the vagus nerve longitudinally, transecting its medial portion, and anastomosing the cut end of its central portion to the cut end of the peripheral portion of the resected RLN. They also reported some recovery in phonation postoperatively. However, the latter procedure is not recommended because of the possibility of vagus nerve paralysis.

ARA is a procedure in which the ansa cervicalis is transected and the cut end of its central portion is anastomosed to the cut end of the peripheral portion of the resected RLN. In 1990, Akira Miyauchi devised ARA based on his own idea and published manuscripts regarding his practice in 1994[4] and 1998.[5] However, this technique had been reported by Dr. RL Crumley in 1986.[6] Ansa cervicalis is a motor nerve forming a loop in front of the internal jugular vein and branching to the sternothyroid, sternohyoid, and omohyoid muscles. The outcome of ARA does not differ from that of DA. The technique requires only one anastomosis, which can be performed in an easy position near the larynx. Additional merit is that the times required for the nerve regeneration and voice recovery are shorter than those with FNG. For these reasons, the ARA is the most frequently adopted procedure for nerve reconstruction in Kuma Hospital. In cases where the ansa cervicalis on the ipsilateral side is not available, the contralateral ansa cervicalis can be used for the reconstruction.[7] We inserted a suction tube between the trachea and the esophagus, suctioned the contralateral ansa cervicalis into the tube, and brought it to the side of the defect to make the anastomosis.

Thyroid carcinoma often partially or completely invades the RLN near the ligament of Berry, making the dissection to preserve or reconstruct the RLN problematic because only the RLN portion central to the invasion can be found in such cases. Miyauchi et al. devised the "laryngeal approach" to the peripheral portion of the RLN that involves dividing the inferior constrictor muscle along the lateral edge of the thyroid cartilage and identifying the nerve behind the thyroid cartilage[8] (Fig. 7.4A–E). They performed this procedure before tumor resection in 10 patients and after tumor resection in 3 patients. Of the former patients, three without preoperative VCP had preserved RLN with sharp dissection and restored nerve function after surgery. The remaining seven patients (five of whom had VCP preoperatively) required nerve reconstruction, which was comparably easy because the peripheral RLN had already been identified. By contrast, one of the three patients who underwent the procedure after tumor resection could not undergo nerve reconstruction because the peripheral stump of the RLN could not be found. Thus, they concluded that

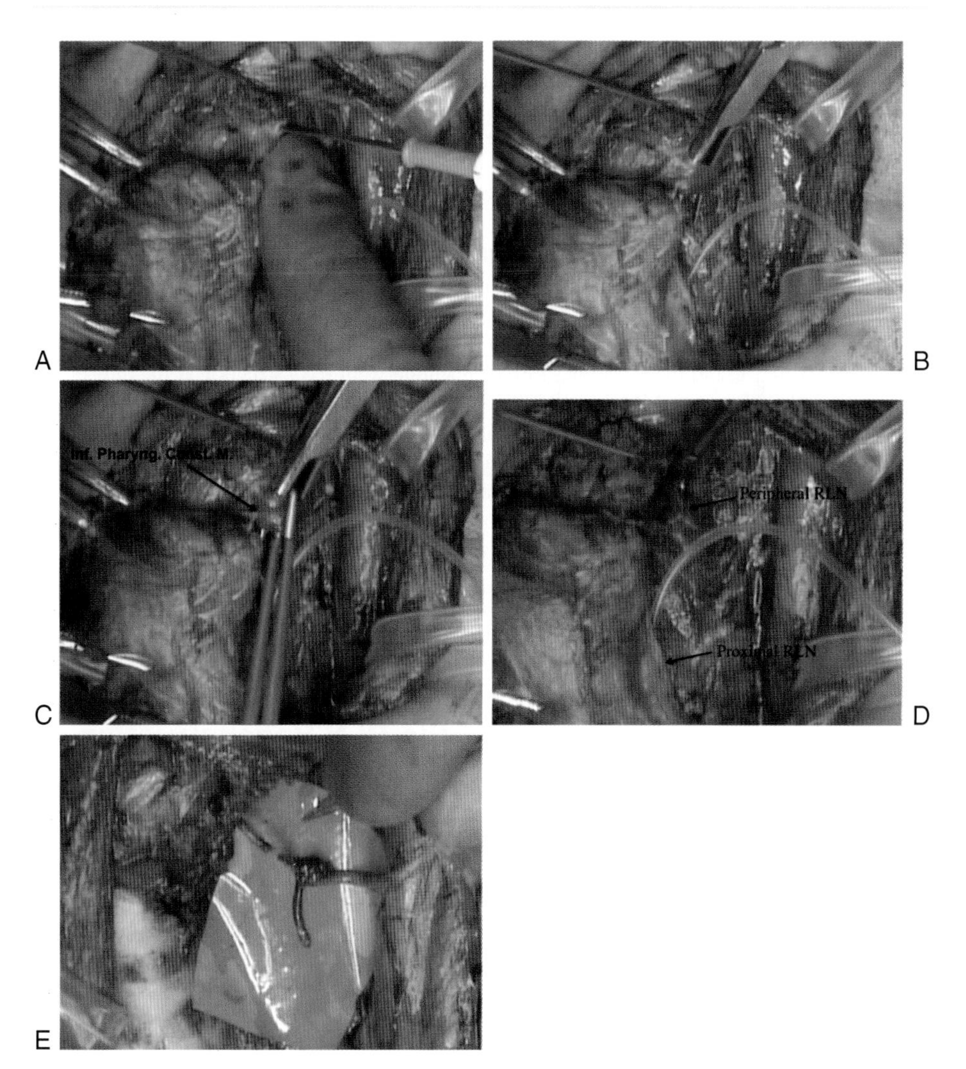

Fig. 7.4 (A) Laryngeal approach: marking a hole in the inferior pharyngeal constrictor muscle at the lateral edge of the thyroid cartilage using electrocautery. (B) Laryngeal approach: dissecting the inferior pharyngeal constrictor muscles along the lateral edge of the thyroid cartilage. (C) Laryngeal approach: cutting the inferior pharyngeal constrictor muscles *(Inf. Pharyng. Const. M.)* along the lateral edge of the thyroid cartilage with a pair of bipolar coagulators. (D) Laryngeal approach: locating the peripheral RLN behind the thyroid cartilage. (E) Laryngeal approach: performing ARA with the distal portion of the RLN found behind the thyroid cartilage. *ARA,* Ansa cervicalis-RLN anastomosis; *RLN,* recurrent laryngeal nerve.

for thyroid carcinoma with invasion of the RLN at or around the ligament of Berry, the laryngeal approach before dissection of the RLN facilitates preservation or, if the RLN is invaded by the carcinoma, reconstruction of the nerve.

When thyroid carcinoma invades the trachea at or near Berry's ligament, requiring resection of the trachea for curative surgery, the RLN can be at risk of injury. The presence of the RLN in the vicinity significantly interferes with tracheal surgeries such as tracheal resection and repair. Miyauchi et al. proposed "lateral mobilization" of the RLN.[9] They divided the inferior pharyngeal constrictor muscle along the lateral edge of the thyroid cartilage to find the peripheral RLN and mobilized the RLN laterally before performing the tracheal surgery. The RLNs in 8 of the 11 patients who underwent this procedure (including 2 patients with RLN paralysis preoperatively) could be preserved and mobilized laterally, and those in the remaining 3 patients were resected and reconstructed with the ansa cervicalis after lateral mobilization of the peripheral stump of the RLN.[9] Tracheal surgery was performed safely for all the patients. Therefore, this technique is proved to be useful for preservation of the RLN when patients undergo tracheal surgery for invading lesions at or near Berry's ligament.

From 1984 to 2007, Miyauchi performed RLN reconstructions during thyroid surgery in 88 patients with thyroid cancer in Kuma Hospital or Kagawa Medical University Hospital (16 men and 72 women, mean age, 55.6 years [range, 18–78 years]). Fifty-one (58%) of the patients had VCP preoperatively. Seven patients underwent RLN reconstruction in the second surgery for carcinoma recurrence, and the remaining 81 patients underwent reconstruction at the time of the initial surgery. In this series, ARA was the most frequently performed procedure (65 cases, 74%). DA and FNG had limited indications as described earlier and were performed in only in 7 and 14 patients, respectively. VRA was performed in only two patients as described earlier. Of the 65 patients who underwent ARA, anastomosis was performed behind the thyroid cartilage in 31 (48%). In eight ARA cases, anastomosis was constructed using the contralateral ansa-cervicalis. Surgical loupes at a magnification of 2.5 times were used in 51 patients, and microscopic operation was performed in 10 patients, while no magnification was used in the remaining 27 patients. The thickness of the thread used for the anastomosis ranged from 6-0 to 9-0, with 8-0 being the mode. The authors usually placed three stitches to make an end-to-end anastomosis of the nerves using microsurgical instruments.

Evaluation of the Outcomes of the RLN Reconstruction

We routinely examine the vocal cords of the patients after RLN reconstruction using a fiber-optic laryngoscope. However, it is not suitable for evaluating vocal cord function because the vocal cords on the side of the reconstruction do not recover their normal movements after reconstruction. Several methods are available for evaluating laryngeal functions after reconstruction, with the easiest and most practical method being to periodically measure the maximum phonation time (MPT). In patients who underwent RLN reconstruction, the serial measurements usually show a sudden increase in MPT around 3 months after surgery. We record the MPT 1 year postoperatively to evaluate the phonatory recovery. Table 7.2 presents the comparison of MPTs between the patients who underwent RLN reconstruction (16 men and 72 women) at 1 year after surgery, healthy subjects (8 men and 26 women), and patients with VCP (9 men and 18 women)

TABLE 7.2 ■ **Maximum Phonation Time in Healthy Subjects, Patients With Vocal Cord Paralysis, and Patients Who Underwent Reconstruction of Recurrent Laryngeal Nerve**

		Healthy Subjects	Patients With VCP	Patients With RLN Reconstruction
Male	No. of Patients	8	9	16
	MPT	28.6 ± 10.8	10.1 ± 4.3	20.9 ± 11.7
Female	No. of Patients	26	18	72
	MPT	16.7 ± 5.1	6.3 ± 2.9	18.8 ± 6.6

The values are presented as mean ± standard deviation (sec).
MPT, Maximum phonation time; *RLN,* recurrent laryngeal nerve; *VCP,* vocal cord paralysis.

TABLE 7.3 ■ **Phonation Efficiency Index in Healthy Subjects, Patients With Vocal Cord Paralysis, and Patients Who Underwent Reconstruction of Recurrent Laryngeal Nerve**

		Healthy Subjects	Patients With VCP	Patients With RLN Reconstruction
Male	No. of Patients	8	9	16
	PEI	6.79 ± 2.52	3.24 ± 1.49	5.53 ± 2.72
Female	No. of Patients	26	18	72
	PEI	6.73 ± 2.04	3.29 ± 1.48	7.59 ± 2.82

The values are expressed as mean ± standard deviation (sec/L).
PEI, Phonation efficiency index; *RLN*, recurrent laryngeal nerve; *VCP*, vocal cord paralysis.

as controls.[10] Although the MPTs of the patients with VCP were much shorter than those of the healthy subjects, the MPTs of the patients who underwent RLN reconstruction reached almost normal MPTs regardless of sex. As shown in Table 7.2, the MPT in the men was much longer than that in the women among the healthy subjects and in patients with VCP. Then, to adjust for such a difference, we divided the MPT by the vital capacity (sec/L), which we designated as "phonation efficacy index" (PEI).[10] PEI should indicate the vocal cord function by converting a unit volume of exhaled air to a certain length of phonation (Table 7.3). The patients with VCP had significantly smaller PEIs than the healthy subjects, and the patients who underwent RLN reconstruction achieved nearly normal PEI values 1 year after surgery. This measurement is suitable for evaluating vocal cord function regardless of sex. We analyzed whether various factors such as age at surgery, presence or absence of VCP preoperatively, RLN reconstruction methods, use of a magnifier, and thickness of the thread are related to the PEI and found that none of these significantly affected the PEI 1 year after surgery. These facts indicate that regardless of vocal cord function, sex, and age, if we reconstruct the resected RLN using any reconstruction procedure with any suture thread thickness, with or without surgical magnifiers, patients' vocal cords would recover to nearly normal.

Yoshioka et al. evaluated 228 patients who underwent RLN resection and reconstruction, and demonstrated that none of the following factors significantly affected phonatory recovery: age, preoperative VCP, reconstruction method, site of the distal anastomosis, use of a magnifier, suture thread thickness, and surgeon experience. Of the patients, only 24 (10.5%) had MPTs of less than 9 seconds at 1 year after surgery, but this insufficiency was not associated with the factors.[11] Therefore, this technique is essential in cases of RLN resection, and all thyroid surgeons should be familiar with these reconstruction techniques and attempt a RLN reconstruction if necessary.

References

1. Nishida T, Nakao K, Hamaji M, Kamiike W, Kurozumi K, Matsuda H. Preservation of recurrent laryngeal nerve invaded by differentiated thyroid cancer. *Ann Surg*. 1997;226:85–91.
2. Kihara M, Miyauchi A, Yabuta T, et al. Outcome of vocal cord function after partial layer resection of the recurrent laryngeal nerve in patients with invasive papillary thyroid cancer. *Surgery*. 2014;155:184–189.
3. Ezaki H, Ushio H, Harada Y, Takeichi N. Recurrent laryngeal nerve anastomosis following thyroid surgery. *World J Surg*. 1982;6:342–346.
4. Miyauchi A, Matsusaka K, Kawaguchi H, Nakamoto K, Maeda M. Ansa-recurrent nerve anastomosis for vocal cord paralysis due to mediastinal lesions. *Ann Thorac Surg*. 1994;57:1020–1021.
5. Miyauchi A Matsusaka A, Kihara M, et al. The role of ansa-to-recurrent-laryngeal nerve anastomosis in operations for thyroid cancer. *Eur J Surg*. 1998;164:927–933.

6. Miyauchi A, Yokozawa T, Kobayashi K, Hirai K, Matsuzuka F, Kuma K. Opposite ansa cervicalis to recurrent laryngeal nerve anastomosis to restore phonation in patients with advanced thyroid cancer. *Eur J Surg*. 2001;167:540–541.
7. Crumley RL, Izdebski K. Vocal quality following laryngeal reinnervation by ansa hypoglossi transfer. *Laryngoscope*. 1986;96:611–616.
8. Miyauchi A, Masuoka H, Tomoda C, et al. Laryngeal approach to the recurrent laryngeal nerve involved by thyroid cancer at the ligament of Berry. *Surgery*. 2012;152(1):57–60.
9. Miyauchi A, Ito Y, Miya A, et al. Lateral mobilization of the recurrent laryngeal nerve to facilitate tracheal surgery in patients with thyroid cancer invading the trachea near Berry's ligament. *World J Surg*. 2007;31:2081–2084.
10. Miyauchi A, Inoue H, Tomoda C, et al. Improvement in phonation after reconstruction of the recurrent laryngeal nerve in patients with thyroid cancer invading the nerve. *Surgery*. 2009;146:1056–1062.
11. Yoshioka K, Miyauchi A, Fukushima M, Kobayashi K, Kihara M, Miya A. Surgical methods and experiences of surgeons did not significantly affect the recovery in phonation following reconstruction of the recurrent laryngeal nerve. *World J Surg*. 2016;40:2948–2955.

CHAPTER 8

Post-Thyroidectomy Emergencies: Management of Tracheal and Esophageal Injuries

Gustavo Romero-Velez ■ Randall P. Owen

CHAPTER OUTLINE

Introduction

The thyroid gland can be affected with benign and malignant diseases that will require thyroid surgery. About 150,000 thyroidectomies are performed each year in the United States. This common procedure has a low morbidity and mortality, especially when performed by intermediate- and high-volume surgeons compared with those who do less than three thyroidectomies per year.[1,2] However, injuries to the esophagus or trachea during thyroidectomy can have serious consequences, including death.

The advances in thyroid surgery have made this a safe operation. Compared to 1850 when the mortality rate was 40%, now it approaches 0%. Although death after a thyroidectomy is a rare event, it can still happen. Gomez-Ramirez in a study including 30,495 thyroidectomies from 26 different centers found 20 deaths.[3] Most of the deaths were attributed to airway complications including tracheal injury and cervical hematoma causing respiratory compromise. Sepsis secondary to esophageal injury was also found as a cause of death in one patient of this cohort.[3] It is important to mention that half of the mortalities in this series had an associated retrosternal goiter.

Morbidity after thyroidectomy is also low, with an overall complication rate between 3% and 5%. Common complications include wound infection (0.02% to 0.5%), hematoma (0.3% to 4.3%), transient recurrent laryngeal nerve palsy (1% to 2%), permanent recurrent laryngeal nerve palsy (less than 1%), transient hypoparathyroidism (1.6% to 50%), permanent hypoparathyroidism (0% to 13%), and chylous fistula (less than 1%).[4]

Tracheal and esophageal injuries can also occur; however, the incidence is so low that only a few case reports and case series exist in the literature that can help us understand, diagnose, and treat these problems. Most of the reports agree that this complication is so infrequent that surgeons would at most encounter one case during their entire career. Nonetheless, it is important to be aware of these complications, including their diagnosis and treatment.

Trachea

ANATOMY

It is important to be conscious of the tracheal anatomy to have a better understanding of the pathophysiology of injuries caused during thyroidectomy.

The trachea is a tubular structure that connects the outside air with the lung's parenchyma. It has an average length of 11.8 centimeters, starting at the cricoid cartilage and ending at the carina. During its course it is composed of 18 to 22 D-rings with an anterior C-shaped cartilage and a posterior membranous wall.[5] The posterior aspect of the trachea is in close relationship with the esophagus, separated by the trachealis muscle.

There are three components of tracheal anatomy that thyroid surgeons should pay close attention to as these factors can play an important role during tracheal injuries. The first factor is the well-known relationship of the trachea with the thyroid gland. The thyroid isthmus crosses anterior to the trachea at the second to third tracheal ring. This close relationship makes the trachea prone to both direct injury during dissection and invasion by tumors of the thyroid that may require en bloc resection.

Together with the close proximity between the trachea and the thyroid comes a joint vascular supply. These two structures are supplied by the inferior thyroid artery. Injury to the vascular supply of the trachea can predispose to tracheal ischemia and with it, perforation. The tracheal branches arising at the proximal inferior thyroid artery approach the tracheal wall laterally and give superior and inferior branches that anastomose with the contralateral side. Given this vascular configuration, circumferential dissection of the trachea of more than 1 to 2 cm predisposes to ischemia.[5]

The last factor of tracheal anatomy that is worth mentioning is its delicate wall; its thickness averages 3 mm. It is critical to understand these anatomic facts and relationships in order to operate on the thyroid gland safely and prevent unnecessary injury.

INCIDENCE AND RISKS FACTORS

The true incidence of tracheal injury during thyroidectomies is not well known. Gosnell et al. in a study including 11,917 thyroidectomies during a 45-year period at a single institution found seven cases, for an incidence of 0.06%.[6] In a study from 2018, performed by Tartaglia et al., an extensive literature review found only 16 patients reported.[4] It is postulated by some authors that although it is a rare complication, it is underreported.

As previously mentioned, the reporting of tracheal injuries comes from case reports and case series. Risk factors for its occurrence have been postulated. Factors attributable to the tracheal wall are: thyrotoxic goiter that causes long-term tracheal compression that over time may cause tracheomalacia[7]; female sex as the trachea wall is thinner; and multi-nodular goiter that will cause intense fibrosis making the dissection plane more difficult. Excessive retraction of the gland while dissecting the ligament of Berry can cause distortion of the trachea, exposing the posterolateral surface to injury.[6] In fact, at times the surgeon can become confused regarding the anatomy when excessive traction and rotation are applied to the thyroid. The membranous portion of the trachea can be exposed and pointing up at the surgeon and can be easily penetrated if the surgeon is not aware.

Factors associated with altered tracheal blood supply are: improper or prolonged intubation; elevated cuff pressure impeding adequate blood supply; and intraoperative bleeding with increased use of electrosurgical devices that can cause thermal injury. Hematoma formation is thought to cause compression and diminished vascular supply. Superinfection of the hematoma or primary deep surgical site infection may also predispose to tracheal necrosis and perforation.

Another contributing factor reported is acute elevation of the intrathoracic pressure with a Valsalva maneuver. This is hypothesized to act at an already weakened tracheal wall leading to perforation. Some authors suggest that patients should abstain from strenuous activities for a few weeks postoperatively and to have adequate control of coughing and sneezing.

CLINICAL PRESENTATION

There are two main presentations of tracheal injury that have been reported: one is the incidental intraoperative finding and the other and more feared is the delayed presentation that can happen days to weeks after surgery. All patients with subcutaneous emphysema after thyroidectomy should be consider to have a tracheal rupture until proven otherwise.

Preoperative findings concerning for malignant tumor invasion into the trachea include cough, hoarseness, hemoptysis, and dyspnea. Fiberoptic laryngoscopy may occasionally demonstrate tracheal invasion, but usually a thin-cut computed tomography (CT) scan through the trachea is necessary to determine invasion. If invasion is still uncertain at the time of surgery, then tracheoscopy should be performed at the outset of the procedure. The author (Owen) finds the best technique to be placement of a laryngeal mask airway (LMA) followed by insertion of a fiberoptic scope through the LMA for examination of the larynx and tracheal wall. This is suitable for a tumor with minimal invasion and widely patent airway, whereas a tumor that has penetrated the trachea widely and is causing near airway obstruction should be handled with an awake tracheostomy below the tumor, or consideration of cardiopulmonary bypass should be entertained if a tracheostomy cannot be placed due to the extensive nature of the tumor.

Well-differentiated thyroid cancer rarely invades other tissues; however, when this occurs it is controversial if the surgical management should include the removal of the affected structures or if the tumor should be "shaved off" with the possibility of leaving microscopically positive margins. In general, shaving tumor off of the trachea is acceptable if no gross disease is left behind and the trachea is not penetrated. In case of en bloc resection of the trachea, primary reconstruction can be attempted if less than six rings are involved. In other cases, flap reconstruction or permanent tracheostomy may be necessary.[8]

Removal of large tumors creates an increased risk for intraoperative damage. Intraoperative findings associated with tracheal injury are ongoing leak from the ventilatory system, bubbling at the surgical field, or even an exposed endotracheal tube. The most common site of injury is the posterolateral tracheal surface and, according to Gosnell et al., that is likely the result of excessive traction while dissecting the ligament of Berry.[6] These injuries can be encountered during the dissection or might be recognized at the end of the procedure while doing a leak test. Given this possibility, it is recommended to perform a leak test at the end of the procedure by filling the surgical site with sterile saline and asking the anesthesiologist to perform a Valsalva maneuver.

A delayed presentation of tracheal injury can happen days or even weeks after the original surgery. This presentation is less common, but given its potential to compromise the airway, it can be lethal. These patients present with dyspnea, hoarseness, facial and neck swelling secondary to subcutaneous emphysema, and wound infection. A story of coughing or sneezing can be reported by the patient prior to the initiation of the symptoms. Once this lesion is encountered, one should be aware of potential concomitant complications including recurrent laryngeal nerve injury.

DIAGNOSIS AND INITIAL TREATMENT

Physicians taking care of these patients should have a high index of suspicion of a delayed presentation. Differential diagnosis includes esophageal injuries, pneumothorax, and necrotizing soft tissue infections. The priority should be to stabilize the patient following the airway, breathing, and circulation (ABC) principles of trauma. One should be prepared to perform an emergency tracheostomy or rapid-sequence endotracheal intubation using a fiberscope. In case of endotracheal intubation, the cuff should be positioned distal to the injury. This principle is also important in case of injuries found intraoperatively to maintain proper ventilation.

Once the patient is stabilized, including a secure airway, a chest X-ray should be done to rule out a pneumothorax. This will not reveal the tracheal injury, but secondary signs such as subcutaneous emphysema can be encountered. A CT scan of the chest and neck with IV contrast can demonstrate the defect. A normal CT scan does not rule out the diagnosis, as false negatives can be found in case of adjacent edema, secretions, or hemorrhage.[9] Bronchoscopy (or tracheoscopy as described previously) can also be done to assess the injury. In case of concomitant sepsis, broad-spectrum antibiotics should be promptly started.

NONOPERATIVE MANAGEMENT

Tracheal injuries encountered intraoperatively should be repaired—surgical repair will be discussed in the following section. For patients with delayed presentation, once the diagnosis is made, the symptoms and most importantly the respiratory status will dictate further management. Even though most patients reported in the literature underwent surgical repair of the injury, a few cases of successful nonoperative management have been described.[10–14]

Conzo et al. were the first to report the nonoperative management of a small tracheal perforation (1.5 mm) following thyroidectomy.[10] Davies et al. followed with another case where a "pinhole"-size defect was managed expectantly with favorable results.[11] Benson et al. also described in their case a pinhole-size defect (1 mm) found on bronchoscopy; his group managed the subcutaneous emphysema with a bedside exploration and a Penrose drain placement, which was removed after a few days.[12] Gonzalez-Sanchez used intravenous antibiotics and bedside wound exploration, which caused a tracheal fistula that closed with conservative management.[13] In all of these cases, the patients were mildly symptomatic from the subcutaneous emphysema, had no respiratory distress, and showed hemodynamic stability.

Mazeh et al. also attempted nonoperative management in their case.[14] Given worsening symptoms 4 days after presentation, they pursued operative management where a 2.5-cm linear tear was found. These five cases suggest that it is reasonable to consider a trial of nonoperative treatment for stable patients with small defects (less than 1 cm).[15]

Prior to discussion of the operative management of tracheal injuries during thyroidectomy, it is worth mentioning that some authors have tried a minimally invasive approach. One author proposed the use of covered stents into the trachea.[16] This novel approach was reported by Han et al., where, at a single institution, two patients developed a tracheal perforation after thyroidectomy. In both cases the diagnosis was confirmed by bronchoscopy, and under fluoroscopic guidance, a 20- × 60-mm covered stent (Sewon Medical Co., Seoul, Korea) was placed. They had no recurrence of perforation at 31- and 35-month follow-up, respectively.

OPERATIVE MANAGEMENT

Urgent surgical management should be considered in those patients exhibiting cardiopulmonary instability, large pneumothorax, large pneumomediastinum, enlarging or symptomatic subcutaneous emphysema, and/or tracheal deviation.[11] As mentioned previously, during the initial management the priority should be to secure an airway and treat based on the principles of trauma, treating any condition that interferes with cardiopulmonary stability (i.e., tamponade, tension pneumothorax).

Common operative findings include necrosis and larger defects, usually greater than 1 cm. Most of the lesions are in the posterolateral aspect of the trachea, but injuries to the anterior surface have also been reported. When necrosis is found, it is necessary to debride the trachea until healthy tissue is encountered. Once it is debrided, the injury size will determine the type of repair needed.[17–22] Different approaches have been reported in the literature, including primary repair with absorbable sutures, primary repair reinforced with a fibrin-thrombin patch, primary repair with muscle flap reinforcement (strap muscles or sternocleidomastoid), circumferential tracheal excision with anastomosis, or tracheostomy placement. Postoperative drain placement after the repair is controversial: there is no evidence that one approach is better compared with another, and given the rarity of this entity, is in unlikely we will have comparative studies between techniques.[4,6]

Concomitant infection can be found at the time of the surgical exploration. It is not clear if the infection predisposes to necrosis and perforation or the perforation causes secondary colonization and infection. Studies reporting associated infection have found *Staphylococcus* and *Streptococcus* species in the cultures. In those cases, broad-spectrum antibiotics should be promptly started and then therapy should be tailored based on cultures. One case also reported the successful treatment of a large infected tracheal defect with a vacuum-assisted closure therapy (VAC).[23]

CONCLUSION

Tracheal injury after thyroidectomy is a rare complication. It can be encountered intraoperatively or weeks after the index operation. There are multiple surgical procedures for its management. A high index of suspicion is needed for those with a delayed presentation, and subcutaneous emphysema should prompt further investigation. Cardiopulmonary stability will dictate the treatment.

Esophagus

ANATOMY

As stated for tracheal injuries, knowledge of esophageal anatomy is crucial and will help understand the mechanism of an injury caused during thyroidectomy.

The esophagus is a muscular tube-like organ that starts at the pharynx at the level of the sixth cervical vertebra. During its course it crosses three anatomical compartments: the neck, the thorax, and the abdomen. Through its course it has relationships with different structures. In the neck, the esophagus lies posterior to the larynx and trachea just left of the midline. The posterior border of the cervical esophagus is marked by the prevertebral cervical fascia.[24] Although the esophagus is not always in direct contact with the thyroid, rarely, large or invasive tumors can sometimes penetrate the esophagus.

Different from other gastrointestinal organs, the esophagus lacks a serosa. Its architecture consists of three layers: mucosa, submucosa, and muscularis. Important anatomical considerations for esophageal repair are that the submucosa is the strongest layer and that the absence of serosa can make repair a challenge.[24] In regard to the muscular layer, the cervical esophagus is composed of skeletal muscle, whereas the lower esophagus is made up of smooth muscle.

Given the long course of the esophagus through three different anatomical regions, the blood supply comes from various branches at each level. The cervical esophagus receives its supply from the inferior thyroid artery. The thoracic and abdominal esophagus are supplied by branches of the thoracic aorta and the left gastric artery, respectively. Just as described in tracheal injuries, proximal ligation of the inferior thyroid artery can predispose to ischemia and perforation. Venous drainage at the neck follows the arterial supply via the inferior thyroid vein; however, the esophagus has an extensive submucosal venous plexus.

INCIDENCE AND RISK FACTORS

Esophageal injury during thyroidectomy is even more rare than tracheal injuries with only a few reported cases in the literature.[10,25–28] No studies have reported the actual incidence of this complication. The incidence of esophageal perforation not associated with thyroidectomy is also low, with only 3.1/1,000,000 per year.[29] Based on the study by Gomez-Ramirez,[3] esophageal perforation during thyroidectomy occurs less than 0.0001% of the time. However, the mortality reported for esophageal perforations can be as high as 29%.[25]

Risks factors identified in the available case reports are reoperation, difficult intubation, and the use of laryngeal mask.[10,25] Esophageal perforations occurring during difficult intubation or nasogastric tube placement can occur even in nonthyroid surgery. It is well known to surgeons the added difficulty of operating in a previously operated field; in cases where a completion thyroidectomy is needed, the surgeon should be extra meticulous, as the normal tissue planes will be disturbed with excessive fibrosis and scar tissue.

One particular circumstance that is important to discuss is that of a patient with anaplastic thyroid cancer. Patients generally present with a rapidly growing irregular mass of the thyroid, often with symptoms of airway compromise and dysphagia. Fine-needle aspiration biopsy is useful to suggest the diagnosis, but definitive diagnosis with core needle biopsy or open biopsy is generally required. Whereas for other varieties of thyroid cancer surgical extirpation is the mainstay of treatment and the best hope for cure, in anaplastic thyroid cancer this is not the case. Rather, aggressive surgery can result in tracheal or esophageal perforation. Esophageal perforation in particular will generally never close in this setting. Thus, a patient with a terrible disease and very limited life span will now have the additional morbidity of an esophageal fistula. This may also prevent the administration of radiation and/or chemotherapy or participation in a clinical trial. Thus, if anaplastic thyroid cancer is suspected, a biopsy should be taken and the incision closed until the result is known and a well-informed plan can be formulated.

CLINICAL PRESENTATION

In patients who will undergo thyroidectomy who complain of dysphagia, a suspicion of esophageal invasion should be raised. Direct invasion into the esophagus by differentiated thyroid carcinoma ranges from 1% to 3.2%.[28] In cases where there is preoperative concern, diagnostic testing should include esophagoscopy with or without endoscopic ultrasound to exclude esophageal involvement prior to undergoing a thyroidectomy.

Esophageal injuries can be recognized intraoperatively by the presence of exposed esophageal mucosa or thick secretions caused by saliva. Excessive traction of the thyroid may lead to esophageal injury. In cases of uncertain location of the esophagus or where its relationship with the thyroid is unsure, a nasogastric tube can be placed by the anesthesiologist to help palpate and better localize its course.[25] Intraoperative esophagoscopy can also be considered in cases where there is concern for injury.[10]

Postoperatively, patients can present with wound discharge, wound infection, or subcutaneous emphysema. In some cases where a drain is left in place, the output will be noted to be turbid, raising the concern of esophageal or lymphatic leak. Other symptoms reported by patients can be vomiting, dysphagia, and dyspnea. Patients can also present with florid sepsis; however, cervical esophageal perforations are much better tolerated, compared with perforations in the thorax and the abdomen.[25] Cervical esophageal perforation can progress to mediastinitis, cervical abscess, and carotid pseudoaneurysm if it is not promptly recognized and treated.[27]

DIAGNOSIS AND INITIAL TREATMENT

A delay in treatment has a direct correlation with mortality in esophageal injuries.[30] The natural history of the disease progresses from contamination of the surrounding spaces to sepsis and death in as quick as 24 to 48 hours.[29] As the mortality of this injury is related to sepsis, resuscitation with crystalloids and early administration of intravenous broad-spectrum antibiotics is key during the initial phase. The patient has to be nothing by mouth (NPO). In association with resuscitation, it is important to obtain source control either with surgical or minimally invasive techniques.

Antibiotic coverage should be targeted toward both aerobic and anaerobic bacteria. Antifungal therapy is controversial. The Infectious Diseases Society of America does not recommend antifungal coverage for community-acquired gastrointestinal perforations, but there is a role for antifungals in health care–associated infections and immunocompromised patients.[31] In a series of 27 patients with esophageal perforation, Elsayed et al. found that patients with positive fungal cultures had the worst outcomes, including increased mortality, hospital stay, and intensive care unit (ICU) stay.[32]

Esophageal perforation can be seen in different imaging studies. Chest and neck X-ray will only show nonspecific findings such as subcutaneous emphysema, pleural effusion, pneumomediastinum, and pneumothorax. Contrast-enhanced CT is proposed by the World Society of Emergent Surgery Guidelines as the test of choice with a sensitivity of 92% to 100%.[30] Esophagogram with gastrografin or barium can also provide valuable information, especially whether the perforation is contained or not. Endoscopy can be used as a diagnostic tool in cases where imaging is inconclusive.

NONOPERATIVE MANAGEMENT

Once the diagnosis is made and the patient has been stabilized, the surgeon has to decide if the patient warrants a reoperation or if the injury can be managed nonoperatively. The risks and benefits of both possibilities have to be compared; reoperation can be challenging, as the planes could be disrupted given the inflammation, increasing the risk of further damage. However, if the patient has sepsis or worsening symptoms, surgery is needed.

Nonoperative treatment can be offered to those patients with an early presentation, a contained perforation, and who show no evidence of systemic symptoms or cardiovascular instability. These patients should be under close surveillance (i.e., ICU).[29,30] Surgical management needs to be considered if these criteria are absent at presentation or during follow-up. One way of making this decision is using the Pittsburgh esophageal perforation severity scoring system. This calculator uses 10 clinical and radiological variables to classify patients into low-, medium-, and high-risk groups.[33] Only low-risk group patients are potential candidates for nonoperative management.

Nonoperative management is similar to the initial treatment of esophageal perforations. It includes having patients NPO, coverage with broad-spectrum antibiotics, and appropriate control of the leak with a drain. If a drain has not been placed during surgery, then a drain should be placed into the area of concern. In addition to these elements, a cornerstone of this management is adequate nutritional support. Nutrition can be given via different routes including total parenteral nutrition, or tube feeds via nasogastric tube or gastrostomy tube. (However, a nasogastric tube can be placed under direct vision at surgery, but should not be attempted blindly in a patient with an esophageal injury.) Proton pump inhibitors should be started as well.[30]

Two of the case reports of esophageal injuries caused by thyroidectomy have described successful nonoperative management.[26,27] In both cases, suction drains were left during the index operation, and turbid discharge was noted postoperatively. The presence of drains provided control of the fistula, avoiding the need for surgical reexploration. In most thyroidectomies the placement of a drain is not routine, but it should be considered if there is concern for an esophageal injury. With control of the fistula, nonsurgical management in selected cases with broad-spectrum antibiotics and nutrition supplementation is an option. Once the drainage decreases and an esophagogram shows no fistula, the drains can be removed.

ENDOSCOPIC MANAGEMENT

As previously mentioned, esophageal perforations can be evaluated with endoscopy when the diagnosis by CT is uncertain. Endoscopic evaluation should be performed with caution, as it can potentially aggravate the injury. Once the injury has been identified, there are therapeutic options that have been described in case series and retrospective studies. The three endoscopic therapeutic options are: endoclips, covered stents, and endoscopic vacuum therapy.

Endoclips come in two different types: through the scope and over the scope. The former are considered for smaller perforations, usually less than 10 mm, whereas the latter can cover areas up to 30 mm.[34] The overall reported success rate for endoscopic clips is between 45% and 95%. Factors implicated in their success include anatomical location, chronicity, type of injury (perforation vs leak vs fistula), and if they are used as primary or as rescue therapy. The best results are achieved with acute perforations where clips are used as the primary intervention.[35]

Covered stents bypass the injury site, allowing it to heal and preventing ongoing contamination of the extraluminal spaces from luminal contents. There is a potential risk of stent migration in 10% to 37% of the cases that will require another procedure for its retrieval.[36] Similar to the experience with endoscopic clips, the results are variable. Factors associated with failure include injuries greater than 6 cm and injuries of the cervical esophagus given that stents at this location are not generally well tolerated.[34] Ozer et al. reported the successful use of a covered stent in combination with surgical exploration and muscle reconstruction in a case of esophageal injury during thyroidectomy.[25] Their patient had no complications or complaints from the stent. However, patients with proximal esophageal stents sometimes report pain and discomfort.

It is worth mentioning the endoscopic vacuum therapy for esophageal perforations. This relatively new technique that was first described in 2006 works similarly to a traditional vacuum device promoting granulation tissue. The sponge is introduced endoscopically into the esophageal perforation or abscess cavity. Möschler et al. reported the successful treatment of two cases with proximal iatrogenic esophageal injuries using endoscopic vacuum therapy.[37]

OPERATIVE MANAGEMENT

Operative management is usually offered to those patients who present with sepsis or have deterioration while undergoing a nonoperative approach. At surgery, definitive repair is preferable but will not always be feasible, and a judgment may be made to minimize damage and drain widely instead. Each case will be different, and treatment should be tailored to the patient based on the presentation, surgeon experience, and comfort.

In a case of thyroidectomy for a T2 papillary thyroid cancer, Conzo et al. encountered a fistula at the pharyngo-esophageal junction on a Gastrografin swallow. The patient exhibited signs of wound infection without systemic signs; they took their patient back for reexploration and drain placement without esophageal repair.[10] The presence of the drain permitted control of the fistula, which healed 15 days later with proper nutritional support and antibiotics. The size and location of the defect are not mentioned.

In cases where an intraoperative esophageal defect is noted either from iatrogenic injury or due to a concomitant resection given tumor invasion, treatment will differ depending on the depth of the injury. Primary repair can be done where the injury is only muscular without affecting the mucosa or submucosa. Full-thickness injuries require muscular flap repair, gastric pull-up, or jejunal free flap repair for circumferential defects.[8] For cases where primary repair is done, surgeons should be careful not to suture the "backwall" of the esophagus. Peng et al. described a case of esophageal stenosis in a case where an esophageal injury during thyroidectomy was primarily repaired.[28]

Multiple procedures have been described to repair cervical esophageal injuries. Some of the possible options include repair over T-tubes, repair with muscle flaps, resection and reconstruction with gastric pull-up, jejunal free flaps, or colon transposition. Esophageal resection is a major operation. The reader should be conscious that these complex reconstruction techniques are not free of risk and should only be attempted by those with proper experience.

More aggressive interventions to achieve control of the fistula include exclusion and diversion with an esophagostomy. Cervical esophagostomy has been in the armamentarium of the surgeon for a long time but is infrequently used.[38] This intervention with a high mortality (15% to 40%)[29] could appear to be radical after a thyroidectomy; however, complete diversion can be lifesaving in cases with ongoing contamination where other techniques have failed. As we have mentioned before, control of sepsis is crucial, and oral secretions have a high concentration of bacteria[39] that can be exteriorized with complete diversion.

The cervical esophagus is better approached via a left incision anterior and parallel to the sternocleidomastoid. The carotid sheet is retracted laterally, and once the esophagus is identified, a Penrose is placed around it to help retract it to the incision. While encircling the esophagus, care should be taken not to injure the recurrent laryngeal nerve. The esophagus is then dissected for mobilization superiorly and inferiorly. Once it is free, it is transected and ligated distally, and the proximal end is exteriorized and matured.[38,39] One of the major disadvantages of this procedure is the need for further and more complex reconstruction.

CONCLUSION

Esophageal injuries are rare and even more rare after thyroidectomies. Despite its low frequency, the injury carries a high rate of mortality. Early treatment includes broad-spectrum antibiotics and source control. Nonoperative management can be considered for stable patients, whereas those with instability should be emergently explored. Surgeons operating on the thyroid should be aware of this complication, including its management.

References

1. Al-Qurayshi Z, Robins R, Hauch A, Randolph GW, Kandil E. Association of surgeon volume with outcomes and cost savings following thyroidectomy: a national forecast. *JAMA Otolaryngol Neck Surg*. 2016;142(1):32. doi:10.1001/jamaoto.2015.2503.
2. Loyo M, Tufano RP, Gourin CG. National trends in thyroid surgery and the effect of volume on short-term outcomes: volume-based trends in thyroid surgery. *The Laryngoscope*. 2013;123(8):2056–2063. doi:10.1002/lary.23923.
3. Gómez-Ramírez J, Sitges-Serra A, Moreno-Llorente P, et al. Mortality after thyroid surgery, insignificant or still an issue? *Langenbecks Arch Surg*. 2015;400(4):517–522. doi:10.1007/s00423-015-1303-1.
4. Tartaglia N, Iadarola R, Di Lascia A, Cianci P, Fersini A, Ambrosi A. What is the treatment of tracheal lesions associated with traditional thyroidectomy? Case report and systematic review. *World J Emerg Surg*. 2018;13(1):15. doi:10.1186/s13017-018-0175-4.
5. Furlow PW, Mathisen DJ. Surgical anatomy of the trachea. *Ann Cardiothorac Surg*. 2018;7(2):255–260. doi:10.21037/acs.2018.03.01.
6. Gosnell JE, Campbell P, Sidhu S, Sywak M, Reeve TS, Delbridge LW. Inadvertent tracheal perforation during thyroidectomy. *Br J Surg*. 2006;93(1):55–56. doi:10.1002/bjs.5136.
7. Golger A, Rice LL, Jackson BS, Young JEM. Tracheal necrosis after thyroidectomy. *Can J Surg*. 2002; 45(6):463–464.
8. Gillenwater AM, Goepfert H. Surgical management of laryngotracheal and esophageal involvement by locally advanced thyroid cancer. *Semin Surg Oncol*. 1999;16(1):19–29.
9. Santiago-Rosado LM, Lewison CS. Tracheal trauma *StatPearls*. Treasure Island, FL: StatPearls Publishing; 2020. http://www.ncbi.nlm.nih.gov/books/NBK500015/.
10. Conzo G, Stanzione F, Della Pietra C, et al. Tracheal necrosis, oesophageal fistula: unusual complications of thyroidectomy Report of two case and literature review. *Ann Ital Chir*. 2012;83(3):259–264.
11. Davies P. Conservative treatment of delayed tracheal perforation following thyroidectomy. *The Otorhinolaryngologist*. 2013;6(2):119–121.
12. Benson M, Dhillon V, Tufano R. Delayed tracheal perforation after hemithyroidectomy. *Ann Clin Case Rep*. 2017;2:1355.
13. González-Sánchez-Migallón E, Guillén-Paredes P, Flores-Pastor B, Miguel-Perelló J, Aguayo-Albasini JL. Late tracheal perforation after total thyroidectomy: conservative management. *Cir Esp Engl Ed*. 2016;94(1):50–52. doi:10.1016/j.cireng.2015.02.007.
14. Mazeh H, Suwanabol P, Schneider D, Sippel R. Late manifestation of tracheal rupture after thyroidectomy: case report and literature review. *Endocr Pract*. 2012;18(4):e73–e76. doi:10.4158/EP11344.CR.
15. Zhao Z, Zhang T, Yin X, Zhao J, Li X, Zhou Y. Update on the diagnosis and treatment of tracheal and bronchial injury. *J Thorac Dis*. 2017;9(1):E50–E56. doi:10.21037/jtd.2017.01.19.
16. Han X, Mu Q, Liu C, et al. Covered stent implantation in the treatment of tracheal rupture after thyroidectomy. *J Vasc Interv Radiol*. 2016;27(11):1758–1761. doi:10.1016/j.jvir.2016.04.017.

17. Jacqmin S, Lentschener C, Demirev M, Gueroult S, Herman P, Ozier Y. Postoperative necrosis of the anterior part of the cervical trachea following thyroidectomy. *J Anesth*. 2005;19(4):347–348. doi:10.1007/s00540-005-0330-4.
18. Chauhan A, Ganguly M, Saidha N, Gulia P. Tracheal necrosis with surgical emphysema following thyroidectomy. *J Postgrad Med*. 2009;55(3):193–195. doi:10.4103/0022-3859.57401.
19. Heavrin BS, Hampson S, Stack LB. Tracheal perforation after thyroidectomy. *J Emerg Med*. 2012; 43(4):e259–e260. doi:10.1016/j.jemermed.2011.03.031.
20. Bertolaccini L, Lauro C, Priotto R, Terzi A. It sometimes happens: late tracheal rupture after total thyroidectomy. *Interact Cardiovasc Thorac Surg*. 2012;14(4):500–501. doi:10.1093/icvts/ivr126.
21. Rosato L, Ginardi A, Mondini G, Sandri A, Oliaro A, Filosso PL. Efficacy of fleece-bound sealing system (TachoSil®) in delayed anterior tracheal lacerations secondary to ischemic tracheal necrosis after total thyroidectomy. *Minerva Chir*. 2012;67(3):271–275.
22. Escott ABJ, Pochin RSB. Repair of a posterior perforation of the trachea following thyroidectomy with a muscle transposition flap. *Ear Nose Throat J*. 2016;95(2):E14–E17. doi:10.1177/014556131609500205.
23. Philippe G, Pichon N, Lerat J, Amiel JB, Clavel M, Mathonnet M. Successful treatment of anterior tracheal necrosis after total thyroidectomy using vacuum-assisted closure therapy. *Crit Care Res Pract*. 2012;2012:1–4. doi:10.1155/2012/252719.
24. Patti MG, Gantert W, Way LW. Surgery of the esophagus. Anatomy and physiology. *Surg Clin North Am*. 1997;77(5):959–970. doi:10.1016/s0039-6109(05)70600-9.
25. Ozer MT, Demirbas S, Harlak A, Ersoz N, Eryilmaz M, Cetiner S. A rare complication after thyroidectomy: perforation of the oesophagus: a case report. *Acta Chir Belg*. 2009;109(4):527–530. doi:10.1080/00015458.2009.11680477.
26. Akbulut G, Gunay S, Aren A, Bilge O. A rare complication after thyroidectomy: esophageal perforation. *Ulus Travma Derg Turk J Trauma Emerg Surg TJTES*. 2002;8(4):250–252.
27. Rabie ME. Hypopharyngeal fistula complicating difficult thyroidectomy for invasive papillary cancer. *Ann R Coll Surg Engl*. 2014;96(7):e24–e26. doi:10.1308/003588414X13946184902640.
28. Peng H, Wang SJ, Li W. Rare complication after thyroidectomy-cervical esophageal stenosis: a case report and literature review. *World J Surg Oncol*. 2014;12(1):308. doi:10.1186/1477-7819-12-308.
29. Søreide J, Viste A. Esophageal perforation: diagnostic work-up and clinical decision-making in the first 24 hours. *Scand J Trauma Resusc Emerg Med*. 2011;19(1):66. doi:10.1186/1757-7241-19-66.
30. Chirica M, Kelly MD, Siboni S, et al. Esophageal emergencies: WSES guidelines. *World J Emerg Surg*. 2019;14(1):26. doi:10.1186/s13017-019-0245-2.
31. Solomkin JS, Mazuski JE, Bradley JS, et al. Diagnosis and management of complicated intra-abdominal infection in adults and children: guidelines by the Surgical Infection Society and the Infectious Diseases Society of America. *Clin Infect Dis*. 2010;50(2):133–164. doi:10.1086/649554.
32. Elsayed H, Shaker H, Whittle I, Hussein S. The impact of systemic fungal infection in patients with perforated oesophagus. *Ann R Coll Surg Engl*. 2012;94(8):579–584. doi:10.1308/003588412X13373405388095.
33. Schweigert M, Santos Sousa H, Solymosi N, et al. Spotlight on esophageal perforation: a multinational study using the Pittsburgh esophageal perforation severity scoring system. *J Thorac Cardiovasc Surg*. 2016;151(4):1002–1011. doi:10.1016/j.jtcvs.2015.11.055.
34. Goenka MK, Goenka U. Endotherapy of leaks and fistula. *World J Gastrointest Endosc*. 2015;7(7):702. doi:10.4253/wjge.v7.i7.702.
35. Haito-Chavez Y, Law JK, Kratt T, et al. International multicenter experience with an over-the-scope clipping device for endoscopic management of GI defects (with video). *Gastrointest Endosc*. 2014;80(4):610–622. doi:10.1016/j.gie.2014.03.049.
36. Salminen P, Gullichsen R, Laine S. Use of self-expandable metal stents for the treatment of esophageal perforations and anastomotic leaks. *Surg Endosc*. 2009;23(7):1526–1530. doi:10.1007/s00464-009-0432-4.
37. Möschler O, Nies C, Mueller M. Endoscopic vacuum therapy for esophageal perforations and leakages. *Endosc Int Open*. 2015;03(06):E554–E558. doi:10.1055/s-0034-1392568.
38. Rush BF. Cervical esophagostomy—a neglected operation. *Arch Surg*. 1970;101(2):145. doi:10.1001/archsurg.1970.01340260049008.
39. Koniaris LG, Spector SA, Staveley-O'Carroll KF. Complete esophageal diversion: a simplified, easily reversible technique. *J Am Coll Surg*. 2004;199(6):991–993. doi:10.1016/j.jamcollsurg.2004.07.024.

CHAPTER 9

Radioactive Iodine (^{131}I) Thyroid Ablation and the Salivary Glands

Louis Mandel

CHAPTER OUTLINE

Introduction

Thyroid cancer, the most common endocrine malignancy, has a worldwide prevalence that continues to increase. It is estimated that 52,000 new cases were reported in the United States in 2019.[1] The increasing use of ultrasound to detect small, nonpalpable, malignant thyroid nodules will cause this incidence to increase in the future. Thyroid cancer is a malignancy of the relatively young, mostly women in the fifth decade of their life at the time of diagnosis.[2] Over 90% of the thyroid cancers are differentiated thyroid cancers (DTC),[3] usually papillary or follicular carcinomas. Standard management of DTC involves total or subtotal thyroidectomy followed by the oral administration of radioactive iodine (^{131}I). The radioactive iodine will be absorbed and concentrated by benign and malignant thyroid cells because iodine is an inherent part of their normal metabolic activity. Because it is radioactive, the ^{131}I will eradicate postsurgical benign and/or malignant thyroid tissue remnants. The ablation also serves to diminish malignant recurrences, and facilitates postoperative surveillance via an improvement in the ability to monitor alterations in serum thyroglobulin. Furthermore, postoperative scanning with radioactive iodine (RAI) for recurrences will be more accurate if it does not have to compete with ^{131}I uptake by any postsurgical residual normal thyroid or neoplastic tissue. This therapeutic approach, thyroidectomy followed by ^{131}I ablation, has proven to be very effective and has a 10-year survival rate exceeding 80%.[4]

Reassessment of ^{131}I Therapy

Unfortunately, the administration of RAI has been associated with adverse effects because of the tissue damage caused by radioactivity's effect on other iodine-avid tissues, most frequently the salivary glands (SGs). Adverse SG reactions commonly include sialadenitis and less commonly taste aberration. Additionally, secondary SG adverse effects include increased occurrences of a primary SG malignancy and rarely, a transient facial nerve palsy. The concerns regarding these reactions originated when all DTC patients were subjected to ^{131}I therapy, mostly in the 100 mCi range. Such levels of radioactive iodine radiation are sufficient to cause secondary SG tissue damage with both subjective and objective symptomatology.

The relatively numerous adverse effects involving the SGs and other iodine-avid tissues have encouraged the reassessment of the use of RAI as a therapeutic tool. The papers of Schlumberger et al.[5] and Mallick et al.[6] have given impetus to the trend to utilize lower doses of ^{131}I for thyroid ablation. A meaningful decrease in the frequency and severity of complications, particularly the reported incidences of sialadenitis, has resulted. The transition to lower doses of radioactive iodine has been rapid and is supported by three observations. First, the published manuscripts of Schlumberger et al.[5] and Mallick et al.[6] have indicated that successful ^{131}I ablation can be achieved with 30 mCi and can be used to treat the low-risk patient. Objections to the finding of these authors have centered around the inadequate follow-up period (6 to 9 months) for their patients. Second, newly published American Thyroid Association guidelines state that the use of ^{131}I is not justifiable in all DTC patients.[7] Although there is little controversy over its benefits in most patients, the use of ^{131}I has uncertain value in low-risk disease. Irradiation with ^{131}I can be avoided in those DTC patients who have no local tumor invasion, no metastases, and no aggressive histology associated with their existing neoplastic thyroid nodule. Third, the introduction of recombinant thyroid-stimulating hormone (rhTSH), as a substitute for the traditional preablation withdrawal of thyroid hormone and dietary iodine, has allowed the patient to remain euthyroid.[8,9] The period of hypothyroidism, with its reduction in quality of life caused by withdrawal of levothyroxine and dietary iodine, is no longer a concern. Renal clearance of serum ^{131}I occurs more rapidly in the euthyroid state than in a hypothyroid state. These three approaches, regarding radioactive iodine thyroid ablation, have succeeded in decreasing SG injury by decreasing the availability of toxic tissue doses of ^{131}I in the circulating serum. Despite a therapeutic trend to lower the RAI dose to a range of 30 to 50 mCi, treatment approaches using 75 to 100 mCi RAI for ablation are generally used. Ablation is considered successful when a scan reflects the absence of ^{131}I uptake by thyroid tissue and serum thyroglobulin is undetectable after TSH administration. Thyroid ablation has been reported to be more effectively achieved when 100 mCi RAI is administered.[10]

Adverse Effects of ^{131}I

Regardless of the new norms in DTC care, secondary SG adverse effects will still be observed, albeit to a lesser extent and intensity. Adverse drug reactions are unintended responses resulting from the use of normal drug dosages that are being used for the therapy of a disease.11 The negative secondary consequences following the therapeutic use of RAI in thyroid cancer patients readily meet this definition. Prompt recognition of the symptomatology associated with these adverse reactions, most commonly SG injury induced by radioiodine, avoids misdiagnoses and leads to effective treatment.

SIALADENITIS

Within 24 to 48 hours after initial RAI therapy, SG pain and swelling often develop. Usually, the parotid glands are involved, often bilaterally. An inflammatory reaction is initiated by the ^{131}I radiation and leads to a vasculitis with endothelial wall injury and increased vascular permeability.[12,13] The escape of vascular constituents, fluid and cells with their cytokines, results in the patient's clinical SG swelling and pain, which are almost always transient.[14] This immediate problem has been reported to occur in as many as 50% of the recipients of this radioiodine ablation.[15] Unfortunately, no data are available regarding low and high RAI dosages and their relationship to the frequency of this immediate post ^{131}I sialadenitis. This period of temporary SG swelling and pain coincides with the period of increased patient radioactivity that in the past required patient isolation.

Renal and salivary excretory activity rapidly come into play and function to lower the serum ^{131}I levels. Within a short time frame, the vascular endothelial wall reestablishes its normal permeability gradient. Abnormal extravasation terminates and the intraglandular elements of inflammation recede. Pain and swelling subside within a few days, and the patient usually enters a symptom-free period,[16] which may be transient or permanent.

Following this early SG reaction, the first gland symptom that usually prompts a voluntary post-RAI therapy visit is a manifestation of ^{131}I-incited duct injury. It is obstructive in nature, and

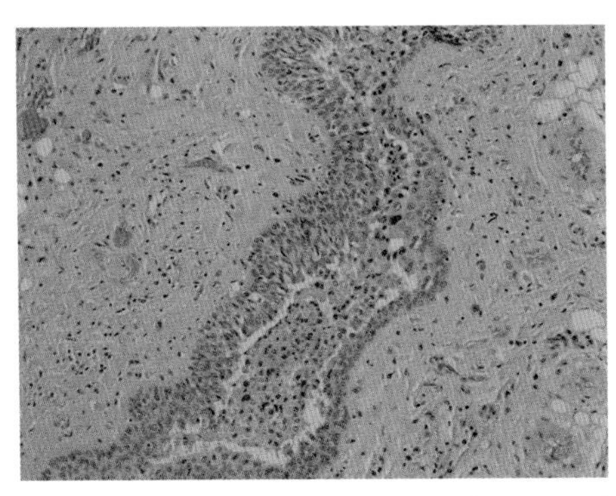

Fig. 9.1 Microscopic view of inflammatory exudate blocking lumen of excretory duct. (Hematoxylin and eosin, magnification ×200.)

tends to occur months after an ablation with 75 mCi or more of radioiodine. The striated ducts of the SGs harbor the transport system for the ^{131}I. The sodium iodide symporter molecule, the transporter of the radioiodine, resides in the basolateral membrane of the striated duct. The SG ducts concentrate iodide by substituting iodide for Cl^- as a substrate in the Na/K/Cl symporter molecule.[17] The concentration of iodine in duct cells will reach a tissue-to-serum concentration gradient of 50:1.[18] Calculations indicate that this extremely high concentration in the ducts is three to four times higher than what occurs in the parenchymal SG-secreting cells.[19] Problems arise because the reproductive capacity for SG cells lies in the stem cells of the ductal system. The high radioactive iodine concentration in the duct damages the DNA of the stem cells that inhabit the ductal system.[20,21] Because the reproductive capacity for SG cells is possessed by these stem cells, delayed and decreased cell production and cell death with scarring are the inevitable consequences. Additionally, the irradiation's effect on the cellular plasma membrane adds to acinar cell death.[20]

All the SGs, particularly the major producers of saliva (two parotid glands [PGs] and two submandibular salivary glands [SMSGs]), are injured by the ^{131}I radioactivity. However, they are asymmetrically involved with any combination of 1 to 4 PGs/SMSGs demonstrating varying degrees of damage. Symptomatology is more often observed in the PGs than in the SMSGs. The relative resistance of the SMSGs as compared to the PGs has been attributed to the fact that the SMSG has a higher proportion of striated ducts than does the PG. These relatively more numerous striated ducts contain the iodide transport molecule that will allow for a higher rate of ^{131}I clearance through the SMSG than that which occurs in the PG.[22] This rapid SMSG transit of the ^{131}I decreases the exposure time available for radiation injury. Additionally, SMSG secretion is uninterrupted even in unstimulated times. The persistent secretion acts to continually and consistently flush out radiation-containing saliva, thus decreasing the gland's exposure to radiation. Simultaneously, the mucus element present in the SMSG secretion, but absent in PG secretions, serves as a protective asset against radiation.

Duct fibrosis with luminal stricturing reflects the end game of radiation-induced duct inflammation. The luminal passage is further narrowed by the development of intraluminal obstructive inflammatory exudates that act as blocking plugs (Fig. 9.1). The duct constriction and inflammatory exudate combine to effectively limit the luminal passageway. Salivary flow is impeded, particularly during periods of increased salivary demand (eating), and SG pain and swelling follow as saliva backs up. In turn, the retained saliva adds to glandular inflammation, with swelling and pain accentuated by the inflammation caused by the physical presence of retained intraglandular saliva. As many as 44% of patients will develop symptoms of obstructive sialadenitis months after having been exposed to RAI ablation.[23] Reported incidences of sialadenitis have varied because the investigations have not had a standardized universal design. Confusion exists because studies have involved different levels of ^{131}I dosages, varied means (objective/subjective) of evaluating the presence of adverse effects, and different follow-up periods.

Although the glandular swellings are exacerbated when saliva is stimulated during meals, they partially subside after eating. The obstruction usually is not complete: a narrowed patent lumen will still be present. Therefore during unstimulated periods (between meals), glandular swelling and discomfort decrease as saliva slowly passes through the narrowed lumen. A diminution in SG swelling and pain is also made possible when the soft intraluminal plug formed by the inflammatory exudate is spontaneously extruded by the effects of increased retrograde hydrostatic salivary pressure. The patient will become aware of a salty taste because the damaged ducts have failed to adequately resorb sodium and chloride ions from the retained exiting saliva. Although some symptom amelioration now occurs, it may not be total. The SG inflammation initiated by the duct obstruction and the retained saliva can persist objectively and/or subjectively for varying periods, with remissions that can vary from weeks to months.

Because obstruction leads to salivary stagnation, an ascending secondary infection from the oral cavity is always a threat. The failure of duct flushing and the favorable media offered by stagnant retained saliva encourage bacterial colonization. The infectious process superimposed upon the already existing obstructed gland will cause a heightening of SG symptomatology that will include a pus-containing cloudy saliva. Continued SG exacerbations of pain and swelling from an infection-scarred and narrowed duct and a decreased salivary lavage can be expected.

Persistent obstructive symptomatology can lead to the development of a long-standing chronic sialadenitis. Diagnosis can readily be accomplished when the patient's history of having received RAI is factored into the patient's clinical complaints. Chronic obstructive sialadenitis has been reported to occur in as many as two-thirds of the patients who received ^{131}I ablation doses of 100 to 150 mCi.[24] The damage to the SGs is in direct proportion to the administered ^{131}I dosage.[18,21,24] In most patients, subjective symptom resolution eventually occurs, with only 5% of patients reporting subjective SG problems when seen 7 years after RAI treatment.[14] Although some ductal strictures from the preexisting duct inflammation are present, the resulting narrowed lumen apparently is wide enough to accommodate the salivary demand and eliminate subjective complaints. Nevertheless, the sensitivity of a scintigraphic examination will usually reflect the presence of objective SG injury in the form of a decreased uptake with or without a secretory delay.

An initially high or repeated ^{131}I dose is required when tumor recurrence or metastases are present. Subjective and objective hyposalivation will then become evident if ^{131}I has been utilized in the range of 300 mCi.[21] Apparently, the high level of radioactive iodine being absorbed by the SG is now sufficient to initiate a significant acinar cell loss. Lipid peroxidation, within the cell membrane from irradiation, precipitates cell death.[20,25] Further acinar cell loss results from DNA radiation damage in the progenitor and stem cells of the SG.[20,21] The decrease in acinar cell numbers results in a decreased salivary production. Gross SG parenchymal destruction with eradication of salivary production can be anticipated when total levels of ^{131}I reach 500 mCi.[24,26] Obstructive symptoms will not be present because parenchymal salivary production has been eliminated. A secondary ascending duct infection may now occur because of the absence of salivary lavage. This infectious inflammatory reaction is superimposed on the previously existing radiation-induced SG inflammation and accentuates it.

Objective authentication of gland function is most accurately determined via scintigraphy. A scintigram has the advantage of simultaneously evaluating in real time the activities of the two PGs and the two SMSGs. The radioisotope technetium 99m pertechnetate (TPT) is administered intravenously, circulates, and is picked up by the SGs. The TPT, a radioisotope of molybdenum, is considered safe because it only has a 6-hour half-life and it does not produce the destructive beta radiation associated with ^{131}I. The TPT emits a nondestructive gamma radiation that can be imaged by a gamma camera. The tracer is effectively concentrated by the SG. The SG is then stimulated with sour candy and its secretion-containing TPT is visualized by a gamma camera and graphed. The graph makes it possible to view the uptake and secretory abilities of individual glands in real time.

Because the damaging effect of ^{131}I on the SGs can best be illustrated via scintigraphy, four case outlines and their scintigraphs are presented to demonstrate the varied effects that different ^{131}I doses have on the SGs. Recombinant thyroid stimulating hormone was used in Cases 9.2 and 9.3.

Case Reports

CASE 9.1

During a routine head and neck examination, a papillary thyroid carcinoma was discovered in a 38-year-old female. Following thyroidectomy, 30 mCi ^{131}I was administered. Although the patient had no SG symptomatology, scintigraphy was performed 5 months after the RAI ablation, to evaluate the effect of the low-dose radioiodine on the SGs. Uptakes in both PGs and both SMSGs were seen to be within normal limits, and the secretion fractions in both PGs and both SMSGs were also normal (Fig. 9.2).

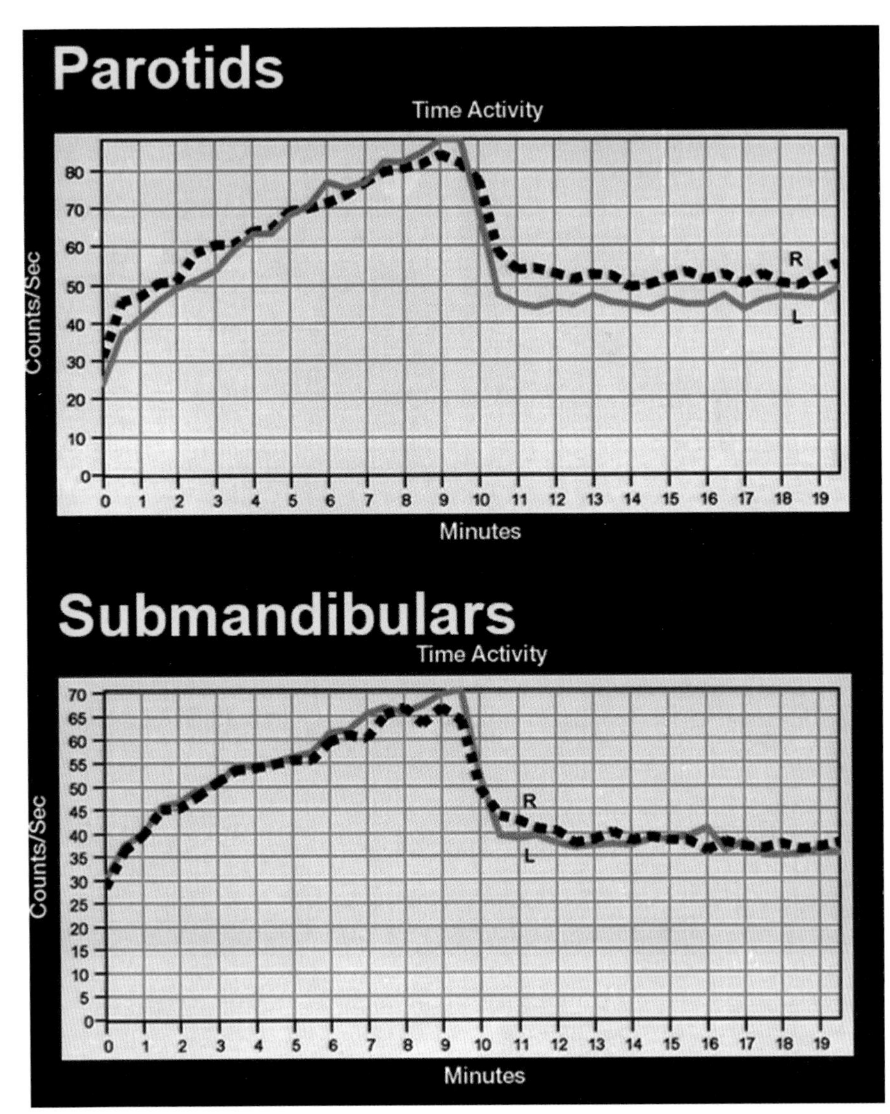

Fig. 9.2 Case 9.1: Scintigraphy performed 5 months after patient received 30 mCi ^{131}I for thyroid ablation. Right *(R)* and left *(L)* parotid and submandibular salivary glands demonstrate normal TPT uptake. After stimulation with lemon candy at the 10-minute mark, secretion from all salivary glands is also seen to be normal.

CASE 9.2

A 32-year-old female was seen because of a persistent painful left PG swelling that worsened with eating (Fig. 9.3A). Eleven months previously, she had been treated with 75 mCi ^{131}I following a thyroidectomy for a papillary carcinoma. She stated that she had one prior episode (2 months beforehand) of left PG swelling that resolved spontaneously after 5 days. Her present PG swelling developed 1 week ago. There have been no problems association with the SMSG. A CT scan confirmed the presence of a left PG inflammation (Fig. 9.3B). Scintigraphy revealed that a left PG duct obstruction was the cause of the PG inflammation (Fig. 9.3C).

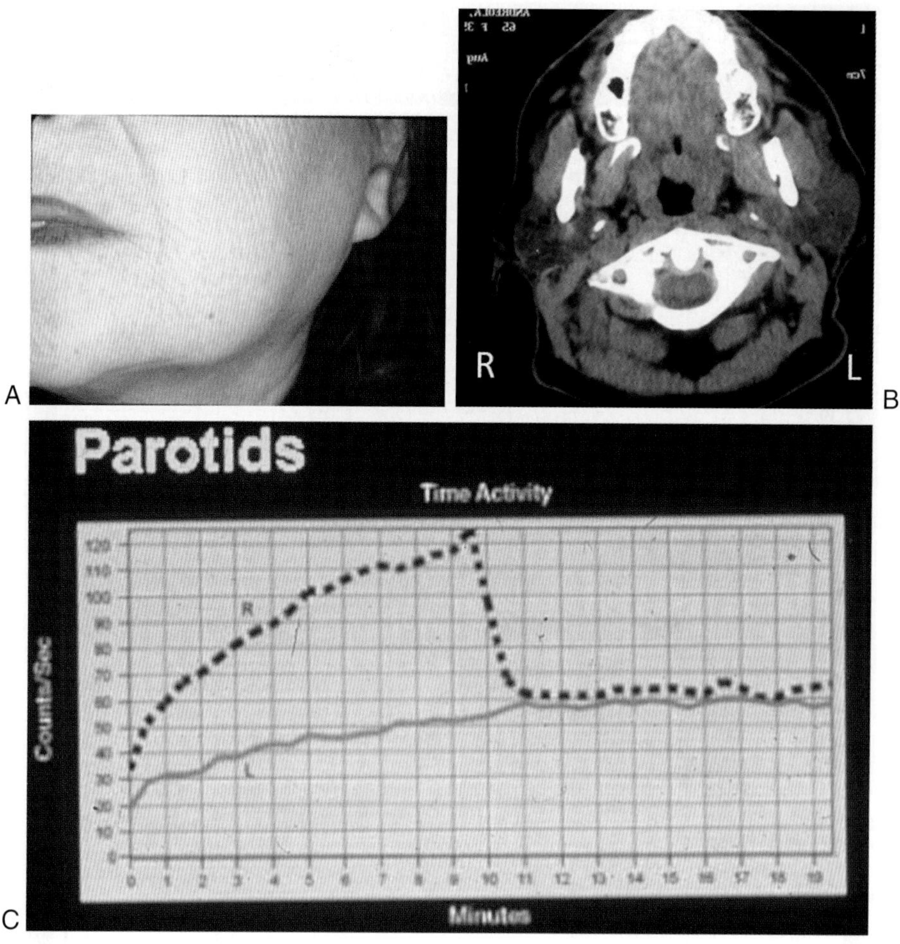

Fig. 9.3 Case 9.2: (A) Patient with left parotid gland swelling 11 months after receiving 75 mCi ^{131}I following thyroidectomy for papillary carcinoma. (B) CT scan demonstrates inflamed left parotid gland. (C) Scintigram: right *(R)* parotid gland demonstrates normal pickup and secretion of TPT. Left *(L)* parotid reveals delayed pickup (from glandular inflammation) and failure to secrete (duct obstruction) TPT at 10-minute mark. *CT,* Computed tomography; *TPT,* technetium 99m pertechnetate.

CASE 9.3

A 42-year-old female was diagnosed as having a papillary thyroid carcinoma. Five weeks post thyroidectomy, 150 mCi radioactive iodine was given for ablation. Seven months later, the patient presented with a 3-month history of sporadic PG swellings, sometimes affecting the right PG and at times the left PG. The swellings usually were initiated by eating and caused moderate discomfort. These episodes would last from one to several days. Periods of remission, lasting from one to several weeks, would intervene, but recurrences would again develop. A scintigram (Fig. 9.4) revealed a mildly delayed uptake of TPT in both PGs with a marked failure of TPT normal secretion at the 10-minute stimulation point, also in both PGs. Duct obstructions had developed from the inflammatory effect of radioactive iodine on the duct epithelium. The scintigram also revealed that the right SMSG function was normal, but no activity was evident in the left SMSG. Nevertheless, the patient had no subjective symptomatology associated with the left SMSG.

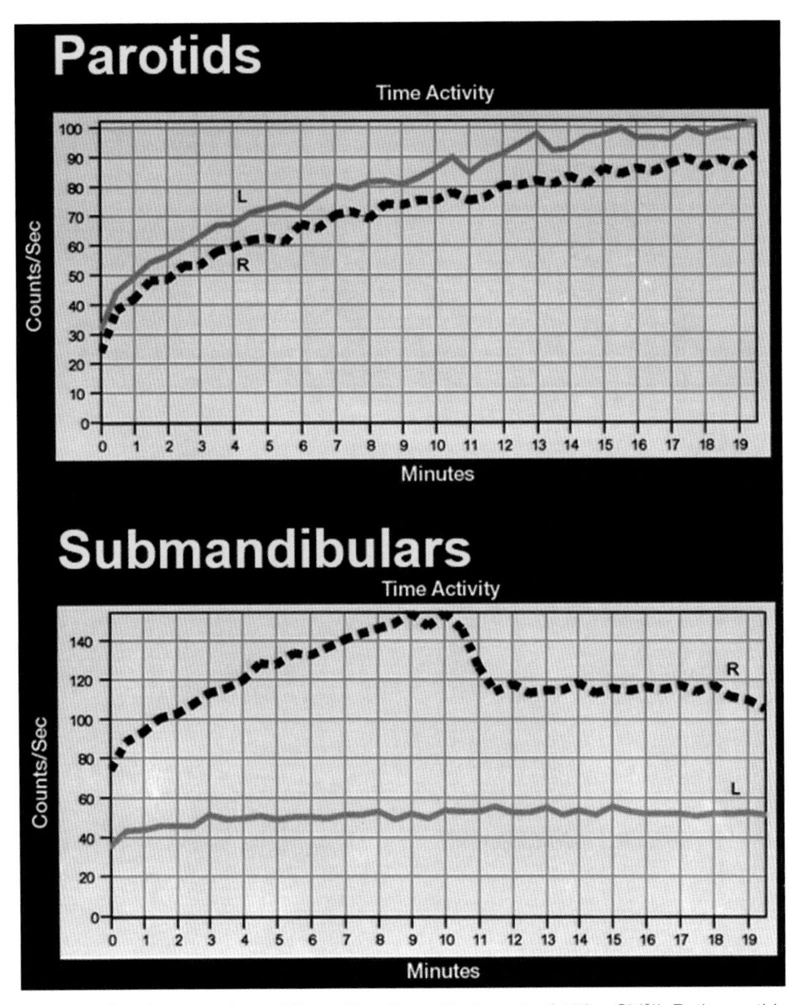

Fig. 9.4 Case 9.3: Scintigram performed 7 months after patient received 150 mCi ^{131}I. Both parotids show a sluggish technetium 99m pertechnetate (TPT) uptake with a failure to secrete TPT. The right *(R)* submandibular gland function is normal, whereas the left *(L)* submandibular gland shows no activity.

CASE 9.4

A 78-year-old female was seen because of a subjective complaint of an extremely dry mouth. She had been treated for a thyroid follicular carcinoma 22 years ago. Initially, 75 mCi ^{131}I was prescribed, but because she developed lung metastasis, two additional doses of ^{131}I (298 mCi and 299 mCi) were given in the following years. The gland irradiation caused by the cumulative ^{131}I (672 mCi) served to effectively destroy SG parenchyma. A scintigraphic study confirmed right and left PG and SMSG inactivity. Uptake and secretion in the four SGs were essentially absent (Fig. 9.5).

A review of these four case outlines and their respective scintigrams serve to highlight the following observations:

1. Damage to the SGs is in direct proportion to the dosage level of ^{131}I.
2. The PGs are more susceptible than the SMSGs to the damaging effect of ^{131}I ionizing radiation.
3. Duct obstruction and SG swelling represent the first signs of ^{131}I-induced gland injury. Parenchymal damage with hyposalivation only develops in relation to high doses of radioiodine.
4. Involvement of the SGs (two PGs and two SMSGs) is asymmetric and can occur in any combination of one to four SGs.

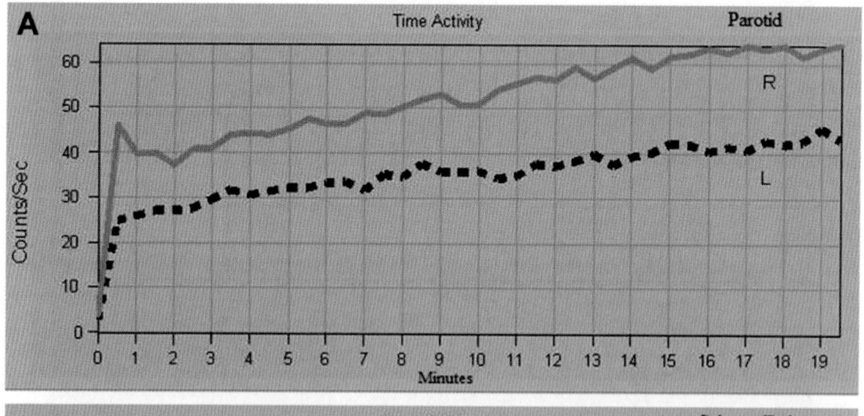

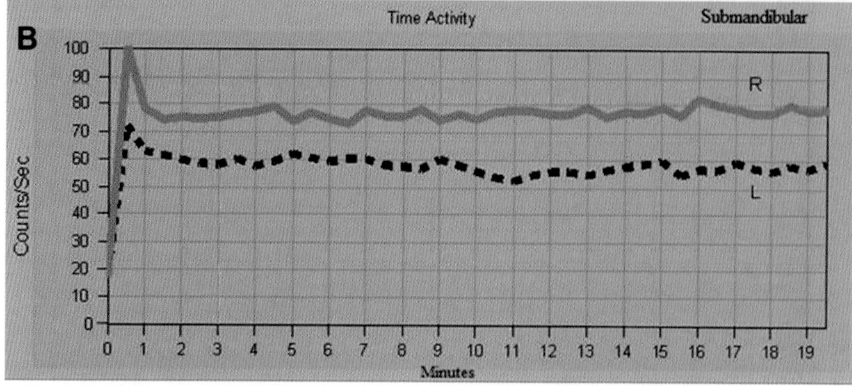

Fig. 9.5 Case 9.4: Because of lung metastasis, patient received a cumulative dose of 672 mCi ^{131}I. Scintigram demonstrates total failure of technetium 99m pertechnetate (TPT) uptake and secretion by both parotid (A) and both submandibular (B) glands.

HYPOSALIVATION

The decreased salivation following ^{131}I ablation may have several origins. Acinar degeneration can occur secondary to the sialadenitis initiated by duct obstruction. A second cause originates from the direct effect irradiation has on the secreting acini. Radioactive iodine dosages in the range of 300 mCi will cause great acinar damage, with almost complete acinar loss occurring when doses of 500 mCi are used. The loss of the secreting cells leads to hyposalivation with subjective and objective oral dryness. Hyposalivation favors SG duct–ascending infections that may further compromise the parenchyma of the SG. Normal salivary protective functions also will be impeded. Dental caries will become prevalent with the loss of the protective properties of saliva. Oral lubrication is diminished, speech may be impaired, and patients can develop stomatodynia. The dry oral mucous membrane is susceptible to candidiasis. The mucosa will be erythematous with adherent debris. Eating can become a problem because saliva is not available for food softening or to ease swallowing.

TASTE

Taste alterations, usually transient, often develop concurrently with the initial ^{131}I ingestion and appear to be dose related. Distorted taste perception has been reported in 16% of the patients who received 150 mCi ^{131}I[27] and 27% of those who received 200 mCi ^{131}I.[28] With higher ^{131}I doses, the loss of taste can become permanent. There is no data available regarding the incidence of dysgeusia in patients exposed to the lower (30 to 100 mCi ^{131}I) dosages that are more frequently utilized.

It is also important to know that RAI-damaged salivary ducts do not adequately resorb sodium and chloride ions from the secreted saliva as it travels through the ducts toward the oral cavity. In such circumstances, a salty taste will be noted by the patient. Taste dysfunction may also be due to a direct radiation effect on oral cavity taste buds. Another explanation for dysgeusia rests with the von Ebner serous glands that are situated in the immediate vicinity of the taste buds present in the circumvallate papilla. These serous cells and their ducts are prone to injury by the radioactivity of ^{131}I. Their secretions can be decreased and an inability to transport chemical food tastants to the taste buds can result.

SECONDARY PRIMARY SALIVARY GLAND MALIGNANCY

An excess of 53 solid malignant tumors in 10,000 patients, who received 150 mCi ^{131}I and were followed for 10 years, has been reported.[29] An increased risk of 30%[30,31] over the general population of any secondary primary cancer, including SG cancer, has also been reported[29,32] to occur following ^{131}I ablation. Pediatric patients have an increased risk of developing a SG cancer of 1 in 588 ^{131}I treated patients.[33] The ability of the SG ducts to concentrate ^{131}I makes them vulnerable to increased incidences of SG malignancy, often a mucoepidermoid carcinoma, secondary to the carcinogenic effect of the absorbed irradiation.[32] The trend toward low-dose radioiodine and the use of rhTSH have combined to lower radiation exposure and reduce the risk of the onset of any secondary primary malignancy. There is a direct relationship between increasing doses of ^{131}I and salivary gland cancers.[29,33] Although the onset of the SG malignancy has been attributed primarily to the radiation injury initiated by the ^{131}I, other factors may be involved. Environmental and genetic factors that act to encourage thyroid malignancy can also play a role in the onset of SG malignancies.[34]

FACIAL NERVE

Anatomically, the facial nerve courses through the PG on its way to innervate the facial musculature. Facial nerve palsy is a rare complication of ^{131}I ablation. A review of the literature found only one report of two cases of facial nerve impairment.[35] The problem is probably related to the PG inflammation that occurs in relation to ^{131}I radioactivity. The glandular inflammation may secondarily involve the facial nerve and temporarily impede transmission of nerve impulses. The palsy tends to recede in tandem with the recession of the SG inflammatory process.[35]

Treatment

Treatment begins with prevention. Rather than accept the salivary gland damage produced by ^{131}I, an early use of sour lemon candy has been recommended to increase salivation. An increased salivary flow will lessen the transit time of ^{131}I through the SGs and theoretically decrease glandular exposure to the radiation produced by ^{131}I. Transit time through the SGs can also be decreased with cholinergic drugs such as pilocarpine or cevimeline, using an empiric 5-day dosage regimen (2 days before, the day of, and 2 days after treatment with ^{131}I). However, the counterargument is that the sour candy or medication stimulation will bring an increased blood flow with increased amounts of ^{131}I into the SG. Nakada et al.[36] suggested that a 24-hour delay in the use of the lemon candy would allow for renal clearance to lower serologic ^{131}I and would serve to lower SG exposure to ^{131}I. However, confirmation of their results has not been realized. Recombinant TSH is administered prior to ablation because it is generally accepted that it allows for the more rapid renal clearance of ^{131}I that will decrease SG radiation exposure.[23] If medically possible, the temporary suspension of the use of any anticholinergic medications is also helpful.

Massaging the PG, the gland most susceptible to injurious effect of the radioactive iodine, is reported to reduce the immediate post-^{131}I incidence of SG dysfunction[15] (Fig. 9.6). The procedure, when properly performed, hastens the evacuation of ^{131}I-containing saliva without increasing the blood flow to the PG. Vitamin E has been reported to have a radioprotective effect on SGs via its ability to scavenge the tissue-damaging free radicals released by radiation.[28] Amifostine also has been advocated as a free radical scavenger, but its value for SG protection has not been replicated.[30]

Following the onset of obstructive symptomatology, sialendoscopy has proven to be beneficial in alleviating SG pain and swelling[37] through its ability to open a luminal pathway. The instrument physically relieves duct obstruction caused by duct constrictions and has a lavaging ability that can flush out luminal debris. Patients who develop PG obstructive symptomatology following ^{131}I

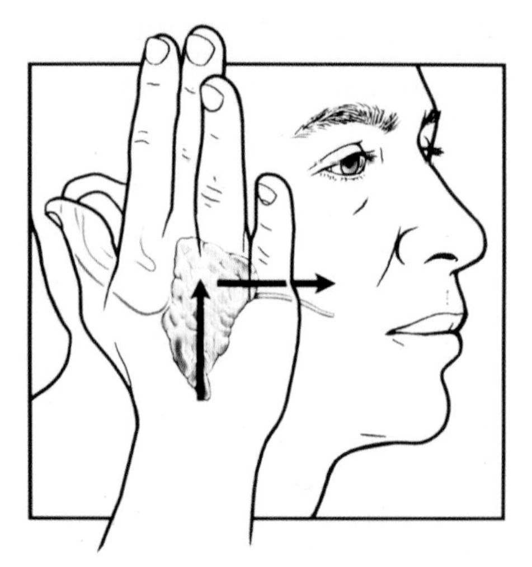

Fig. 9.6 Method for parotid gland massage.

administration can also be treated via aggressive massage to maintain salivary flow. The patient should also encourage salivary lavage with sialagogic agents to prevent salivary stagnation and formation of luminal debris. The avoidance of any form of dehydration and the maintenance of an acceptable daily fluid intake should be emphasized. Caution must be practiced when using prescribed anticholinergic agents.

Patients who have received the higher dosages of ^{131}I often present themselves with varying degrees of dry mouth. If residual glandular parenchyma is present, some saliva will be produced and cholinergic agents can then serve to increase salivation and ameliorate the symptoms of dry mouth. Because radioactive iodine dosages of 300 mCi or more have a very severe destructive effect on SG parenchyma, salivary production can drop to minuscule levels. In such situations, cholinergic agents will prove to be of no value because secreting parenchyma is absent. Treatment must be palliative in these cases. The use of artificial salivas has met with limited success. Commercial products are available to moisten and lubricate the oral cavity. Fluoride therapy in the form of mouth washes, toothpaste, and topical applications should be instituted as a prophylactic measure to combat the anticipated increase in dental caries.

References

1. Siegel AL, Miller KD, Jemal A. Cancer statistics, 2019. *CA Cancer J Clin.* 2019;69:7–34.
2. Hayat MJ, Howlader N, Reichman ME, Edwards BK. Cancer statistics, trends, and multiple primary cancer analyses from the Surveillance, Epidemiology, and End Results (SEER) Program. *Oncologist.* 2007;12:20–37.
3. Sunavala-Dossabhoy G. Radioactive iodine: an unappreciated threat to salivary gland function. *Oral Dis.* 2018;24:198–201.
4. Links TP, van Tol KM, Jager PL, et al. Life expectancy in differentiated thyroid cancer: a novel approach to survival analysis. *Endo Rel Canc.* 2005;12:273–280.
5. Schlumberger M, Catargi B, Borget I, et al. Strategies of radioiodine ablation in patients with low-risk thyroid cancer. *N Engl J Med.* 2012;366:1663–1673.
6. Mallick V, Harmer C, Yap B, et al. Ablation with low-dose radioiodine and thyrotropin alfa in thyroid cancer. *N Engl J Med.* 2012;366:1674–1685.
7. Haugen BR, Alexander KC, Bible GM, et al. 2015 American Thyroid Association on management guidelines for adult patients with thyroid nodules and differentiated thyroid cancer: The American Thyroid Association Guidelines Task Force on thyroid nodules and differentiated thyroid cancer. *Thyroid.* 2016;26:1–133.
8. Menzel C, Kranert WT, Dobert N, et al. rhTSH stimulation before radioiodine therapy in thyroid cancer reduces the effective half-life of ^{131}I. *J Nucl Med.* 2003;44:1065–1068.
9. Hanscheid H, Lassmann M, Luster M, et al. Iodine biokinetics and dosimetry in radioiodine therapy of thyroid cancer: procedures and results of a prospective international controlled study of ablation after rhTSH or hormone withdrawal. *J Nucl Med.* 2006;47:648–654.
10. Doi SAR, Woodhouse NJ, Thalib L, Onitilio A. Ablation of thyroid remnant and I-131 dose in differentiated thyroid cancer: a meta-analysis revisited. *Clin Med Res.* 2007;5:87–90.
11. Hedinger CC, William ED, Sobin LH. *WHO Histologic Typing of Thyroid Tumors.* 2nd ed. Berlin/Heidelberg/New York: Spinger Verlag; 1988.
12. Iakovou I, Goulis DG, Tsinaslanidou Z, Giannoula E, Katsikaki G, Konstantinidis I. Effect of recombinant human thyroid-stimulating hormone on levothyroxine withdrawal on salivary gland dysfunction after radioactive iodine administration for thyroid remnant ablation. *Head Neck.* 2016;38:E227–E230.
13. Canzi P, Cacciola S, Cappaccio P, et al. Interventional sialendoscopy for radio-iodine-induced sialadenitis; quo vadis? *Acta Otorhinolaryngol Ital.* 2017;37:155–159.
14. Grewal RK, Larson SM, Pentlow CE, et al. Salivary gland side effects commonly develop several weeks after initial radioactive iodine ablation. *J Nucl Med.* 2009;50:1605–1610.
15. Son SH, Lee C-H, Jung J-H, et al. The preventive effect of parotid gland massage on salivary gland dysfunction during high-dose radioactive iodine therapy for differentiated thyroid cancer. *Clin Nucl Med.* 2019;44:625–633.
16. Mandel SJ, Mandel L. Radioactive iodine and the salivary glands. *Thyroid.* 2003;13:265–271.

17. Almeida JP, Sanabria AE, Lima ENP, Konalski LP. Late side effects of radioactive iodine on salivary gland function in patients with thyroid cancer. *Head Neck.* 2011;33:686–690.
18. Caglar M, Tuncel M, Alpar R. Scintigraphic evaluation of salivary gland dysfunction in patients with thyroid cancer after radioiodine treatment. *Clin Nucl Med.* 2002;27:767–771.
19. Zanzonico P. Radiation dose to patients and relatives incident to ^{131}I therapy. *Thyroid.* 1997;7:199–204.
20. Konings AWT, Coppes RP, Vissink A. On the mechanism of salivary gland radiosensitivity. *Int J Radiat Oncol Biol Phys.* 2005;62:1194–2005.
21. Raza H, Khan AU, Hameed A, Khan A. Quantitative evaluation of salivary gland dysfunction after radioiodine therapy using salivary gland scintigraphy. *Nucl Med Com.* 2006;27:495–499.
22. La Perle KMD, Kim DC, Hall NC, et al. Modulation of sodium/iodide symporter expression in the salivary glands. *Thyroid.* 2013;23:1029–1036.
23. An Y-S, Yoon J-K, Lee SJ, et al. Symptomatic late-onset sialadenitis after radioiodine therapy in thyroid cancer. *Ann Nucl Med.* 2013;27:386–391.
24. Jeong SY, Kim HW, Lee S-W, Ann B-C, Lee J. Salivary gland function 5 years after radioactive iodine ablation in patients with differentiated thyroid cancer: direct comparison of pre-and postablation scintigraphies and their relation to xerostomia symptoms. *Thyroid.* 2013;23:609–616.
25. Nagler RM. The enigmatic mechanism of irradiation-induced damage to the major salivary glands. *Oral Dis.* 2002;8:141–146.
26. Spiegel W, Reiners C, Borner W. Sialadenitis following iodine ^{131}I therapy for thyroid carcinoma (letter). *J Nucl Med.* 1985;26:816.
27. Brown AP, Greening WP, McCready VR, Shaw HJ, Harmer CL. Radioiodine treatment of metastatic thyroid carcinoma: The Royal Marsden Hospital experience. *Br J Radiol.* 1984;57:323–327.
28. Alexander C, Bader JB, Schaefer A, Finke C, Kirsh CM. Intermediate and long-term side effects of high-dose radioiodine therapy for thyroid carcinoma. *J Nucl Med.* 1998;39:1551–1554.
29. Rubino C, de Vathaire F, Dottorini ME, et al. Secondary primary malignancies in thyroid cancer patients. *Br J Canc.* 2003;89:1638–1644.
30. Maenpaa HO, Heikkonen J, Vaalavirta L, Tenhunen M, Joensuu H. Low vs. high radioiodine activity to ablate the thyroid after thyroidectomy for cancer: a randomized study. *PLoS ONE.* 2008;3:e1885–e1892.
31. Iyer NG, Morris LGT, Tuttle RM, Shah AR, Ganly I. Rising incidence of second cancers in patients with low-risk (TiNo) thyroid cancer who receive radioactive iodine therapy. *Cancer.* 2011;117:4439–4446.
32. Saluja K, Butler RT, Pytynia KB, et al. Mucoepidermoid carcinoma post-radioactive iodine treatment of papillary thyroid carcinoma: unique presentation and putative etiologic association. *Human Pathol.* 2017;68:189–192.
33. Marti JL, Jain KS, Morris LGT. Increased risk of second primary malignancy in pediatric and young adult patients treated with radioactive iodine for differentiated thyroid cancer. *Thyroid.* 2015;25:681–687.
34. Brown AP, Chen J, Hitchcock YJ, Szabo A, Shrieve DC, Tward JD. The risk of second primary malignancies up to three decades after treatment of differentiated thyroid cancer. *J Clin Endocrinol Metab.* 2008;93:504–515.
35. Levenson D, Gulec S, Sonenberg M, Lai E, Goldsmith SJ, Larson SM. Peripheral facial nerve palsy after high-dose radioiodine therapy in patients with papillary thyroid carcinoma. *Ann Int Med.* 1994;120:576–578.
36. Nakada K, Ishibashi T, Takei T, et al. Does lemon candy decrease salivary gland damage after radioiodine therapy for thyroid cancer? *J Nucl Med.* 2005;46:261–266.
37. Bhayani MK, Acharya V, Kongkiatkamon S, et al. Sialendoscopy for patients with radioiodine-induced sialadenitis and xerostomia. *Thyroid.* 2015;25:834–838.

PART 3

Parathyroid

CHAPTER 10

Hypercalcemic Crisis

Tariq Chukir ■ Azeez Farooki ■ John P. Bilezikian

CHAPTER OUTLINE

Introduction

Calcium, the most abundant mineral in the human body, has an essential role in many cellular processes such as enzymatic reactions and neuromuscular functions. It is also one of the building blocks of bone. Most of the body's calcium, in fact, is in the skeleton, but the 0.3% that is found in the circulation is a critically important regulator of the function of other organs such as the nervous system and the heart. Calcium in the circulation is partitioned into three compartments: 40% is bound to proteins, mainly albumin; about 10% is complexed to ions such as citrate; and 50% is free or ionized, which reflects the physiologically active moiety. The total serum calcium concentration accurately reflects the ionized fraction unless there is an abnormality in the serum albumin or in pH. When the serum albumin is reduced, a correction is made by increasing the measured calcium value by 0.8 mg/dL for every 1 g/dL reduction in the serum albumin. Symptoms of hypercalcemia reflect, in part, the corrected serum calcium concentration. Hypercalcemia is defined by serum calcium levels above the normal range (e.g., 8.4 to 10.2 mg/dL). Most clinicians classify hypercalcemia into three grades: mild (less than 12 mg/dL), moderate (12 to 14 mg/dL), or severe greater than 14 mg/dL). The estimated prevalence of hypercalcemia in the general population is 1% to 3%.[1,2]

Etiology/Pathophysiology

Parathyroid hormone (PTH) and vitamin D play important roles in calcium homeostasis. Secretion of PTH is regulated by the ionized calcium concentration. An increase in the ionized calcium concentration will abruptly reduce the synthesis and secretion of PTH. The vast majority of patients who present with hypercalcemia, about 90%, will have primary hyperparathyroidism (PHPT) or hypercalcemia of malignancy (HOM). In these two situations, the parathyroid system either recognizes (HOM) or does not recognize (PHPT) that the serum calcium is elevated, and PTH is either responsible for the hypercalcemia (PHPT) or is not responsible for the hypercalcemia (HOM). We refer to these two entities as PTH-dependent (PHPT) or PTH-independent (HOM) hypercalcemia. The remaining 10% of hypercalcemic individuals comprise a long list of other etiologies. As is the case for the two most common causes of hypercalcemia, the remaining etiologies are either dependent or independent of PTH.

PTH-DEPENDENT HYPERCALCEMIA

Besides PHPT, hypercalcemia due to excessive PTH secretion can be seen in the following conditions: chronic use of thiazide diuretics or lithium, end-stage renal disease (tertiary hyperparathyroidism), parathyroid cancer, or, very rarely, a tumor that secretes authentic PTH.

PHPT accounts for more than 90% of the cases of hypercalcemia in ambulatory settings. In the United States, PHPT has an estimated prevalence of 23 cases per 10,000 in women and 8.5 per 10,000 in men. PTH excess can arise from a benign, neoplastic change of one or more of the four parathyroid glands. Single parathyroid adenomas are the most common etiology of PHPT, accounting for approximately 80% of cases. Other causes include multiple adenomas (~10%), hyperplasia of all four glands (less than 10%), and parathyroid carcinoma (less than 1%). Four-gland parathyroid disease is due to parathyroid cell hyperplasia. It can be sporadic or part of inherited syndromes, such as multiple endocrine neoplasia type 1 (MEN1), MEN2A, familial isolated hyperparathyroidism, and hereditary-jaw tumor syndrome.[3,4]

Tertiary hyperparathyroidism is characterized by elevated serum calcium and PTH in patients with end-stage, chronic kidney disease. Decreased phosphorus excretion, failure of the kidneys to synthesize 1,25-dihydroxyvitamin D, and hypocalcaemia in patients with kidney disease are together responsible for secondary hyperparathyroidism. At this stage, particularly when the creatinine clearance falls below 40 mL/minute, the PTH level will be elevated but the serum calcium will be normal. The chronic and progressive effects of these biochemical imbalances may lead to a semi-autonomous condition, akin to PHPT, with hyperplasia of all four parathyroid glands and eventual emergence of frank hypercalcemia. When the serum calcium rises in this setting, the terminology changes from secondary (high PTH but no hypercalcemia) to tertiary hyperparathyroidism (high PTH and hypercalcemia).[5] The estimated prevalence of secondary or tertiary hyperparathyroidism in patients with a glomerular filtration rate below 20 mL/minute per 1.73 m^2 is 80%.[6] Tertiary hyperparathyroidism is reported in up to 30% of patients who are candidates for and have received kidney transplants.[7]

Familial hypocalciuric hypercalcemia (FHH) is a clinical syndrome characterized by exceedingly low urinary calcium excretion in the setting of elevated serum calcium with inappropriately normal or elevated PTH. The genetic etiology in FHH, a mutation in the calcium-sensing receptor (CaSR) with reduced sensitivity to extracellular calcium, leads to a higher "set point" for calcium. Poor sensing by the mutant CaSRs in the kidney leads to excessive renal conservation and markedly reduced urinary calcium excretion. Three variants with generally similar phenotypes are known as FHH1, FHH2, and FHH3. FHH1 follows an autosomal dominant pattern of inheritance with complete penetrance, typically by the age of 30. Over 200 inactivating mutations in the CaSR have been described in FHH1. FHH2 is due to inactivating mutations in the GNA11 gene encoding the G-protein subunit α11. FHH3 is due to inactivating mutations in the AP2S1 gene encoding the adaptor-related protein complex 2, sigma 1 subunit (AP2σ).[8] It is unusual for patients with FHH to develop end organ damage. The differentiation between PHPT and FHH usually rests with the familial inheritance pattern, the surfacing of the disease in young adulthood or before, and a urinary clearance ratio of Ca/Cr that is below 0.01. A cautionary note here is that many patients with PHPT, particularly those with low intake of calcium, can have urinary Ca to creatinine clearance ratios below 0.01. The diagnosis is unequivocally established by genetic analysis. It is important to recognize this genetic disease because patients with FHH should not undergo parathyroid surgery. It is not curative.

Lithium-induced hypercalcemia is characterized by elevated serum calcium levels with inappropriately normal or elevated PTH in patients. The mechanism remains elusive, but it has been suggested that lithium may alter the set point of CaSR.[9] Thiazide-related hypercalcemia can also mimic PHPT. In both situations, stopping the drug, if possible, may lead to normalization of these biochemical indices. More often, however, the hypercalcemia and elevated PTH levels remain after stopping therapy for 3 to 6 months. The diagnosis of PHPT is then established. Some experts believe now that lithium and thiazides unmask latent PHPT that was not evident clinically prior to the administration of the drug. The majority of patients who are discovered to have hypercalcemia in the setting of lithium or thiazide use will be shown to have PHPT.

PTH-INDEPENDENT HYPERCALCEMIA

Suppressed PTH levels in the setting of hypercalcemia are consistent with non–PTH-mediated hypercalcemia as seen in patients with HOM, granulomatous diseases, milk alkali syndrome, hypervitaminosis D, and immobility.

HOM is a common complication of advanced cancer, with an estimated incidence of 20% to 30%.[10] PTH-independent HOM is mediated through various mechanisms, including the development of focal osteolytic lesions; the secretion of parathyroid hormone-related peptide (PTHrP), also known as humoral HOM; or overproduction of 1,25-dihydroxyvitamin D (calcitriol). PTHrP-mediated HOM is usually associated with limited survival.[11]

Overproduction of calcitriol is a well-recognized complication of lymphomas and granulomatous diseases and is thought to be driven by increased activity of 1-alpha-hydroxylase in macrophages.[12,13] Hypercalcemia in the setting of elevated calcitriol levels in patients with solid tumors has been described recently and was shown to be associated with failure to normalize serum calcium after antiresorptive therapy.[14] Hypercalcemia, independent of PTH, can also be due to vitamin D toxicity as was reported in patients who took excessive amounts of an over-the-counter product, Soladek.[15]

Presentation, Evaluation, and Diagnosis

The clinical presentation of hypercalcemia varies according to the degree of hypercalcemia and ranges from patients who are virtually asymptomatic to those who have severe symptoms. Often, the rapidity of onset of hypercalcemia rather than the absolute value of serum calcium determines the severity of symptoms related to hypercalcemia. The most likely etiology for asymptomatic, chronic hypercalcemia in the ambulatory setting is PHPT. The clinical manifestations of symptomatic hypercalcemia include polyuria, polydipsia, dehydration, neuropsychiatric disturbances, changes in sensorium, shortening of the QT interval, gastrointestinal symptoms, osteoporosis, kidney stones, and/or renal insufficiency.[3] Although PHPT normally causes chronic mild (less than 12 mg/dL) hypercalcemia, some patients may be affected with severe symptoms. At times, these patients, against a backdrop of mild hypercalcemia, can become markedly hypercalemic. "Parathyroid crisis" is the term applied to these individuals. It is important to note that patients with PHPT can present with life-threatening hypercalcemia. This point is often not recalled in the setting of acute, symptomatic hypercalcemia in view of the fact that most patients with PHPT have only mildly elevated serum calcium levels. However, in a patient with an antecedent history of mild hypercalcemia, the emergence of acute, symptomatic hypercalcemia is most likely to be due to PHPT.

The first step after confirming the presence of hypercalcemia is to measure serum PTH levels. If serum PTH is elevated or inappropriately normal, it suggests PTH-mediated hypercalcemia. In patients without advanced kidney disease, and not taking thiazides or lithium, the differential diagnosis is rapidly narrowed to PHPT, FHH, or, rarely, a tumor producing authentic PTH. The latter possibility is so rare that it is practically not a consideration. A 24-hour urine measurement of the clearance ratio between calcium and creatinine usually settles any uncertainty between PHPT and FHH. This differential becomes important in younger individuals, particularly if there is a family history. Two points are worth repeating in this regard. FHH is a rare disease and there is almost 100% penetrance before the age of 30. In the typical postmenopausal woman who presents with mild hypercalcemia and an elevated PTH, it is all but certain that the correct diagnosis is PHPT. Measurements of vitamin D metabolites in PHPT will typically show levels of 25-hydroxyvitamin D that are in the low normal range. The 1,25-dihydroxyvitamin level will be in the high normal range or frankly elevated. It is usually not necessary to measure 1,25-dihydroxyvitamin D in the evaluation of PHPT.[3] The serum phosphorus is typically in the low normal range, and in contrast to an earlier time, it is not often frankly low.[3,16] The evaluation in PHPT proceeds with bone mineral density, 24-hour urinary calcium and stone risk profile, and renal imaging to rule out nephrocalcinosis or nephrolithiasis. Guidelines for parathyroidectomy include any one of the following: serum calcium greater than 12.0 mg/dL; bone density T-score at lumbar spine, hip, or distal 1/3 radius less than or equal to 2.5; renal involvement (stones, renal calcifications, creatinine clearance less than 60 cc/minute); or age younger than 50.[17] In patients who meet any one of these criteria and are planning to undergo parathyroidectomy, parathyroid localization studies are needed to identify abnormal parathyroid tissue. Localizing radiographic studies include sestamibi scintigraphy, sestamibi scintigraphy combined with single photoemission tomography (SPECT), SPECT combined with computed tomography (SPECT-CT fusion), and four-dimensional computed tomography (4D-CT).[18–20]

HOM is the most common cause of PTH-independent hypercalcemia. Although HOM occurs in patients with cancer, it is uncommon to find patients with symptomatic hypercalcemia in whom the cancer is not known. After confirming PTH-independent hypercalcemia (i.e., the PTH level is undetectable), the next step is to determine the etiology of HOM by measuring PTHrP and 1,25-dihyroxyvitamin D in addition to a radiographic evaluation for osteolytic bone lesions.[10]

Milk alkali syndrome is another cause of PTH-independent hypercalcemia that is due to ingestion of large amounts of calcium carbonate. Obtaining a thorough medical history of medications and supplements (including antacids) should be obtained during the evaluation of hypercalcemia.

PATHOPHYSIOLOGY OF SYMPTOMATIC HYPERCALCEMIA

The sequence of pathophysiologic events that lead to symptomatic hypercalcemia is common to virtually all causes of hypercalcemia. The central mechanism is the activated osteoclast, the bone-resorbing cell. It is activated in PHPT, in HOM, and even in vitamin D toxicity. The activated osteoclast excessively resorbs bone and releases calcium into the circulation. In patients with normal renal function who are not dehydrated, the calcium challenge will initially be met by increasing urinary calcium excretion. The hypercalcemia also impairs the kidneys' water-conserving mechanisms, leading to polyuria. In turn, polydipsia follows. As the serum calcium rises further, the polydipsia cannot keep up with the polyuria, and anorexia develops. Dehydration follows and is worsened by vomiting, at times. Rapidly worsening hypercalcemia follows as the kidneys can no longer keep up with the need to excrete the additional calcium presented to them. Central nervous system features become prominent with lethargy and other indices of altered mental status.

MANAGEMENT

The degree of hypercalcemia along with associated symptoms determines the urgency of therapy. Symptoms are determined both by the level of the corrected serum calcium per se as well as its rate of rise. For the same hypercalcemic value, if the serum calcium has risen slowly, symptoms tend to be less severe.

Patients with mild hypercalcemia, such as in the typical patient with PHPT, tend to be asymptomatic. If symptoms are present, they tend to be nonspecific and do not require immediate treatment. In contrast, most patients with moderate to severe hypercalcemia present urgently and require immediate attention. The first step in the management of symptomatic hypercalcemia is to address the dehydration that inevitably accompanies symptomatic hypercalcemia. Intravenous fluid with isotonic saline is the fluid of choice because it helps to facilitate urinary calcium excretion. Within the first few hours 500 mL can be administered, followed by a more moderate rate of 150 to 200 mL/hour. Once hypovolemia is corrected, administration of furosemide can be considered in certain situations to further increase urinary calcium excretion.[21] Furosemide is often not necessary in someone whose renal and cardiac functions are normal, but if there are concerns about the ability of the patient to handle the fluid load, the loop diuretic can be helpful. Another useful initial step is subcutaneous or intramuscular calcitonin, given as 200 units every 8 to 12 hours. Calcitonin reduces bone resorption, the central pathophysiologic feature of most severe hypercalcemic states. Although calcitonin works rapidly, within 12 hours, it is not very potent and will reduce the serum calcium by no more than 1 to 2 mg/dL. In addition, the effects of calcitonin are short-lived. Patients with severe hypercalcemia typically require more potent and long-lasting agents.[21]

As the major "culprit" inciting the severe hypercalcemic state is the osteoclast, the most specific management approach is to use an inhibitor of osteoclast-mediated bone resorption. The bisphosphonates are the classic drugs used in this setting. Because intravenous or parenteral therapy is required, the two choices are pamidronate (30, 60, or 90 mg) or zoledronic acid (4 mg). Both agents are effective and generally follow the same time course, with the serum calcium falling 24 to 48 hours after administration. In the study of Major et al., zoledronic acid had a greater effect both in terms of the reduction of the serum calcium and the duration of the effect.[22] Both agents do carry a warning about their use in patients with renal insufficiency. However, in the setting of acute hypercalcemia, and without preexisting renal disease, the renal dysfunction is usually "pre-renal" due to dehydration. It is not, therefore, an absolute contraindication to the use of bisphosphonates. However, renal function should be taken into consideration in the decision to use a bisphosphonate.[23]

Another mechanism by which hypercalcemia is induced is by RANK ligand, a powerful bone-resorbing cytokine. It is often stimulated in the context of acute hypercalcemia. The RANK ligand inhibitor, denosumab, is, therefore, another option.[24,25] An advantage of denosumab (60 or 120 mg given subcutaneously; 120 mg is the approved dose for HOM) over the bisphosphonates is that renal dysfunction is not a contraindication. Denosumab, like the bisphosphonates, requires 24 to 48 hours for an effect to be appreciated.

Because both the bisphosphonates and denosumab are not immediately acting, a standard of many practitioners faced with this situation is to use combination therapy with calcitonin *and* either a bisphosphonate or denosumab. In this way one takes advantage of the rapid but weak effects of calcitonin while waiting for the more delayed but more powerful anticalcemic effects of pamidronate, zoledronic acid, or denosumab to manifest themselves.

If hypercalcemia is associated with elevated 1,25 dihydroxyvitamin D, such as occurs in some lymphomatous malignancies or granulomatous diseases, corticosteroids or other inhibitors of 1-alpha-hydroxylase (e.g., ketoconazole) can be considered. Multiple myeloma and some breast cancers may be responsive to glucocorticoids. In extreme situations, hemodialysis can be used in patients with life-threatening hypercalcemia, refractory to the approaches listed above.[26]

Summary

Hypercalcemia is a common medical problem, occurring in 1% to 3% of the population. It can be classified into mild (less than 12 mg/dL), moderate (12 to 14 mg/dL), or severe (greater than 14 mg/dL). The causes are conveniently divided into those in which the hypercalcemia is due to PTH excess and those in which the hypercalcemia is an independent process associated with suppressed PTH. More than 90% of hypercalemia is due to primary hyperparathyroidism or hypercalcemia of malignancy. They both can be associated with life-threatening hypercalcemia.

The approaches to the management of severe hypercalcemia include intravenous hydration with saline, furosemide (if necessary), and calcitonin with an intravenous bisphosphonate or subcutaneous denosumab.

References

1. Palmér M, Jakobsson S, Akerström G, Ljunghall S. Prevalence of hypercalcaemia in a health survey: a 14-year follow-up study of serum calcium values. *Eur J Clin Invest.* 1988;18(1):39–46.
2. Frølich A. Prevalence of hypercalcaemia in normal and in hospital populations. *Dan Med Bull.* 1998; 45(4):436–439.
3. Insogna KL. Primary hyperparathyroidism. *N Engl J Med.* 2018;379(11):1050–1059.
4. Bilezikian JP, Cusano NE, Khan AA, Liu JM, Marcocci C, F. Bandeira. Primary hyperparathyroidism. *Nat Rev Dis Primers.* 2016;2:16033.
5. van der Plas WY, Noltes ME, van Ginhoven TM, Kruijff S. Secondary and tertiary hyperparathyroidism: a narrative review. *Scand J Surg.* 2019:1457496919866015.
6. Levin A, Bakris GL, Molitch M, et al. Prevalence of abnormal serum vitamin D, PTH, calcium, and phosphorus in patients with chronic kidney disease: results of the study to evaluate early kidney disease. *Kidney Int.* 2007;71(1):31–38.
7. Pitt SC, Sippel RS, Chen H. Secondary and tertiary hyperparathyroidism, state of the art surgical management. *Surg Clin North Am.* 2009;89(5):1227–1239.
8. Lee JY, Shoback DM. Familial hypocalciuric hypercalcemia and related disorders. *Best Pract Res Clin Endocrinol Metab.* 2018;32(5):609–619.
9. Szalat A, Mazeh H, Freund HR. Lithium-associated hyperparathyroidism: report of four cases and review of the literature. *Eur J Endocrinol.* 2009;160(2):317–323.
10. Stewart AF. Clinical practice. Hypercalcemia associated with cancer. *N Engl J Med.* 2005;352(4): 373–379.
11. Mundy GR, Edwards JR. PTH-related peptide (PTHrP) in hypercalcemia. *J Am Soc Nephrol.* 2008; 19(4):672–675.
12. Fuss M, Pepersack T, Gillet C, Karmali R, Corvilain J. Calcium and vitamin D metabolism in granulomatous diseases. *Clin Rheumatol.* 1992;11(1):28–36.
13. Hewison M, Kantorovich V, Liker HR, et al. Vitamin D-mediated hypercalcemia in lymphoma: evidence for hormone production by tumor-adjacent macrophages. *J Bone Miner Res.* 2003;18(3):579–582.
14. Chukir T, Liu Y, Hoffman K, Bilezikian JP, Farooki A. Calcitriol elevation is associated with a higher risk of refractory hypercalcemia of malignancy in solid tumors. *J Clin Endocrinol Metab.* 2020;105(4):e1115–e1123.
15. Lowe H, Cusano NE, Binkley N, Blaner WS, Bilezikian JP. Vitamin D toxicity due to a commonly available "over the counter" remedy from the Dominican Republic. *J Clin Endocrinol Metab.* 2011;96(2):291–295.
16. Donovan PJ, Achong N, Griffin K, Galligan J, Pretorius CJ, Mcleod DS. PTHrP-mediated hypercalcemia: causes and survival in 138 patients. *J Clin Endocrinol Metab.* 2015;100(5):2024–2029.
17. Bilezikian JP, Brandi ML, Eastell R, et al. Guidelines for the management of asymptomatic primary hyperparathyroidism: summary statement from the Fourth International Workshop. *J Clin Endocrinol Metab.* 2014;99(10):3561–3569.
18. Eslamy HK, Ziessman HA. Parathyroid scintigraphy in patients with primary hyperparathyroidism: 99mTc sestamibi SPECT and SPECT/CT. *Radiographics.* 2008;28(5):1461–1476.
19. Rodgers SE, Hunter GJ, Hamberg LM, et al. Improved preoperative planning for directed parathyroidectomy with 4-dimensional computed tomography. *Surgery.* 2006;140(6):932–940.
20. Yeh R, Tay YD, Tabacco G, et al. Diagnostic performance of 4D CT and sestamibi SPECT/CT in localizing parathyroid adenomas in primary hyperparathyroidism. *Radiology.* 2019;291(2):469–476.
21. Suki WN, Yium JJ, von Minden M, Saller-Hebert C, Eknoyan G, Martinez-Maldonado M. Acute treatment of hypercalcemia with furosemide. *N Engl J Med.* 1970;283(16):836–840.
22. Major P, Lortholary A, Hon J, et al. Zoledronic acid is superior to pamidronate in the treatment of hypercalcemia of malignancy: a pooled analysis of two randomized, controlled clinical trials. *J Clin Oncol.* 2001;19(2):558–567.

23. Bilezikian JP. Clinical review 51: management of hypercalcemia. *J Clin Endocrinol Metab*. 1993;77(6): 1445–1449.
24. Dellay B, Groth M. Emergency management of malignancy-associated hypercalcemia. *Adv Emerg Nurs J*. 2016;38(1):15–25.
25. Thosani S, Hu MI. Denosumab: a new agent in the management of hypercalcemia of malignancy. *Future Oncol*. 2015;11(21):2865–2871.
26. Cardella CJ, Birkin BL, Rapoport A. Role of dialysis in the treatment of severe hypercalcemia: report of two cases successfully treated with hemodialysis and review of the literature. *Clin Nephrol*. 1979; 12(6):285–290.

CHAPTER 11

Hypocalcemic Crisis: Acute Postoperative and Long-Term Management of Hypocalcemia

Stuart Campbell ■ Tara Corrigan ■ John P. Bilezikian ■ Alexander Shifrin

CHAPTER OUTLINE

Introduction

Calcium is an essential cofactor for numerous enzymatic reactions and is an essential cation for muscle function. Hypocalcemia is a major, potentially life-threatening complication following thyroid and parathyroid surgery. Hypocalcemia is defined as total serum calcium levels below the normal range (generally 8.5 to 10.5 mg/dL). However, defining hypocalcemia by the total calcium value assumes that the several forms of circulating calcium are in the usual proportions. Under these circumstances, the physiologically active form of calcium, namely ionized calcium, is represented accurately by the total calcium measurement. The ionized calcium consists of approximately 50% of the total plasma calcium: 40% of plasma calcium is bound to plasma proteins, mostly albumin, and 10% is complexed with anions such as bicarbonate, sulfate, phosphate, lactate, and citrate. A reduced albumin concentration will lower the total calcium concentration without affecting the ionized calcium concentration and, thus, be associated with signs or symptoms of hypocalcemia.[1] Under these circumstances, the total calcium measurement does not accurately reflect the ionized fraction and a correction factor is applied. For every g/dL the albumin is below a standardized value, 4 g/L, the total calcium is adjusted upward by 0.8 mg/dL. To circumvent this calculation, the ionized calcium can be measured directly, but it requires special handling and a calibrated ionized calcium electrode. Most laboratories are not equipped on a routine basis to measure the ionized calcium directly; thus the corrected calcium concentration is more frequently determined. Magnesium levels also play a critical role in this discussion because this cation is required for normal secretion of parathyroid hormone (PTH). When low, PTH secretion is inhibited. Such patients can present with the biochemical abnormalities of hypoparathyroidism, namely hypocalcemia and undetectable levels of PTH. In addition, hypomagnesemia is associated with peripheral resistance to renal and skeletal actions of PTH.[2–4] Measuring serum magnesium levels and replacing magnesium to normal levels if low (greater than 1.7 mg/dL) is a critical component in the treatment of hypocalcemic patients.

Calcium levels are normally regulated by a feedback mechanism whereby PTH is secreted in response to low calcium levels, which stimulates the kidney to reabsorb calcium, activate vitamin D to promote intestinal absorption of dietary calcium, and stimulate bone resorption of calcium. Conversely, but much less important from a physiologic point of view, calcitonin is secreted by thyroid C cells in response to high calcium levels stimulating bone deposition of calcium and reduced gastrointestinal and kidney resorption of calcium. More important is the response of the parathyroid axis to hypercalcemia in which PTH is immediately inhibited and those physiologic properties are reversed.

The mechanism behind a transient postoperative hypocalcemia following parathyroidectomy is the dysregulation of the calcium feedback loop due to long-standing hyperparathyroidism that may not immediately recover. Postoperative hypocalcemia after parathyroid surgery is typically transient. More prolonged hypocalcemia after parathyroid surgery can be due to "hungry bone syndrome." This syndrome describes a period of rapid skeletal calcium accrual in patients who have preexisting parathyroid bone disease. The hypocalcemia associated with the hungry bone syndrome lasts as long as it takes for the skeletal system to replenish itself with calcium. It can take several days or months.

In their review of 1112 bilateral neck dissections over a 17-year period, Allendorf et al.[5] reported transient hypocalcemia in 1.8% of patients. More recent data from the Collaborative Endocrine Surgery Quality Improvement Program (CESQIP) estimates postoperative hypocalcemia in primary hyperparathyroidism to be 10.5% after recurrent parathyroid surgery but only 2.4% after the initial operation.[6] At its extreme, postoperative hypocalcemia can be permanent due to removal of all parathyroid tissue and/or sacrifice of its vascular supply. Permanent hypoparathyroidism is said to occur in 1.6% of patients who undergo neck surgery.[7,8]

As thyroid surgery is a more common procedure, transient or permanent hypoparathyroidism occurs more often than after parathyroid surgery. The etiology of postoperative hypocalcemia following thyroidectomy is due to "stunning" or ischemia to all four parathyroid glands or inadvertent removal or devascularization, or failed autotransplantation of parathyroid glands. With specific reference to thyroid surgery, transient hypoparathyroidism occurs in approximately 23% to 38% of patients undergoing total thyroidectomy, with about 7% to 14% requiring a long-term calcium supplementation. Permanent hypoparathyroidism was reported to be between 0.12% and 5.8%.[6,7,9–11] Risk factors for postoperative hypocalcemia after thyroid surgery include surgery for Graves' disease, lymphocytic thyroiditis (Hashimoto's thyroiditis), bilateral neck dissections, repeat operations, and surgery for malignancy as well as surgeon's expertise and experience.[1,6,9,12,13] The experience of the surgeon has the most important role in the success of the surgery and lowering the rate of hypoparathyroidism after thyroidectomy or parathyroidectomy. Studies by Sosa et al.[12] and Aspinall et al.[13] demonstrated that a high-volume surgeon is the one who performs more than 50 parathyroidectomies and thyroidectomies per year.

Clinical Presentation

The classic symptom of hypocalcemia is neuromuscular irritability of both sensory and motor nerves. Hypocalcemia decreases the threshold for neuron firing, resulting in hyperexcitability and muscle spasm (tetany). Symptoms of neuronal hyperexcitability can range from relatively benign findings, such as paresthesia, numbness, tingling, and muscle spasms, to life-threatening tetany, namely cardiac bronchospasm, laryngospasm, and cardiac dysrhythmias.[14] In order to prevent the development of life-threatening sequela of hypocalcemia, it is important to recognize and treat the milder and initial symptoms of hypocalcemia such as circumoral facial tingling and twitching, numbness, and tingling weakness of the hands and feet. If not corrected, these symptoms rapidly progress to muscle cramps and spasm in the extremities with lightheadedness, bradycardia, and seizures. Accompanying cognitive symptoms of confusion, anxiety, irritability, and hallucinations are also observed.[14] Cardiovascular symptoms are also common in hypocalcemia, such as bradycardia, hypotension, and arrhythmias. Additional clinical presentations include seizures, papilledema, and psychiatric disturbances.[14]

Physical Examination

Postoperative hypocalcemia can be detected on physical examination by seeing the manifestations of neuromuscular hyperexcitability, cardiovascular abnormalities, and psychiatric disturbances. Neuromuscular hyperexcitability often presents with the classic findings of Chvostek's sign and Trousseau's sign. Chvostek's sign is performed by manually tapping the facial nerve about 2 cm anterior to the external auditory meatus. Ipsilateral twitching of the face results. Trousseau's sign is elicited by inflating a blood pressure cuff slightly over the systolic pressure for 2 to 3 minutes. A positive result will be seen by carpal spasm, manifest by flexion of the wrist and metacarpophalangeal joints with adduction of thumb and fingers. Whereas Chvostek's sign can be seen in as many as 10% of normocalcemic individuals, Trousseau's sign is much more specific for hypocalcemia. Cardiovascular changes can be seen by hypotension and electrocardiographic (ECG) changes. The prolonged QT interval is the most classic sign by ECG but the ST segment can also be increased. Rarely, hypocalcemia can lead to *torsades de pointes*, a form of polymorphic ventricular tachycardia. Psychiatric disturbances can also be detected with irritability and depression. Rarely, psychosis is associated with hypocalcemia.[14]

Diagnostic Tests

Although the history and physical examination can point toward postoperative hypocalcemia, the diagnosis is made mainly by detecting serum calcium levels that are below normal. Postoperative hypocalcemia can be diagnosed by serum calcium levels below 8.5 mg/dL; however, serum calcium levels must be interpreted appropriately. Serum calcium binds proteins within the blood, mainly albumin, and only ionized calcium within the blood contributes to physiologic activity. Serum calcium should be corrected for albumin levels with the formula: corrected calcium (Ca) = serum Ca level + [0.8 × (normal albumin − patient's albumin)]. The normal albumin level is defaulted to 4 mg/dL Standard Units (40 g/L SI Units); therefore, the formula can be changed to that default value in the calculator: corrected Ca = serum Ca + 0.8 × (4 − serum albumin). Ionized calcium can be measured directly and is the most accurate level of calcium activity within the blood. Ionized calcium should be greater than 1.1 mmol/L (4.4 mg/dL). Hypocalcemia is often associated with hypomagnesemia, and magnesium levels should be checked and replaced to a level above 1.7 mEq/L. Measurement of serum PTH also should be included to confirm the diagnosis of acute postoperative hypoparathyroidism. The PTH level is actually a very important diagnostic element. If the patient is experiencing postoperative hypoparathyroidism, the PTH level will be low. If, however, the patient is experiencing the hungry bone syndrome (see earlier), their PTH level may actually be elevated, reflecting not hypoparathyroidism but a normal physiologic response to skeletal calcium demand.

Prevention of Postoperative Hypocalcemia

Prevention of postoperative hypocalcemia starts with preoperative patient counseling. Patients should be taught to recognize early signs and symptoms of hypocalcemia. In addition, the importance of medical adherence and compliance to calcium supplementation postoperatively should be stressed to prevent severe hypocalcemia and its potential for life-threatening symptoms. Patients are instructed to begin calcium supplementation while in recovery on the day of surgery and to continue at regular intervals even during the night. They are advised to notify their surgical team once hypocalcemic symptoms begin so that dose adjustments of oral calcium supplementation can be implemented prior to the development of more severe symptoms. Patients that are high risk for hypocalcemia following parathyroidectomy or thyroidectomy should be monitored more cautiously, with repeat laboratory testing within a few days of discharge to ensure supplementation with calcium is appropriate to avoid either under- or overdosing.

The most effective way to treat postoperative hypocalcemia is through preventative measures with prophylactic supplementation of calcium preoperatively and postoperatively, and operative strategies to preserve the parathyroid glands. Preoperative vitamin D levels, which should always be measured, will dictate whether vitamin D repletion should be given prior to surgery. Most experts recommend 25-hydroxyvitamin D levels greater than 30 ng/mL in patients with metabolic bone diseases such as primary hyperparathyroidism.[9,15] This recommendation is eminently reasonable, although it has not been clearly shown that low vitamin D levels contribute to postoperative hypocalcemia.[9,16] A preoperative supplementation strategy to reduce postoperative hypocalcemia includes vitamin D optimization preoperatively by aggressively replacing vitamin D deficiency if the 25-hydroxyvitamin D level is less than 20 ng/mL with 50,000 IU of oral ergocalciferol once per week for 8 weeks.[17,18] Vitamin D levels of 20 to 30 ng/mL can be treated less aggressively with 1000 IU of ergocalciferol per day from either dietary or supplementary sources.[17,18]

Intraoperative strategies to avoid postoperative hypocalcemia include measuring PTH levels intraoperatively during parathyroidectomy, careful parathyroid gland preservation during a thyroidectomy, and parathyroid gland autotransplantation in the event that postoperative hypoparathyroidism is a concern (e.g., glands are incidentally removed, devascularized, and appeared to be nonviable). Parathyroid gland devascularization during thyroid surgery can lead to post-thyroidectomy hypoparathyroidism. Parathyroid preservation surgical techniques are used to decrease the incidence of post-thyroidectomy hypoparathyroidism, which include careful identification of parathyroid glands and meticulous dissection. Parathyroid autotransplantation can also be used to reconstitute parathyroid function after devascularization. Parathyroid autotransplantation involves implanting slices of viable parathyroid tissue into the ipsilateral sternocleidomastoid muscle, or subcutaneously into the muscle in the forearm. Fresh autografts or cryopreserved parathyroid tissue can be used for implantation, with the success rate being approximately 70% for cryopreserved tissue and 90% for fresh, autotransplanted tissue.[19,20] The parathyroid autotransplantation technique into the ipsilateral sternocleidomastoid muscle is performed as follows. The devascularized or accidently removed parathyroid gland is placed into a container with sterile normal saline solution until it is ready to be reimplanted. Then, the gland is crushed into small pieces with a scalpel. A pocket is created in the ipsilateral sternocleidomastoid muscle, ensuring there is no hematoma development, as this would impede the survival of the implanted parathyroid gland. Nonabsorbable nylon or an absorbable Vicryl (Ethicon Inc, NJ) suture is placed the same way so as to close the opening through both sides of the muscle pocket, and an air-node is created. The crushed fragments of the parathyroid gland are placed into the pocket and the air-node is tied down. A small, 5-mm, titanium clip is placed either on the node or on the end of the suture to mark the area of reimplantation in order to preserve the implant in case of future surgery in this area. Autotransplantation into the muscle or subcutaneous reimplantation into a forearm is performed for parathyroid hyperplasia. In the case of recurrence, the transplanted parathyroid gland can be easily removed from the arm under local anesthesia, avoiding re-exploration of the previously operated neck.

Prophylactic Postoperative Calcium and Vitamin D Replacement

It is much more difficult and takes longer to treat hypocalcemia symptoms than to prevent their development. Thus recent statements from the American Association of Clinical Endocrinologists and the American College of Endocrinology recommend routine, prophylactic treatment with oral calcium with or without calcitriol for all patients after a parathyroidectomy to prevent transient hypocalcemia.[9] Oral calcium supplementation appears to be the most cost-effective approach. Calcium carbonate is the medication of choice, given as 500 to 1000 mg three times a day. This approach has been demonstrated to reduce postoperative hypocalcemia to approximately 10%.[9] Our replacement protocol consists of oral calcium carbonate with vitamin D (OsCal, GSK, USA) starting with 500 to 1000 mg every 6 hours for the first week, then 500 to 1000 mg every 8 hours for the second week, then 500 to 1000 mg every 12 hours for the third week, and then 500 mg every 12 hours for the fourth week. We usually follow patients 2 weeks after the surgery with serum calcium and PTH levels. If the levels are within normal ranges, we stop calcium replacement earlier. Also, we modify our empiric replacement protocol based on intraoperative findings, such as the viability of the parathyroid glands during the thyroidectomy, or the number of parathyroid glands removed during the parathyroidectomy. We also decrease the dose of calcium in patients with impaired renal function and in elderly patients.

Another strategy is more objective and based on immediate postoperative PTH levels, within 1 hour of the surgery. If the PTH level is above 15 pg/mL (detected but at the lower limit of normal), the patient can be discharged home on prophylactic oral dose of 500 to 1000 mg of calcium three times a day. If the PTH level is less than 15 pg/mL, calcitriol at a dose of 0.5 to 1.0 μg per day should be started in addition to calcium. Magnesium supplementation should be considered if the serum magnesium level is below normal. It may take up to 72 hours for calcitriol to be effective.[9] The patient can be observed in the hospital overnight, or, if reliable, compliant, and close by, they can be sent home with clear instructions on symptoms and when to call the doctor.

An alternative to calcium carbonate is calcium citrate (2000 to 6000 mg per day) administered orally in divided doses for those patients on proton pump inhibitors, elderly patients with achlorhydria, and those who had a gastric bypass.[9,21] Calcium carbonate requires an acidic environment for absorption, whereas calcium citrate does not. The advantage of calcium carbonate is that it is about 40% elemental calcium, whereas calcium citrate is only 21% elemental calcium. For enhanced absorption, both preparations of calcium should be taken with meals. It is important to administer oral calcium dosing separate from oral thyroid hormone replacement due to the binding of levothyroxine by calcium and inhibiting levothyroxine absorption. Levothyroxine should be taken 1 hour before or 3 hours after calcium is taken.[21] In some patients who are very sensitive to fluctuations in the serum calcium, an "every 6 hours" or "every 8 hours" dosing regimen is preferred over a QID (four times a day) or TID (three times a day) in order to avoid the prolonged fasting period that occurs during sleep and which can result in morning hypocalcemia.[21]

Measuring calcium levels postoperatively has been used to predict who can be safely discharged and who will require post-thyroidectomy calcium and vitamin D supplementation.[22] If the serum calcium level is less than 8.5 mg/dL, or the ionized calcium level is less than 1.1 mmol/L, replacement should be considered. The pitfall with this protocol is in the timing of the measurement as studies have failed to demonstrate the reliability of the immediate postoperative calcium measurements to predict the development of hypoparathyroidism. Postoperatively, the decrease in serum calcium level can be delayed by as much as 48 to 72 hours and only materialize after the patient is home.

Medical Management of Acute and Chronic Postoperative Hypocalcemia

Management of postoperative hypocalcemia, either from post-thyroidectomy or post-parathyroidectomy, focuses on calcium supplementation. The severity of the symptoms and the degree of hypocalcemia guide the aggressiveness and modality of calcium supplementation. Guidelines for the postoperative management of hypoparathyroidism[9] recommend measuring PTH and calcium levels postoperatively, and supplementing with oral calcium (1 to 3 g daily of elemental calcium) if calcium levels are less than 7 mg/dL or ionized calcium levels less than 1.1 mmol/L, or if symptomatic with carpopedal spasm, perioral numbness, or positive Chvostek's sign. If calcium levels remain below 7 mg/dL despite calcium supplementation, 0.5 μg of calcitriol twice daily can be added. Additional algorithms for measuring and treating postoperative hypocalcemia caused by postoperative hypoparathyroidism involve measuring PTH hormone and calcium levels to determine calcium dosage, calcitriol dosage, and adding intravenous calcium if severe symptoms are present.[23] Supplementation can be escalated to include up to 6000 mg calcium per day, 2 μg/day calcitriol, or intravenous magnesium of 1 mg/kg per hour if patients remain symptomatic and hypocalcemic.[23] In severe cases of hypocalcemia, refractory to oral supplementation or with severe symptoms, intravenous calcium should be administered as an initial bolus of 1 to 2 g of calcium in 50 mL of 5% dextrose infused over 20 minutes. If symptoms of severe hypocalcemia persist, an intravenous calcium infusion of a solution composed of 11 g of calcium gluconate added to normal saline or 5% dextrose water, to provide a final volume of 1000 mL, is administered at 50 mL/hour and adjusted to maintain the calcium level in the low normal range.[9] The formula, however, is weight-based (15 mg calcium/kg weight). It is important to include continuous ECG monitoring during intravenous calcium replacement, as rapid replacement can elicit cardiac arrythmias. Patients should then be transitioned to oral calcium plus oral calcitriol to ensure calcium levels remain normal and symptoms do not recur. Magnesium levels should also be checked, especially in patients who are not responding to calcium supplementation. If the serum magnesium level is below 1.7 mEq/L, then 1 to 2 mg intravenous magnesium should be given in addition to calcium supplements.

In our outpatient protocol, we initiate calcitriol therapy at 0.25 μg once or twice a day for moderate, and 0.5 μg once or twice a day for severe hypocalcemia, or if 1-hour postoperative PTH level is less than 15 pg/mL. We recommend rechecking calcium and PTH levels in 2 to 3 days after the initiation of calcitriol therapy and then every 3 days thereafter to avoid an overdose and development of rebound hypercalcemia. A cautionary note to all providers is to be very cautious with administration of calcitriol in combination with calcium in patients with borderline renal function or the elderly. In these latter two situations, hypercalcemia can occur rather quickly.

SUMMARY

Transient postoperative hypocalcemia is a relatively common complication occurring in roughly 23% to 38% of patients undergoing total thyroidectomy. Permanent hypoparathyroidism is much less common, occurring between 0.12% and 5.8%. The best way to treat postoperative hypocalcemia is through preventative measures with patient education, prophylactic supplementation of calcium postoperatively, and operative strategies to preserve the parathyroid glands. Medical management of acute postoperative hypocalcemia include vigorous oral calcium supplementation with addition of oral calcitriol. If the patient is refractory to oral therapy, hospitalization is required to administer intravenous calcium, followed by initiation of an intravenous calcium infusion protocol.

Chronic Management of Hypocalcemia

Although most patients who develop postoperative hypocalcemia recover, some do not. In fact, the most common cause of permanent hypoparathyroidism is after neck surgery, occurring in about 75% of all patients with hypoparathyroidism.[24,25] Chronic hypoparathyroidism is defined as well-documented reductions in the corrected serum calcium and PTH concentrations over a 6-month period.[26] This time point is useful because some patients who develop hypoparathyroidism after parathyroid surgery will regain parathyroid function within 6 months.[27] Other causes of hypoparathyroidism are due to an autoimmune destruction of the parathyroid glands, to genetic etiologies (e.g., DiGeorge syndrome, autosomal dominant hypoparathyroidism), or very rarely to infiltration of the parathyroid glands with iron, copper, or metastatic cancer.[28]

It has already been mentioned, but is worth repeating, that hypomagnesemia, of any etiology, can masquerade as hypoparathyroidism. It is always important to consider this possibility because it is reversible.[29] When administered magnesium, these patients will demonstrate rapid increases in the circulating PTH level and eventual sensitivity to PTH. Although the secretory block is rapidly overcome by magnesium administration, patients will remain hypocalcemic until peripheral resistance to PTH is relieved, several days later. Measures taken to deal with acute hypocalcemia, thus, should be applied to patients with hypomagnesemia, when symptomatic, in the same manner as any other acutely symptomatic hypocalcemic state.

By far the most common cause of chronic hypocalcemia is hypoparathyroidism. It is true that other chronic conditions can be associated with chronic hypocalcemia such as gluten enteropathy and other malabsorption syndromes, such as bariatric surgery. Nutritional, severe vitamin D deficiency is virtually unheard of in the developed world, but it can also be associated with hypocalcemia.

The pathophysiology of chronic hypoparathyroidism is related to the lack of PTH's actions on its target organs, the skeleton and the kidneys, and to its indirect gastrointestinal actions.[30] Without PTH, the skeleton becomes inactive and no longer serves as a useful reservoir for calcium when there is need. Without PTH, the kidneys do not conserve filtered calcium and, thus, a relative hypercalciuria ensues. In addition, the renal tubules lose the phosphaturic actions of PTH, thus leading to hyperphosphatemia. Without PTH, the activation of vitamin D through the actions of PTH on the renal hydroxylase that converts 25-hydroxyvitamin D to 1,25-dihyroxyvitamin D is impaired. The deficiency in active vitamin D leads to malabsorption of calcium.

GOALS IN THE MANAGEMENT OF ACUTE AND CHRONIC HYPOPARATHYROIDISM

There are seven therapeutic goals[31]:

1. Prevention of symptomatic hypocalcemia. Although the actual serum calcium is related to symptomatology, two other factors are important. The rate at which the serum calcium has fallen can be a key determinant even if the serum calcium is not markedly low. This is an important point in patients who become hypocalcemia after parathyroid surgery. In someone whose preoperative serum calcium is very high, a precipitous postoperative decline can be associated with symptoms even though the serum calcium is not remarkably low. Another important variable is the patient's own sensitivity to a given serum calcium level. For the same hypocalcemic value, a patient may or may not be similarly symptomatic.
2. Maintenance of a serum calcium that is in the lower range of normal or slightly below. The general recommendation is for the serum calcium to range between 8.0 and 9.0 mg/dL. In these patients, who generally are very sensitive to the serum calcium level, levels above 9.5 mg/dL are not always tolerated well, with patients complaining of symptoms of hypercalcemia even though the value itself is within the normal range.

3. Maintenance of the calcium × phosphate product below 55 mg^2/dL^2. This value is ingrained in the literature and certainly should be regarded as the very highest tolerable level. The concern for a chronically elevated Ca × P product relates to the risk of ectopic soft tissue calcifications in the kidneys, vasculature, and brain. Many experts are recommending that the Ca × P product be maintained as close to normal as possible (e.g., 35 to 45 mg^2/dL^2).
4. Avoid hypercalciuria. As noted previously, the lack of the calcium-conserving actions of PTH leads to absolute or relative hypercalciuria. To a certain extent, the magnitude of the hypercalciuria will depend upon how much oral calcium is required to control the serum calcium. The concern for chronic hypercalciuria relates to the risk of kidney stones, nephrocalcinosis, and a reduction in renal function per se.[32]
5. Avoid hypercalcemia. It goes without saying that frank hypercalcemia is to be avoided. But, as noted above, the cautionary note is related to two related advisories, namely to keep the serum calcium in the lower range of normal and to minimize the Ca × P to the extent possible.
6. Control of the serum phosphate. Again, this advice is related to the goal of controlling the Ca × P product, although there is some evidence that hyperphosphatemia per se can be associated with soft tissue calcifications.[32] Patients with hypoparathyroidism will present variably with levels of the serum phosphate that are in the upper range of normal of frankly elevated. Dietary measures are usually sufficient to reach this goal, but rarely phosphate binders are needed.
7. Prevention of renal, vascular, and other soft tissue calcifications. This goal again relates specifically to control of the biochemical manifestations of hypoparathyroidism.

CONVENTIONAL MANAGEMENT

Calcium Supplements

Calcium supplements are a requirement for virtually all patients with hypoparathyroidism.[33] The diet simply cannot provide sufficient amounts of calcium, although it should be emphasized that dietary calcium is more readily bioavailable than supplemental sources of calcium. The range of calcium needed varies enormously from as little as 500 mg daily (rare) to as much as 9 g (rare). The most common dosage range is between 1 and 2 g daily, given in doses of no more than 500 to 600 mg at a time. The reason for not providing more than that amount of calcium at a time is because absorption of calcium becomes less efficient. In view of the large amounts of calcium typically required, calcium carbonate is most attractive because it contains by molecular weight a greater percentage of elemental calcium, 40%, than calcium citrate, which is only 21% elemental calcium. The disadvantage of calcium carbonate is that it has to be given in the presence of a source of acid.[34] If the patient does not have normal gastric acid production, a protein-based meal will provide the proper acidic environment. Another disadvantage of calcium carbonate is that it can be associated with gas and constipation. These disadvantages of calcium carbonate are not so evident with calcium citrate, which does not require gastric acid and is less likely to be associated with gas and constipation. However, the use of calcium citrate will require more pills because it contains only about half the amount of elemental calcium than the carbonate form. In patients who require large of amounts of oral calcium, this can be a significant drawback.[35]

Vitamin D Supplements

Active vitamin D is the other mainstay of therapy. The two formulations are active vitamin D, 1,25-dihydroxyvtamin D (calcitriol), or an active analogue, 1-alpha hydroxycholecalciferol. These forms of vitamin D are administered in multiple daily doses because their half-life is only 4 to 6 hours. Most patients will require, on average, 0.5 to 1.0 μg of calcitriol or 1.0 to 2.0 μg of the 1-alpha analogue. Experts vary as to whether they emphasize active formulations of vitamin D, and thus reduce the need for calcium supplements, or emphasize calcium supplements, and thus reduce the need for active vitamin D. In our opinion, this is more a matter of practice style rather than accompanied by evidentiary support.

Cholecalciferol (Vitamin D3) or Ergocalciferol (Vitamin D2)

Whereas the need for active vitamin D is virtually always a requirement, arguments in favor of using parent vitamin D are less so. It is clear that these patients do not easily convert 25-hydroxyvitamin D to active vitamin D. This point leads some away from using vitamin D at all. On the other hand, vitamin D sufficiency is defined by the level of 25-hydroxyvitamin D[36,37] and not 1,25-dihydroxyvitamin D. Moreover, as we do not know whether other products of the hepatic metabolism of vitamin D are important for other putative actions of vitamin D, many experts seek normal levels of 25-hydroxyvitamin D as a therapeutic goal.[7] Recently, Streeten et al.[38] have advanced another argument, namely better control is achieved in these patients when vitamin D is used. In order to achieve a normal level of 25-hydroxyvitamin D, greater than 20 ng/mL, virtually all patients will require a vitamin D supplement, with recent studies preferring vitamin D3 over vitamin D2.[39]

Thiazide Diuretics

The concern of chronic hypercalciuria leads, in some patients, to the use of thiazide diuretics.

NEWER APPROACHES TO THE MANAGEMENT OF CHRONIC HYPOPARATHYROIDISM

Parathyroid Hormone

Lack of PTH is the fundamental problem in chronic hypoparathyroidism. Without PTH, normal calcium homeostasis will always be abnormal even though conventional management can often deal with the biochemical challenge of maintaining reasonably normal serum calcium levels. Until recently, it was said that hypoparathyroidism was the last classic endocrine deficiency disease for which the missing hormone was not available. Attempts to utilize PTH as a therapy for this disorder started in the modern era with the work of Winer and her colleagues. They and others did not use the full length intact PTH molecule, but rather the foreshortened but fully active amino-terminal fragment known as teriparatide [PTH(1-34)].[40–42] These studies demonstrated that better control than conventional therapy could be achieved with reductions in amounts of supplemental calcium and vitamin D. These studies did not consistently demonstrate a reduction in urinary calcium excretion.

More recently, the intact recombinant native 84-amino acid PTH molecule [rhPTH(1-84)] has been studied.[43–47] The pivotal clinical trial, known as REPLACE,[44] demonstrated that over a titration range of 50 to 100 μg of rhPTH(1-84), supplemental calcium and active vitamin D requirements fell by over 50%, while serum calcium levels were maintained. Almost the same percentage of patients were able to eliminate all active vitamin D and reduce their supplemental calcium needs to 500 mg or less.[46]

As chronic hypoparathyroidism is a life-long disorder, the long-term use of rhPTH(1-84) is of particular importance both with regard to efficacy and safety.[48,49] The 8-year longitudinal data confirmed reductions in supplemental calcium needs by 57% and active vitamin D by 76%.[48] Over time, but not in the near term, urinary calcium declined by 38%, an observation also confirmed in the 5-year follow-up study of the REPLACE trial.[49] Renal function was stable.

Safety of rhPTH(1-84)

The well-known oncogenic effects of high-dose PTH molecules in rats[50,51] have not been seen with any PTH molecules administered to human subjects. Surveillance with teriparatide extends now to over 17 years with no signals being seen.[52–54] In fact, the Food and Drug Administration approval of rhPTH(1-84) in hypoparathyroidism has no time limit as to duration of use. Other safety indices, such as the incidence of hypercalcemia and hypercalciuria, are favorable.[48]

Indications for the use for rhPTH(1-84)

rhPTH(1-84) is approved for patients with hypoparathyroidism who cannot be well controlled on conventional therapy. Several groups, considering the evidence that is available, have offered management guidelines.[7,8,55] Two of these reports deal specifically with rhPTH(1-84).[7,55] Many experts would categorize patients who are not well controlled in at least six different ways:

1. Poor control of the serum calcium (less than 7.5 mg/dL or clinical symptom of hypocalcemia);
2. Needs for oral calcium exceeding 2.5 g/day or active vitamin D by greater than 1.5 μg (or the active vitamin D analogue greater than 3 μg/day);
3. Hypercalciuria, nephrolithiasis, nephrocalcinosis, reduced creatinine clearance or eGFR (less than 60 mL/minute), or increased stone risk by urinary biochemical analysis;
4. Hyperphosphatemia or elevated calcium × phosphate product greater than 55 mg^2/dL^2;
5. Gastrointestinal tract dysfunction with malabsorption or after bariatric surgery;
6. Reduced quality of life.

The starting dose of rhPTH(1-84) is 50 μg/day, administered subcutaneously in the thigh. Either active vitamin D or calcium is reduced by 50% at the same time. In a stepwise fashion, active vitamin D and calcium are gradually reduced with the optimal goal to eliminate active vitamin D and reduce the amount of supplemental calcium to 500 mg/day or lower. rhPTH(1-84) is increased, as needed, in 25 μg steps. If therapy is discontinued, patients often require more calcium and active vitamin D than they did prior to rhPTH(1-84). The skeleton, now activated, is the reason for the enhanced requirements.[7,54]

References

1. Shifrin AL. Brief overview of calcium, vitamin d, parathyroid hormone metabolism and calcium sensing receptor function. In: Shifrin AL, ed. *Advances in Treatment and Management in Surgical Endocrinology*. Oxford: Elsevier; 2019:63–70.
2. Rude RK, Oldham SB, Sharp CF Jr, Singer FR. Parathyroid hormone secretion in magnesium deficiency. *J Clin Endocrinol Metab*. 1978;47:800–806.
3. Allgrove J, Adami S, Fraher L, Reuben A, O'Riordan JL. Hypomagnesaemia: studies of parathyroid hormone secretion and function. *Clin Endocrinol (Oxf)*. 1984;21:435–449.
4. Schlingmann KP, Konrad M. Magnesium homeostasis. In: Bilezikian JP, Clemens TL, Martin J, Rosen CJ, eds. *Principles of Bone Biology*. San Diego: Academic Press; 2020:509–526.
5. Allendorf J, DiGorgi M, Spanknebel K, et al. 1112 Consecutive bilateral neck explorations for primary hyperparathyroidism. *World Journal of Surgery*. 2007;31:2075–2080.
6. Kazaure HS, Thomas S, Scheri RP, Stang MT, Roman SA, Sosa JA. The devil is in the details: assessing treatment and outcomes of 6,795 patients undergoing remedial parathyroidectomy in the Collaborative Endocrine Surgery Quality Improvement Program. *Surgery*. 2019;165(1):242e249.
7. Brandi ML, Bilezikian JP, Shoback D, et al. Management of hypoparathyroidism: summary statement and guidelines. *J Clin Endocrinol Metab*. 2016;101(6):2273–2283.
8. Bollerslev J, Rejnmark L, Marcocci C, et al. European Society of Endocrinology clinical guideline: treatment of chronic hypoparathyroidism in adults. *Eur J Endocrinol*. 2016;173(2):G1–G20.
9. Stack BC, Bimston DN, Bodenner DL, et al. American Association of Clinical Endocrinologists and American College of Endocrinology Disease state clinical review: postoperative hypoparathyroidism–definitions and management. *Endocr Pract*. 2015;21(6).
10. Chadwick D. Hypocalcaemia and permanent hypoparathyroidism after total/bilateral thyroidectomy in the BAETS Registry. *Gland Surg*. 2017;6(Suppl 1):S69–S74.
11. Akram S, Elfenbein D, Chen H, Schneider D, Sippel R. Assessing American Thyroid Association guidelines for total thyroidectomy in Graves' disease. *J Surg Res. Author manuscript. J Surg Res*. 2020;245:64–71.

12. Sosa J, Powe N, Levine M, Udelsman R, Zeiger M. Profile of a clinical practice: thresholds for surgery and surgical outcomes for patients with primary hyperparathyroidism: a national survey of endocrine surgeons. *J Clin Endocrinol Metab*. 1998;83(8):2658–2665.
13. Aspinall S, Oweis D, Chadwick D. Effect of surgeons' annual operative volume on the risk of permanent hypoparathyroidism, recurrent laryngeal nerve palsy and haematoma following thyroidectomy: analysis of United Kingdom registry of endocrine and thyroid surgery (UKRETS). *Langenbecks Arch Surg*. 2019;404(4):421–430.
14. Cusano NE, Bilezikian JP. Signs and symptoms of hypoparathyroidism. *Endocrinol Metab Clin North Am*. 2018;47(4):759–770.
15. Bilezikian JP. Primary hyperparathyroidism. *J Clin Endocrinol Metab*. 2018;103:3993–4004.
16. Lin Y, Ross HL, Raeburn CD, et al. Vitamin D deficiency does not increase the rate of postoperative hypocalcemia after thyroidectomy. *Am J Surg*. 2012;204:888–894.
17. Holick MF. Vitamin D deficiency. *N Engl J Med*. 2007;357(3):266–281.
18. Bordelon P, Ghetu MV, Langan R. Recognition and management of vitamin D deficiency. *Am Fam Physician*. 2009;80(8):841–846.
19. Cohen MS, Dilley WG, Wells Jr SA, et al. Long-term functionality of cryopreserved parathyroid autografts: a 13-year prospective analysis. *TC Surgery*. 2005;138(6):1033–1040; discussion 1040-1041.
20. Barczyński M, Gołkowski F, Nawrot I. Parathyroid transplantation in thyroid surgery. *Gland Surg*. 2017;6(5):530-536. doi:10.21037/gs.2017.06.07.
21. Orloff LA, Wiseman SM, Bernet VJ, et al. American Thyroid Association statement on postoperative hypoparathyroidism: diagnosis, prevention, and management in adults. *Thyroid*. 2018;28(7):830–841.
22. Nahas ZS1, Farrag TY, Lin FR, Belin RM, Tufano RP. A safe and cost-effective short hospital stay protocol to identify patients at low risk for the development of significant hypocalcemia after total thyroidectomy. *Laryngoscope*. 2006;116(6):906–910.
23. Mejia MG, Gonzalez-Devia D, Fierro F, Tapiero M, Rojas L, Cadena E. Hypocalcemia post thyroidectomy: prevention, diagnosis and management. *J Transl Sci*. 2018;4(2):1–7. doi:10.15761/JTS.1000212.
24. Cusano NE, Anderson L, Rubin MR, et al. Recovery of parathyroid hormone secretion and function in postoperative hypoparathyroidism: a case series. *J Clin Endocrinol Metab*. 2013;98(11):4285–4290.
25. Hadker N, Egan J, Sanders J, et al. Understanding the burden of illness associated with hypoparathyroidism reported among patients in the Paradox study. *Endo Pract*. 2014;20:671–679.
26. Clarke BL, Brown EM, Collins MT, et al. Epidemiology and diagnosis of hypoparathyroidism. *J Clin Endocrinol Metab*. 2016;101:2284–2299.
27. Powers J, Joy K, Ruscio A, Lagast H. Prevalence and incidence of hypoparathyroidism in the United States using a large claims database. *J Bone Miner Res*. 2013;28(12):2570–2576.
28. Gordon RJ, Levine MA. Genetic disorders of parathyroid development and function. *Endocrinol Metab Clin North Am*. 2018;47(4):809–823.
29. Siraj N, Hakami Y, Khan A. Medical hypoparathyroidism. *Endocrinol Metab Clin North Am*. 2018;47(4):797–808.
30. Mannstadt M, Bilezikian JP, Thakker RV, et al. Hypoparathyroidism. *Nat Rev Dis*. 2017;3:1–20.
31. Babey M, Brandi ML, Shoback D. Conventional treatment of hypoparathyroidism. *Endocrinol Metab Clin North Am*. 2018;47(4):889–900.
32. Peacock M. Hypoparathyroidism and the kidney. *Endocrinol Metab Clin North Am*. 2018;47(4):839–853.
33. Bilezikian JP, Brandi ML, Cusano NE, et al. Management of hypoparathyroidism: present and future. *J Clin Endocrinol Metab*. 2016;101(6):2313–2324.
34. Heaney RP, Smith KT, Recker RR, Hinders SM. Meal effects on calcium absorption. *Am J Clin Nutr*. 1989;49(2):372–376.
35. Cusano NE, Rubin MR, McMahon DJ, et al. Therapy of hypoparathyroidism with PTH(1-84): a prospective four-year investigation of efficacy and safety. *J Clin Endocrinol Metab*. 2013;98(1):137–144.
36. Ross AC, Manson JE, Abrams SA, et al. The 2011 report on dietary reference intakes for calcium and vitamin D from the Institute of Medicine: what clinicians need to know. *J Clin Endocrinol Metab*. 2011;96(1):53–58.
37. Sempos CT, Heijboer AC, Bikle DD, et al. Vitamin D assays and the definition of hypovitaminosis D: results from the 1st International Conference on Controversies in Vitamin D. *Br J Clin Pharmacol*. 2018;84(10):2194–2207.

38. Streeten EA, Mohtasebi Y, Konig M, Davidoff L, Ryan K. Hypoparathyroidism: less severe hypocalcemia with treatment with vitamin D2 compared with calcitriol. *J Clin Endocrinol Metab.* 2017;102(5):1505–1520.
39. Martineau AR, Thummel KE, Wang Z, et al. Differential effects of oral boluses of vitamin D2 vs vitamin D3 on vitamin D metabolism: a randomized controlled trial. *J Clin Endocrinol Metab.* 2019;104(12):5831–5839.
40. Winer KK, Yanovski JA, Sarani B, Cutler Jr GB. A randomized cross-over trial of once-daily versus twice-daily parathyroid hormone 1-34 in treatment of hypoparathyroidism. *J Clin Endocrinol Metab.* 1998;83(10):3480–3486.
41. Winer KK, Sinaii N, Reynolds J, Peterson D, Dowdy K, Cutler BB Jr. Long-term treatment of 12 children with chronic hypoparathyroidism: a randomized trial comparing synthetic human parathyroid hormone 1-34 versus calcitriol and calcium. *J Clin Endocrinol Metab.* 2010;95(6):2680–2688.
42. Palermo A, Santonati A, Tabacco G, et al. PTH(1-34) for surgical hypoparathyroidism: a 2-year prospective, open-label investigation of efficacy and quality of life. *J Clin Endocrinol Metab.* 2018;103(1):271–280.
43. Rubin MR, Sliney Jr J, McMahon DJ, Silverberg SJ, Bilezikian JP. Therapy of hypoparathyroidism with intact parathyroid hormone. *Osteoporosis Int'l.* 2010;26(11):1927–1934.
44. Mannstadt M, Clarke BL, Vokes T, et al. Efficacy and safety of recombinant human parathyroid hormone (1-84) in hypoparathyroidism (REPLACE): a double-blind, placebo-controlled, randomized, phase 3 study. *Lancet Diabetes Endocrinol.* 2013;1(4):275–283.
45. Lakatos P, Bajnok L, Lagast H, Valkusz Z. An open-label extension study of parathyroid hormone rhPTH(1-84) in adults with hypoparathyroidism. *Endocr Pract.* 2016;22(5):523–532.
46. Clarke BL, Vokes TJ, Bilezikian JP, Shoback DM, Lagast H, Mannstadt M. Effects of parathyroid hormone rhPTH(1-84) on phosphate homeostasis and vitamin D metabolism in hypoparathyroidism: REPLACE phase 3 study. *Endocrine.* 2017;55(1):273–282.
47. Tabacco G, Bilezikian JP. New directions in treatment of hypoparathyroidism. *Endocrinol Metab Clin North Am.* 2018;47(4):901–915.
48. Tay YD, Tabacco G, Cusano NE, et al. Therapy of hypoparathyroidism with rhPTH(1-84): a prospective eight year investigation of efficacy and safety. *J Clin Endocrinol Metab.* 2016;104(11):5601–5610.
49. Mannstadt M, Clarke BL, Bilezikian JP, et al. Safety and efficacy of 5 years of treatment with recombinant human parathyroid hormone in adults with hypoparathyroidism. *J Clin Endocrinol Metab.* 2019;104(11):5136–5147.
50. Vahle JL, Sato M, Long GG, et al. Skeletal changes in rates given daily subcutaneous injections of recombinant human parathyroid hormone (1-34) for 2 years and relevance to human safety. *Toxicol Pathol.* 2002;30(3):312–321.
51. Jolette J, Wilker CE, Smith SY, et al. Defining a non-carcinogenic dose of recombinant human parathyroid hormone 1-84 in a 2-year study in Fischer 344 rats. *Toxicol Pathol.* 2006;34(7):929–940.
52. Cipriani C, Irani D, Bilezikian JP. Safety of osteoanabolic therapy: a decade of experience. *J Bone Min Res.* 2012;27(12):2419–2428.
53. Andrews EB, Gilsenan AW, Midkiff K, et al. The US postmarketing surveillance study of adult osteosarcoma and teriparatide: study design and findings from the first 7 years. *J Bone Miner Res.* 2012; 27(12):2429–2437.
54. Hypoparathyroidism Bilezikian JP. *J Clin Endocrinol Metab.* 2020;105(6):1722–1736.
55. Khan AA, Koch CA, van Uum S, et al. Standards of care for hypoparathyroidism in adults: a Canadian and international consensus. *European J Endocrinol.* 2019;180:P1–P23.

PART 4

Adrenal Glands

CHAPTER 12

Acute Adrenal Hypertensive Emergencies: Pheochromocytoma, Cushing's, Hyperaldosteronism

Monika Akula ■ Raquel Kristin S. Ong ■ Alexander L. Shifrin ■ William F. Young, Jr.

CHAPTER OUTLINE

Introduction

Hypertensive emergency is defined as a rapid and significant elevation of blood pressure with systolic blood pressure greater than 180 mm Hg and/or diastolic blood pressure greater than 120 mm Hg in association with evidence of neurologic, cardiovascular, renal, and other end organ damage.[1] Hypertensive emergencies due to endocrine and metabolic conditions rather than the more common essential hypertension is seen in less than 5% of cases, but, when present, can be the cause of severe morbidity and mortality. Prompt recognition is important to initiate targeted therapy and to avoid life-threatening complications such as stoke and myocardial infarction. A detailed history and physical examination should be taken regarding the onset of hypertension (HTN), contributing family history, medications, and symptoms associated with end organ damage.[2] The most common endocrine conditions that can cause hypertensive emergencies include:

1. Pheochromocytoma/paraganglioma syndrome (PPGL)
2. Primary hyperaldosteronism
3. Cushing's syndrome (CS), including Cushing's disease (CD)

Pheochromocytoma/Paraganglioma (PPGL)

PPGLs comprise about 0.1% cases of HTN. Pheochromocytomas are adrenal tumors arising from the chromaffin cells of the adrenal medulla (80% to 85% of PPGLs), whereas paragangliomas are extra adrenal tumors that arise from the sympathetic chain ganglia in the thorax, abdomen, or pelvis (15% to 20% of PPGLs). The prevalence of pheochromocytoma is about 3% in incidentally discovered adrenal tumors.[3,4] Adrenal medullary tumors have the potential to produce epinephrine with varying amounts of norepinephrine and dopamine, whereas extra adrenal catecholamine-secreting tumors from the thorax, abdomen, and pelvis produce norepinephrine, less frequently dopamine, but not epinephrine. This is an important differential diagnostic factor in determining the source of catecholamines, as phenylethanolamine-N-methyl transferase, the enzyme responsible for the conversion from norepinephrine to epinephrine, is primarily synthesized in the adrenal medulla and not in extra-adrenal chromaffin cells. Epinephrine, otherwise known as adrenaline, primarily increases cardiac output and increases glucose in response to an acute stress to prepare an individual for the "fight or flight" response. Similarly, norepinephrine also increases cardiac output but uniquely also increases vasoconstriction. PPGLs that result in the overproduction of these hormones can cause life-threatening HTN.[3,4]

Paragangliomas originating in the skull base and neck have parasympathetic origin, and do not produce catecholamines except in the rare cases where they produce dopamine and its metabolite 3-methoxytyramine.[4] They are typically benign, but in 17% of cases they can transform into malignant tumors.[3] Risk of malignancy is 30% to 40% higher in patients with germline succinate dehydrogenase subunit B (*SDHB*) pathogenic variants. Germline *SDHB* pathogenic variants are also associated with extra-adrenal location, large tumor size, tumor invasion, young age, positive family history, multifocal tumors, and dopaminergic biochemical phenotype.[4]

CLINICAL FEATURES

Clinical features of PPGLs that secrete excessive catecholamines are variable. The classic triad of headache, palpitations, and excessive sweating is now a more unusual presentation. In earlier stages, some individuals may have minimal, nonspecific symptoms and some may have no symptoms at all. Hypertension is seen in 90% of cases; paroxysmal hypertension in otherwise healthy, young individuals is seen in 50% of cases, and can be the first indication of catecholamine excess. Paroxysmal hypertension can subsequently present as episodic severe acute chest pain due to cardiac vasospasm, and can be mistaken for myocardial infarction or acute aortic dissection. Pheochromocytoma crisis is a rare emergency defined as hypertensive crisis or hypotension with hyperthermia (greater than 104°F), encephalopathy, multiorgan failure, with pulmonary edema and circulatory collapse.[5]

Indications for Testing for Pheochromocytoma/Paragangliomas[4,5]

1. Episodic signs and symptoms of catecholamine excess
2. Lipid poor adrenal incidentaloma, even in normotensive patients
3. Unexpected blood pressure response to surgery, drugs (e.g., β-adrenergic blocker, corticosteroids), or anesthesia
4. Unexplained blood pressure variability
5. Difficult to control blood pressure
6. Hereditary risk of PPGL in family members

7. Syndromic features related to pheochromocytoma-related hereditary syndrome
8. Previous treatment for PPGL

DIAGNOSIS

According to recent Endocrine Society guidelines, the initial screening test is biochemical testing – plasma free or urinary fractionated metanephrines using liquid chromatography with electrochemical or mass spectrometric laboratory methods.[3,4,6] Plasma fractionated metanephrines along with dopamine metabolite 3-methoxy tyramine has higher sensitivity (95%) compared to urinary fractionated metanephrines. Symptomatic PPGL can be excluded if plasma fractionated metanephrine levels are within the normal reference range.[4,6] Specificities of plasma and urine fractionated metanephrines are 96% and 89%, respectively. When measuring plasma fractionated metanephrines, blood work should be done with the patient in supine position for at least 20 minutes using reference standards using the same position to minimize false positive results.[3,4,6] False-positive test results are more common than true positives. The most common causes of false positives are medications such as levodopa, tricyclic antidepressants, and antipsychotics that falsely elevate fractionated metanephrine levels.[3] Biochemical false positives are also common in extremely stressful conditions such as severe pain, cardiac ischemia, and hypoglycemia, and in patients in intensive care units. Therefore, in these settings if the clinician has a high suspicion for PPGL, computed cross-sectional imaging of the abdomen and pelvis may be indicated.[4]

For appropriate interpretation of test results, one has to take into account the pretest probability of disease and extent of elevation above the upper limit of normal.[7] If levels are elevated more than two fold the upper limit of normal, then it is high likely that the patient has PPGL (assuming interfering medications are excluded). But, if levels are less than twice the upper limit of normal, then it is difficult to distinguish between false positives versus true positives. In those cases, the clinician should consider the medications and conditions that can cause false-positive results. If clinical suspicion is high and plasma normetanephrine is elevated, a clonidine suppression test can be done to exclude a catecholamine-secreting tumor.[6]

IMAGING

After clear biochemical evidence of PPGL is established, the next step is to localize the tumor. A computed tomography (CT) scan is preferred over magnetic resonance imaging (MRI) because of its superior spatial resolution in the thorax, abdomen, and pelvis.[3,4] An MRI is preferred in those cases with neck or skull base paragangliomas, pregnancy, or concern for metastatic disease.[4,5] An adrenal lesion with an unenhanced CT attenuation value of less than 10 Hounsfield units (HU) can reliably rule out a pheochromocytoma.[8] Even though a CT scan has higher sensitivity (greater than 90%), it has lower specificity (75% to 80%). A CT scan provides only the anatomic location of the tumor but does not provide any information on the functionality of the tumor. Pheochromocytoma size can vary anywhere from 1 to 15 cm and average approximately 4 to 6 cm upon diagnosis. Smaller tumors consist of solid, homogeneous tissue, whereas in larger tumors it is typical to see central necrosis with a peripheral rim of tumor tissue. Pheochromocytomas are usually spherical in shape, with smooth borders and morphologically can mimic other adrenal masses. Differential diagnosis should include lipid-poor adenoma, adrenal carcinoma, and metastasis.[9] Unlike lipid-rich adenomas, pheochromocytoma attenuation is always 10 HU or higher due to the absence of intracytoplasmic lipids. In targeted adrenal CT protocols, which include late enhancement scans, adenomas express rapid washout. Unfortunately, unenhanced CT attenuation and washout characteristics cannot distinguish between adrenal carcinoma and metastasis.[9]

In patients with suspicion for metastatic PPGL, functional imaging is the next step.[4,10] Functional imaging is not necessary if patients are over 40 years of age, have no family history, an adrenal tumor size less than 3 cm mainly secreting metanephrines, or have negative genetic testing.[1] In extra-adrenal tumors, regardless of tumor size or genetic testing, functional imaging is needed to stage the tumor and determine if there are additional paragangliomas. Iodine-123-metaiodobenzylguanidine (^{123}I-MIBG) scintigraphy and gallium 68 (68-Ga) 1,4,7,10-tetraazacyclododecane-1,4,7,10-tetraacetic acid (DOTA)-octreotate (DOTATATE) positron emission tomography (PET) CT can be used to identify additional PPGLs and stage the known PPGL.[3,10] ^{18}F-fluorodeoxyglucose (^{18}F-FDG) PET CT is also useful in detecting sites of metastatic disease and is preferred over ^{123}I-MIBG scintigraphy in patients with known metastatic PPGL.

GENETIC TESTING

Approximately 40% of PPGLs are inherited or familial and are associated with pathogenic variants in 15 susceptibility genes.[11] The most commonly mutated genes are *RET* proto-oncogene (multiple endocrine neoplasia type 2), von Hippel–Lindau (*VHL*), succinate dehydrogenase subunits B (*SDHB*), C (*SDHC*), D (*SDHD*), and neurofibromatosis type 1 (*NF1*) (Table 12.1). *SDHB* pathogenic variants are associated with aggressive metastatic disease (40% to 60%).[11]

Genetic testing is recommended for all patients with PPGLs, especially those with a positive family history, bilateral adrenal tumors, paraganglioma, and of younger age.[3,4] It is also recommended to counsel family members for the possibility of genetic PPGLs and recommend the evaluation of first-degree relatives.[11]

PREOPERATIVE MEDICAL MANAGEMENT

Preoperative medical management and preparation for surgery is essential to minimize the risks of a catecholamine surge during surgery, which can be fatal. Focus is aimed at controlling volume

TABLE 12.1 ■ **Common Genetic Mutations Associated With PPGL**

Syndrome	Gene	Tumor Type
MEN2a and MEN2b: Multiple Endocrine Neoplasia	*RET*	Pheochromocytoma; adrenergic biochemical phenotype; association with medullary thyroid cancer and in MEN2a with primary hyperparathyroidism
VHL: Von Hippel Lindau	*VHL*	Pheochromocytoma or paraganglioma; noradrenergic biochemical phenotype; association with clear cell renal cell carcinoma and hemangioblastomas of the central nervous system
Familial Paraganglioma, Type 1	*SDHD*	Paraganglioma (sympathetic, parasympathetic) or pheochromocytoma
Familial Paraganglioma, Type 2	*SDHAF2*	Paraganglioma (parasympathetic)
Familial Paraganglioma, Type 3	*SDHC*	Paraganglioma (parasympathetic, rarely sympathetic)
Familial Paraganglioma, Type 4	*SDHB*	Paraganglioma (parasympathetic or sympathetic) associated with renal cell cancer and thyroid tumors
Carney-Stratakis Syndrome	*SDHB* *SDHC* *SDHD*	Paraganglioma (sympathetic and parasympathetic); associated with gastrointestinal stromal tumors
Neurofibromatosis Type 1	*NF1*	Pheochromocytoma; neurofibromas; gliomas

expansion, hypertension, and tachycardia to avoid intraoperative hemodynamic instability. An electrocardiogram should be done as part of the preoperative evaluation; an echocardiogram should be ordered if there are any concerns about cardiac function. Perioperative α-adrenergic blocking agent starting at least 7 to 14 days prior to surgery is recommended. The period of α-adrenergic blockade should be longer in patients with organ damage due to long-standing catecholamine excess.[3]

The most commonly used α-adrenergic blocking agents are phenoxybenzamine and doxazosin. Phenoxybenzamine is a noncompetitive, nonselective α-adrenergic blocking agent that binds to alpha-1 and alpha-2 receptors, has a long half-life (24 to 48 hours), and is not easily overcome by catecholamine tumor burden. The initial dose is 10 mg once or twice orally daily and can be increased by 10 to 20 mg every 2 to 3 days. The final dose is usually 1 mg/kg per day but can be as high as 240 mg/day. Side effects include orthostasis, tachycardia, dizziness, fatigue, and retrograde ejaculation in males, and severe nasal congestion.[12] Phenoxybenzamine is slightly better in controlling systolic blood pressure than selective alpha-1 blockade, and it can be associated with postoperative hypotension 24 to 48 hours following treatment discontinuation; therefore, vasopressor support and intravenous fluids may be needed following surgery.[13]

Doxazosin, prazosin, and terazosin are selective alpha-1 blocking agents, which preferentially bind to alpha-1 receptors, subsequently causing vasodilation. Because these agents do not bind to alpha-2 receptors, tachycardia occurs less often compared to phenoxybenzamine. Due to their short half-life, the last dose should be given on the morning of surgery as they have a risk of inadequately controlling catecholamine release intraoperatively. Conversely, compared to phenoxybenzamine, postoperative hypotension is less likely. Side effects include vertigo, headache, gastrointestinal symptoms, and postural hypotension. Doxazosin has a 12-hour half-life and is usually administered one to two times daily with the initial dose being 1 to 2 mg/day and the maximum dose being 16 mg/day. Prazosin is initiated as a 0.5- to 1-mg dose every 4 to 6 hours and titrated to an average of 2 to 5 mg two to three times a day with a maximum total of 20 to 24 mg/day. Terazosin can be initiated at a dose of 1 mg/day, with an average of 2 to 5 mg/day and maximum dose of 20 mg/day.[13]

Calcium channel blocking agents such as nicardipine, amlodipine, nifedipine, and verapamil can also be used as an add-on therapy in controlling blood pressure preoperatively.[3,12] Calcium channel blockers inhibit norepinephrine-mediated transmembrane influx of calcium into smooth muscle cells/myocardium and therefore significantly assist in controlling hypertension and tachyarrhythmia, without the burden of causing hypotension during a normotensive state. They are useful as adjunct therapy for patients with inadequate blood pressure control to prevent the need for increasing α-adrenergic blockade agents. Calcium channel blockers can be used as an alternative for those patients who cannot tolerate α-adrenergic blockade due to its side effects or in patients with intermittent hypertension. Calcium channel blockers are also very useful in preventing catecholamine-driven coronary vasospasm.[12,13]

β-Adrenergic blockers can be used to counteract tachycardia induced by α-adrenergic blocking agents but should never be used before the initiation of α-adrenergic blockade as an unopposed α-adrenergic effect could cause severe vasoconstriction with subsequent acute cardiac failure, hypertensive crisis, and pulmonary edema. Metoprolol (starting at 12.5 mg extended release once daily and titrated for a target heart rate of 80 beats per minute) and atenolol (starting at 12.5 mg daily) are cardio-selective β-adrenergic antagonists and have less side effects than nonselective β-adrenergic antagonists.[14]

Target blood pressure should be low-normal for age and comorbidities. For example, in a 20-year-old, a systolic blood pressure of 100 mm Hg is reasonable, whereas in a 75-year-old patient with chronic kidney disease, a systolic blood pressure of 130 mm Hg would be a reasonable target. Orthostatic hypotension is not a goal of therapy, but rather a side effect of adrenergic blockade. Orthostasis can be reversed in part by a high sodium diet (5000 mg/day). There is a risk of postoperative hypotension from α-adrenergic blocking agents, hence a high-sodium diet (mentioned previously) and increased fluid intake to increase volume is recommended to decrease perioperative morbidity and mortality.[5,14]

ACUTE MEDICAL MANAGEMENT OF PPGL CAUSING HYPERTENSIVE EMERGENCY

Hypertensive emergency due to PPGL should be managed in the intensive care unit setting with intravenous drugs with a short half-life. The drug of choice for hypertensive emergency due to PPGL is the α-adrenergic blocker phentolamine (half-life of 19 minutes), which can be initiated as a 5-mg intravenous bolus, and additional boluses can be given every 10 minutes to reduce blood pressure to the target level.[14] In addition, an intravenous calcium channel blocker (e.g., intravenous nicardipine) may be used due to its peripheral and coronary vasodilation properties and ability to prevent coronary vasospasm. The initial infusion rate of intravenous nicardipine is 5 mg/hour, increased by 2.5 mg/hour every 15 minutes, with a maximum dose of 30 mg/hour. Clevidipine is also a calcium channel blocker available for intravenous use (initial dose 1 to 2 mg/hour), which has a shorter half-life; however, it is expensive and less widely available, but can achieve tighter blood pressure control with less risk of overshoot hypotension. Finally, IV sodium nitroprusside is a vasodilator with a rapid onset and short duration of effect and can be initiated at a very low rate (0.3 μg/kg per minute) and titrated every few minutes until target blood pressure is achieved; the maximum recommended infusion rate is 10 μg/kg per minute.[12,14]

SURGERY

The best surgical approach for pheochromocytomas is minimally invasive laparoscopic adrenalectomy, unless the tumor is greater than 6 cm or is invasive, in which case open resection is recommended. Posterior retroperitoneoscopic adrenalectomy is the most favorable and direct approach to the adrenal gland with the shortest surgery time due to the elimination of intraperitoneal dissection. Patient satisfaction is higher, and recovery is quicker with the retroperitoneal approach. This is due to less pain and avoidance of the major intraabdominal dissection (such as liver dissection on the right side, or spleen and colon on the left side) required to reach the adrenal glands if surgery is performed through the abdominal transperitoneal approach. Nevertheless, if there are any concerns over the possibility of malignant pheochromocytoma, based on radiologic studies, surgery should be performed through the abdominal approach, starting with laparoscopic and conversion to open if necessary. For paragangliomas, open resection is usually recommended. Partial adrenalectomy (cortical sparing) is suggested for patients with bilateral disease, or hereditary pheochromocytomas, such as MEN2 syndrome, due to a high possibility of bilateral tumors.[15,16] By sparing healthy adrenocortical tissue, it may be possible to avoid life-long glucocorticoid and mineralocorticoid replacement.

Postoperatively, the patient should be monitored closely for hemodynamic instability and hypoglycemia for 24 to 48 hours. Intravenous infusion of normal saline with dextrose as well as vasopressors/inotrope agents may be needed for volume expansion. Sudden catecholamine withdrawal following tumor removal also leads to rebound hyperinsulinemia and subsequent rebound hypoglycemia. Frequent blood glucose monitoring in the first 24 hours after surgery is needed.[12]

PATHOLOGY

All PPGLs have malignant potential. About 10% of pheochromocytomas and 20% of catecholamine-secreting paragangliomas become metastatic. The most utilized scoring system to stratify malignancy risk is the Pheochromocytoma of Adrenal Gland Scales Score (PASS) proposed by

Thompson in 2002. A PASS score of greater than or equal to 4 suggests malignant lesion. One point is given for capsular invasion, vascular invasion, profound nuclear pleomorphism, or hyperchromasia, and two points are given for invasion of periadrenal adipose tissue, focal or confluent necrosis, high cellularity, large nests or diffuse growth, spindling of tumor cells, 4+ mitotic figures per 10 high-power field (hpf), atypical mitotic features, or cellular monotony.[17]

FOLLOW-UP

Plasma or 24-hour urine fractionated metanephrines should be measured at 2 to 6 weeks postsurgery to confirm whether the tumor has been resected successfully. In the case of persistently elevated fractionated metanephrines, further imaging is recommended. The European Society of Endocrinology Clinical Practice Guideline recommends following up on plasma or urine fractionated metanephrine levels every year for at least 10 years. However, many experts recommend life-long follow-up.[18] A metaanalysis showed the risk of recurrence is around 5% during 5-year follow up.[19]

Primary Aldosteronism

Adrenal zona glomerulosa cells produce aldosterone. Aldosterone plays a significant role in hypertension in that it not only binds to mineralocorticoid receptors at renal epithelial cells to promote sodium and water reabsorption and potassium secretion but also binds to mineralocorticoid receptors at cardiomyocytes, cardiac fibroblasts, and vascular smooth muscle cells to cause vasoconstriction and subsequent hypertension. Primary aldosteronism (PA), otherwise known as Conn's syndrome, was first described by Jerome Conn in 1954 in a patient with resistant HTN with hypokalemia due to an aldosterone-producing adrenal adenoma (APA). PA is one of the most common causes of secondary hypertension.[20] PA is most commonly caused by bilateral adrenal hyperplasia (BAH) in approximately 60% to 65% of patients and by unilateral APA in 30% to 40% of patients. Very rarely, it is produced from unilateral adrenal hyperplasia, adrenocortical carcinoma, ectopic aldosterone-producing adenoma, or inherited conditions of familial hyperaldosteronism.[21]

CLINICAL FEATURES

Patients with PA can present with nonspecific symptoms such as fatigue, muscle weakness, muscle cramps, nocturia, and headaches. Clinically, patients will have hypertension but not always hypokalemia. PA can rarely present as a hypertensive emergency, with uncertain prevalence, as there are few cases reported.[20] Early diagnosis of PA is essential, as long-standing PA causes an increase in fibrosis and collagen production at the cardiac intraventricular septum and peripheral vasculature and is subsequently associated with left ventricular hypertrophy, cardiovascular disease, myocardial infarction, and stroke (the most common causes of mortality).

The Endocrine Society recommends screening for PA in patients[20] who meet one of the following criteria:

1. Sustained blood pressure above 150/100 mm Hg in three separate measurements taken on three different days
2. Resistant HTN (greater than 140/90 mm Hg) on three conventional antihypertensive medications, one including a diuretic
3. Controlled HTN (less than 140/90 mm Hg) with four or more medications
4. HTN associated with hypokalemia or adrenal incidentaloma or sleep apnea
5. HTN and family history of early onset of HTN or stroke before 40 years of age
6. HTN with first-degree relatives with PA

DIAGNOSIS

Screening for PA includes measurement of the plasma aldosterone and renin levels in the morning hours in an ambulant patient in the seated position. Plasma aldosterone concentration (PAC) greater than 10 ng/dL associated with a suppressed plasma renin concentration less than 1 ng/mL per hour or a renin concentration below the lower limit of the reference range is a positive case detection test for PA.

However, case detection testing lacks sensitivity and specificity. All patients with positive case detection testing should have PA confirmed with an additional test. Confirmatory testing can be completed using one of the four recommended methods: oral sodium loading with measurement of 24-hour urine aldosterone excretion, the saline infusion test (SIT) over 4 hours, the fludrocortisone suppression test (FST), or the captopril challenge test (CCT). No test is superior to another, and the test is usually chosen based on patient preference, cost, and local expertise. However, in patients with spontaneous hypokalemia with undetectable renin levels and PAC greater than 20 ng/dL, further confirmatory testing is not needed.[20,22]

For the oral sodium loading test, salt intake is increased to 5 g/day for 3 days (confirmed by 24-hour urine sodium content greater than 200 mmol) and slow-release potassium chloride is given to maintain plasma potassium in the normal range. Urinary aldosterone is measured in the 24-hour urine collection between the mornings of day 3 to day 4. An aldosterone level greater than 12 μg/24-hour in a patient with suppressed renin confirms the diagnosis of PA. The SIT should be done in the seated position with 2 L of normal saline infused over 4 hours starting at 8:00 a.m. Levels of renin, aldosterone, cortisol, and plasma potassium are drawn at time 0 and 4 hours. PAC greater than 10 ng/dL confirms PA and levels above 5 ng/dL but less than 10 ng/dL represent a gray zone and are highly suggestive of PA.[20,22]

The FST requires hospitalization for 4 days and is rarely performed anymore.[20,22]

For the CCT, the patient receives 25 or 50 mg of captopril orally while seated. Plasma renin, aldosterone, and cortisol levels are drawn at time 0 and 2 hours after captopril administration. In patients with PA, aldosterone remains elevated and renin remains suppressed following the challenge.[20,22]

IMAGING

After the diagnosis of PA is confirmed, all patients should undergo an adrenal CT scan to localize the tumor as an initial subtype testing. The CT scan also provides details about the size of the adrenal adenoma and any characteristics of malignancy such as irregular borders, delayed washout, local invasion, etc. In bilateral adrenal hyperplasia, the CT scan may show normal-appearing adrenal glands or nodular changes, whereas unilateral APA usually present as microadenomas (less than 1 cm) and may not be visible on CT. Hence, the CT scan can be inaccurate in nearly half of the cases with risk of missing APA or BAH. If a nodule is found on a CT scan, it may be nonfunctioning and unrelated to the diagnosis of PA. Multiple studies have demonstrated that the CT or MRI scan should be used in conjunction with adrenal venous sampling (AVS) to localize the source of PA accurately. Hence, in almost all patients, AVS is a prerequisite before proceeding to surgery. Even though there was an exception not to use AVS in patients younger than 40 years of age with confirmed PA and hypokalemia with normal kidney function, more recent reports recommended to use AVS in all patients with PA.[23–25]

ADRENAL VENOUS SAMPLING

AVS should be done by an experienced interventional radiologist. It can be done either simultaneously or sequentially with or without cosyntropin administration. Cosyntropin increases the blood supply to the adrenal glands, and therefore the adrenal veins can be more easily catheterized. AVS test results are interpreted by measuring adrenal vein aldosterone to cortisol (A/C) concentration in bilateral adrenal veins and A/C concentration in the peripheral vein. The A/C ratio of the dominant to nondominant side is termed the *aldosterone lateralization index* (LI). If AVS is done following cosyntropin, an LI of greater than 4 indicates a unilateral source of aldosterone hypersecretion. If the LI is less than 2, then there is no lateralization, which indicates bilateral adrenal hyperplasia. If AVS is done without cosyntropin, then an aldosterone LI ratio of greater than 2 is used as positive lateralization by some experts. When the nondominant adrenal A/C is lower than the peripheral vein A/C, it is called *contralateral suppression* and is typically found in patients with unilateral adrenal disease. When the aldosterone LI is between 2 and 4, if there is contralateral suppression, patients would likely benefit from unilateral adrenalectomy.[20,22,26]

TREATMENT

Treatment is based on multiple factors including the patient's preference, comorbidities, age, and unilateral versus bilateral PA. For unilateral adrenal hyperplasia or unilateral APA, laparoscopic unilateral adrenalectomy is preferred if the patient is willing to undergo surgery with an acceptable risk. The anterior laparoscopic approach is the most commonly performed method, although some specialized centers also perform retroperitoneoscopic approaches, which is the most direct approach to the adrenal gland with a shorter surgery time and quicker patient recovery (see prior section on surgical treatment of PPGL).[27] In nearly half of all patients, HTN is cured after unilateral adrenalectomy and HTN improved in 100% of patients.[20,22]

For BAH or poor surgical candidates, medical therapy with mineralocorticoid receptor (MR) antagonists is recommended.[20,21] Spironolactone and eplerenone are two available MR antagonists. The starting dose for spironolactone should be 12.5 mg to 25 mg daily; gradual titration upward is needed to find the lowest effective dose. The starting dose for eplerenone should be 25 mg twice daily. The dose of the MR antagonist should be titrated for a target serum potassium concentration of 4.5 mmol/L without the aid of potassium supplementation. With each change in the dosage of the MR antagonist, serum potassium and creatinine should be checked 7 to 10 days later. Caution should be used if MR antagonists are used in patients with chronic kidney disease and should be avoided in patients with stage IV or higher kidney disease due to the risk of life-threatening hyperkalemia.[20,26,28] Hypervolemia can be prohibitive in the use of MR antagonists as monotherapy, and in approximately 50% of patients, a second agent, such as low-dose thiazide diuretic, calcium channel blockers, angiotensin-converting enzyme inhibitors, and angiotensin receptor blockers, have been employed as secondary agents in PA.[20,26,28]

ACUTE MEDICAL MANAGEMENT OF HYPERTENSIVE EMERGENCY CAUSED BY PRIMARY HYPERALDOSTERONISM

The choice of therapy in the case of hypertensive emergency depends on the end organ damage involved. Close monitoring in the intensive care unit setting is necessary and continuous infusion of titratable, short-acting intravenous antihypertensive agents are used to reduce blood pressure in order to limit further end organ damage. Intravenously administered nicardipine (5 to 30 mg/hour) is a calcium channel blocker that can prevent vasospasm and is useful in cases of hypertensive encephalopathy and hemorrhagic stroke. Labetalol (20 to 80 mg administered as an intravenous bolus every 10 minutes or a continuous infusion at a rate of 0.5 to 2 mg/minute) or nitroprusside (0.25 to 10 μg/kg per minute) are also preferred agents. In the setting of acute myocardial infarction, nitroglycerin (5 to 100 μg/minute), labetalol (20 to 80 mg intravenous bolus every 10 minutes or continuous infusion 0.5 to 2 mg/minute), or nitroprusside (0.25 to 10 μg/kg per minute) could be used to increase coronary perfusion and decrease afterload. Lowering the diastolic blood pressure to less than 60 mm Hg can risk a decrease in coronary and renal perfusion and worsening of myocardial ischemia and acute kidney injury, respectively. For acute left ventricular heart failure, nitroglycerin (5 to 100 μg/minute), nitroprusside (0.25 to 10 μg/kg per minute), or enalaprilat (1.25 to 5 mg every 6 hours) are used to decrease afterload. In acute heart failure, β-adrenergic blockers should be avoided.[14,21]

Cushing's Syndrome

CS is another rare endocrine cause of hypertensive emergency. It is a result of hypercortisolism, most commonly caused by iatrogenic or exogenous administration of glucocorticoids. Endogenous production is rare, with an estimated incidence of 2 to 3 cases per million people per year.[29] Endogenous hypercortisolism is caused most commonly by corticotropin (ACTH)-producing tumors in the pituitary gland (CD) in 70% to 85% of cases.[29,30] Endogenous CS is caused by ectopic ACTH production in 15% of cases and by ACTH-independent adrenal pathology in 15% of cases.

CLINICAL PRESENTATION

Clinical features vary from patient to patient, which may include central adiposity, moon faces, supraclavicular fat distribution, wide purple-red striae, proximal muscle weakness, osteoporosis, glucose intolerance, HTN, dyslipidemia, obesity, easy bruising, psychiatric disturbances, amenorrhea, hirsutism, and decreased libido. HTN is prevalent in 75% to 80% of cases of CS.[30] Proposed mechanisms for HTN include increased production of deoxycorticosterone, increased sensitivity to catecholamines, angiotensin II, enhanced cardiac output, increased hepatic production of angiotensinogen, and mineralocorticoid effects of cortisol. Hypertension in CS is significantly correlated with the duration of hypercortisolism and early recognition is important.[30] Cardiovascular disease, infections, and venous thrombosis are the most common causes of mortality in CS.[29] Very rarely, CS presents with hypertensive emergency, which may be associated with acute pulmonary edema and hypertensive encephalopathy, with only a few cases reported.[31]

DIAGNOSIS

Screening for CS should be considered in patients with signs and symptoms consistent with hypercortisolism. In addition, all patients with incidentally discovered adrenal masses should be screened for autonomous glucocorticoid secretion. The Endocrine Society recommends one of four tests as an initial screening test: 1-mg overnight dexamethasone suppression test (DST); 24-hour urine free cortisol (UFC, two measurements); late-night salivary cortisol (LNSC, two measurements); and formal 2-day low-dose DST (0.5 mg dexamethasone every 6 hours × 8). The overnight DST requires the administration of 1 mg of dexamethasone between 11:00 p.m. and midnight and the cortisol level to be drawn at 8:00 a.m. the following morning. LNSC can be performed at home using a designated lab cotton Salivette (multiple manufacturers) for the patient to collect a saliva sample at 11:00 p.m. at night on two separate nights. Serum cortisol at 8:00 a.m. after the 1-mg DST greater than 1.8 μg/dL, LNSC greater than 145 ng/dL, or 24-hour UFC level above the upper limit of normal are considered positive case detection results. If one of the aforementioned test results are positive, consider performing one or two other tests and repeating the abnormal test. False-positive test results can be seen in pregnancy, depression, alcohol dependence, poorly controlled diabetes mellitus, physical stress, intense exercise, etc. If two tests are positive, then further testing to establish the cause of CS is recommended.[29] The first step is to check serum ACTH. Suppressed ACTH levels (less than 10 pg/mL) suggest ACTH-independent CS caused by primary adrenal gland pathology. A CT or MRI of the abdomen is performed in such cases to identify unilateral or bilateral adrenal lesions and to help differentiate between benign versus malignancy. ACTH-independent CS is caused by a unilateral cortisol-secreting adrenal adenoma in 60% and adrenocortical carcinoma (ACC) in 40% of cases, and very rarely by primary pigmented nodular adrenal disease (PPNAD) and bilateral macronodular adrenal hyperplasia (BMAH). On CT, cortisol-secreting adrenal adenomas are typically round to oval with smooth borders and are frequently lipid poor (greater than 10 HU). Features of ACC on a CT scan include: large size (mean diameter 9 cm) with irregular borders; intratumoral necrosis; hemorrhage and calcifications (30% of cases); and lipid poor (greater than 20 HU). In 9% to 19% of cases, ACC may invade the renal vein or inferior vena cava.[32] On contrast-enhanced CT, an absolute contrast washout of greater than 60% and relative contrast washout of greater than 40% indicate adrenal adenoma with high sensitivity and specificity. PPNAD presents as normal or slightly enlarged adrenal glands with multiple small nodules of less than 6 mm,[33] whereas BMAH presents with massively enlarged and multinodular adrenal glands.

Inappropriately normal or elevated ACTH levels greater than 20 pg/mL in a patient with hypercortisolism are consistent with ACTH-dependent CS. Serum ACTH levels of 10 to 20 pg/mL are considered indeterminate and could be from cyclical or mild CS or falsely detectable due to lab error or heterophile antibodies.

Dehydroepiandrosterone sulfate (DHEA-S) is an adrenal androgen that is regulated by ACTH. Hence, serum DHEA-S concentrations are normal or high in CD, whereas it is low in the benign causes of ACTH-independent CS. Measuring DHEA-S level is particularly useful in patients with subclinical hypercortisolism (SH) with adrenal incidentalomas[34] or indeterminate ACTH levels. SH is a condition with hypercortisolism but without the typical symptoms and signs of hypercortisolism. In one study, DHEA-S was found to be significantly low in SH patients compared to age-matched controls, and low DHEA-S levels (less than 40 μg/dL) can be used as a diagnostic marker for SH.[35]

Once ACTH-dependent CS is confirmed, the clinician must localize the source of ACTH secretion. Pituitary-dependent CS typically occurs in women and is slow in onset and relatively mild in degree of signs and symptoms and cortisol excess (e.g., 24-hour UFC less than 500 μg), whereas ectopic ACTH-dependent CS occurs equally in men and women and is typically more rapid in onset, with more severe signs and symptoms and cortisol excess (e.g., 24-hour UFC greater than 1000 μg). A pituitary-directed MRI scan is the first step in distinguishing pituitary-dependent CS from ectopic ACTH. When a clear-cut pituitary adenoma is detected in a woman with slow onset and mild-to-moderate CS, no further localization studies may be needed, whereas if a small pituitary adenoma is detected in a patient with severe CS, it may be a nonfunctioning pituitary tumor and additional testing is needed.[36,37] Bilateral inferior petrosal sinus sampling (BIPSS) is the gold-standard test to distinguish between pituitary-dependent CS and ectopic ACTH syndrome; sensitivity and specificity are greater than 95%. Based on BIPSS results, if there is a central to peripheral ACTH gradient of 2.0 or greater before corticotrophin-releasing hormone (CRH) administration and 3.0 or greater post-CRH, CD is confirmed.[36,37]

CT or MRI of chest and abdomen and pelvis is the first step in imaging to localize the source of ectopic ACTH secretion (EAS). CT or MRI do not reveal any source in around 50% of cases and functional imaging with an octreotide scan or ^{68}Ga-DOTATATE PET/CT is the next step.[36,38] ^{68}Ga-DOTATATE PET/CT imaging has shown promising results in identifying source of EAS in 18 of 22 patients in a recent study.[32,36]

TREATMENT

Surgery

Pituitary surgery is the recommended initial treatment for CD with overall remission rates of 80%,[29,36] whereas adrenal-directed surgery is the treatment of choice for all primary adrenal forms of CS. If there is a suspicion for adrenocortical carcinoma, the anterior laparoscopic approach should be attempted with a low threshold of conversion to open adrenalectomy. The surgeon should be prepared for more extensive surgical resection in the case of invasion into the surrounding organs such as the inferior vena cava (IVC) or liver (on the right), and spleen pancreas, stomach, or colon (on the left). In the case of obvious cortisol-producing adrenocortical carcinoma, the possibility of IVC thrombus extension up to the right atrium should be evaluated prior to surgery by imaging studies. If present, a cardiac surgeon should be involved with the understanding that removal of the atrium thrombus may require a cardiac bypass. Unilateral adrenalectomy is the preferred treatment of choice in patients with cortisol-secreting adrenal adenoma. Bilateral laparoscopic adrenalectomy might be needed for those patients with pituitary-dependent disease when the patient is not cured with pituitary surgery or in those patients with ectopic ACTH syndrome when the ACTH-secreting neoplasm cannot be localized or cannot be resected. In those cases, life-long replacement of glucocorticoid and mineralocorticoid replacement is essential. In patients with pituitary-dependent disease and those with unilateral adrenal dependent disease, postoperative glucocorticoid replacement is necessary until the hypothalamic pituitary adrenal axis recovers (usually 6 to 12 months).

Radiation Therapy

When pituitary surgery is not curative in patients with CD, radiation therapy can be considered if the degree of CS is mild. Radiation therapy is optimally administered with a stereotactic method. Medical therapy is required until radiation therapy becomes effective. A side effect of pituitary radiation therapy is varying degrees of hypopituitarism.[36]

Medical Therapy

Medical therapy is a second-line option of treatment in patients where surgery was not curative or for those who are poor surgical candidates. Available medical treatments include: steroidogenesis inhibitors (e.g., ketoconazole, metyrapone, mitotane, etomidate); somatostatin receptor agonists; dopamine agonists; and glucocorticoid receptor antagonists (e.g., mifepristone). Combination therapy is required in some cases at low doses to achieve cortisol control. Patients treated with medical therapy are at risk of adrenal insufficiency and should be counseled about the risks of adrenal crisis and emergency use of glucocorticoids.[36] Table 12.2 shows different medications, their mechanism of action, dosage, and effect on cortisol and blood pressure.[39]

ACUTE MEDICAL MANAGEMENT OF HYPERTENSIVE EMERGENCY CAUSED BY HYPERCORTISOLISM

Acute pulmonary edema or hypertensive encephalopathy, although very rare, are the more common presentations of hypertensive emergency in patients with CS. In these cases, management in the intensive care unit is necessary to prevent further end organ damage. Intravenous hypertensive medications for acute pulmonary edema and hypertensive encephalopathy include: nicardipine (5 to 30 mg/hour), which can decrease vasospasm; labetalol (20 to 80 mg intravenous bolus every 10 minutes or continuous infusion of 0.5 to 2 mg/minute); and nitroprusside (0.25 to 10 μg/kg per minute). Nitroglycerin (5 to 100 μg/minute), nitroprusside (0.25 to 10 μg/kg per minute), or enalaprilat (1.25 to 5 mg every 6 hours) can be used to decrease afterload.[13]

There have been studies reporting the continuous infusion of etomidate for the control of severe CS. Etomidate, an imidazole derivative similar to ketoconazole, which is usually used as an induction agent for intubation, rapidly decreases steroidogenesis by inhibiting 11β-hydroxylase and inhibiting the side cleavage enzyme. In one study, etomidate was initiated at a rate of 0.02 to 0.04 mg/kg per hour (up-titrated in increments of 0.01 to 0.02 mg/kg per hour) and serum cortisol was measured every 6 hours to target a cortisol concentration of 10 to 20 μg/dL and as a bridge to surgery.[40,41]

TABLE 12.2 ■ **Common Medications for Endogenous Hypercortisolism**

Drug	Mechanism of Action	Dose	Hormone Control	BP Control
Cabergoline	Dopamine agonist	Oral 0.5–7 mg/week	25%–40%	Decrease
Pasireotide	Somatostatin analog, SSRT5	SC 0.3–1.8 mg/day Twice a day	20%–62%	Decrease
Metyrapone	11β-hydroxylase inhibitor	Oral, 0.5–6 g/day 3–4 times/day	45%–100%	Neutral
Ketoconazole	11β-hydroxylase and 17α-hydroxylase inhibitor	Oral 200–1200 mg/day 2–3 times/day	~50%	Decrease
Osilodrostat	11β-hydroxylase and aldosterone synthase inhibitor	Oral, 4–60 mg/day 2 times/day	~90%	Neutral
Mitotane	Inhibits steroid synthesis, adrenolytic agent	Oral, 2–5 g/day 2–3 times/day	~70%	Decrease
Mifepristone	Glucocorticoid receptor antagonist	Oral, 300–1200 mg/day once daily	NA	Increase/decrease

BP, Blood pressure; *SC*, subcutaneous.

References

1. Brathwaite L, Reif M. Hypertensive emergencies: a review of common presentations and treatment options. *Cardiol Clin.* 2019;37(3):275–286.
2. Pappachan JM, Buch HN. Endocrine hypertension: a practical approach. *Adv Exp Med Biol.* 2017; 956:215–237.
3. Davison AS, Jones DM, Ruthven S, Helliwell T, Shore SL. Clinical evaluation and treatment of phaeochromocytoma. *Ann Clin Biochem.* 2018;55(1):34–48.
4. Jacques WML, Graeme E. Update on modern management of pheochromocytoma and paraganglioma. *Endocrinol Metab.* 2017;32(2):152–161.
5. Pappachan JM, Tunn NN, Arunagirinathan G, Sodi R, Hanna FWF. Pheochromocytomas and hypertension. *Curr Hyperten Rep.* 2018;20(1):3.
6. Eisenhofer G, Peitzsch M. Laboratory evaluation of pheochromocytoma and paraganglioma. *Chem.* 2014;60:1486–1499.
7. van Berkel A, Lenders JW, Timmers HJ. Diagnosis of endocrine disease: biochemical diagnosis of phaeochromocytoma and paraganglioma. *Eur J Endocrinol.* 2014;170(3):R109–R119.
8. Buitenwerf E, Berends AMA, van Asselt ADI, et al. Diagnostic accuracy of computed tomography to exclude pheochromocytoma: a systematic review, meta-analysis, and cost analysis. *Mayo Clin Proc.* 2019;94(10):2040–2052.
9. Filip C, Pavel K, Schovneck J. Current diagnostic imaging of pheochromocytomas and implications for therapeutic strategy. *Exp Ther Med.* 2018;15(4):3151–3160.
10. Taieb D, Timmers HJ, Hindie E, et al. EANM 2012 guidelines for radionuclide imaging of phaeochromocytoma and paraganglioma. *Eur J Nucl Med Mol Imaging.* 2012;39:1977–1995.
11. Dahia PL. Pheochromocytoma and paraganglioma pathogenesis: learning from genetic heterogeneity. *Nat Rev Cancer.* 2014;14(2):108–119.
12. Challis BG, Casey RT, Simpson HLD, Gurnell M. Is there optimal preoperative management strategy for phaeochromocytoma/paraganglioma? *Clin Endocrinol (Oxf).* 2017;86(2):163–167.

13. van der Zee PA, de Boer A. Pheochromocytoma: a review on preoperative treatment with phenoxybenzamine or doxazosin. *Neth J Med.* 2014;72:190–201.
14. Muiesan ML, Salvetti M, Amadoro V, et al. An update on hypertensive emergencies and urgencies. *J Cardiovasc Med.* 2015;16(5):372–382.
15. Neumann HPH, Tsoy U, Bancos I, et al. International Bilateral-Pheochromocytoma-Registry Group. Comparison of pheochromocytoma-specific morbidity and mortality among adults with bilateral pheochromocytomas undergoing total adrenalectomy vs cortical-sparing adrenalectomy. *JAMA Netw Open.* 2019;2(8):e198898.
16. Walz MK, Alesina PF, Wenger FA, et al. Laparoscopic and retroperitoneoscopic treatment of pheochromocytomas and retroperitoneal paragangliomas: results of 161 tumors in 126 patients. *World J Surg.* 2006;30(5):899–908.
17. Thompson LD. Pheochromocytoma of the adrenal gland scaled score (PASS) to separate benign from malignant neoplasms: a clinicopatholoci and immunopheotypic study of 100 cases. *Am J Surg Pathol.* 2002;26(5):551–566.
18. Plouin PF, Amar L, Dekkers OM, et al. European Society of Endocrinology clinical practice guideline for long-term follow-up of patients operated on for a phaeochromocytoma or a paraganglioma. *Eur J Endocrinol.* 2016;174:G1–G10.
19. Amar L, Lussey-Lepoutre C, Lenders JW, Djadi-Prat J, Plouin PF, Steichen O. Management of endocrine disease: recurrence or new tumors after complete resection of pheochromocytomas and paragangliomas: a systematic review and meta-analysis. *Eur J Endocrinol.* 2016;175:R135–R145.
20. John WF, Robert MC, Franco M, et al. The management of primary aldosteronism: case detection, diagnosis, and treatment. *J Clin Endocrinol Metab.* 2016;101:1889–1916.
21. Aronova A, Fahey III TJ, Zarnegar R. Management of hypertension in primary aldosteronism. *World J Cardiol.* 2014;6(5):227–233.
22. Vaidya A, Malchoff CD, Auchus RJ. An individualized approach to the evaluation and management of primary aldosteronism. *Endocr Pract.* 2017;23(6):680–689.
23. Mathur A, Kemp CD, Dutta U, et al. Consequences of adrenal venous sampling in primary hyperaldosteronism and predictors of unilateral adrenal disease. *J Am Coll Surg.* 2010;211(3):384–390.
24. Rossi GP, Rossitto G, Amar L, et al. Clinical outcomes of 1625 patients with primary aldosteronism subtyped with adrenal vein sampling. *Hypertension.* 2019;74(4):800–808.
25. Asmar M, Wachtel H, Yan Y, Fraker DL, Cohen D, Trerotola SO. Reversing the established order: should adrenal venous sampling precede cross-sectional imaging in the evaluation of primary aldosteronism? *J Surg Oncol.* 2015;112(2):144–148.
26. Vilela LAP, Almeida MQ. Diagnosis and management of primary aldosteronism. *Arch Endocrinol Metgab.* 2017;61(3):305–312.
27. Walz MK, Gwosdz R, Levin SL, et al. Retroperitoneoscopic adrenalectomy in Conn's syndrome caused by adrenal adenomas or nodular hyperplasia. *World J Surg.* 2008;32(5):847–853.
28. Williams TA, Reincke M. Management of endocrine disease: diagnosis and management of primary aldosteronism: the Endocrine Society guideline 2016 revisited. *Eur J Endocrinol.* 2018;179(1):R19–R29.
29. Nieman LK, Biller BMK, Findling JW, et al. Treatment of Cushing's syndrome: an Endocrine Society clinical practice guideline. *J Clin Endocrinol Metab.* 2015;100(8):2807–2831.
30. Young Jr WF, Calhoun DA, Lenders JWM, Stowasser S, Textor SC. Screening for endocrine hypertension: an Endocrine Society scientific statement. *Endocrine Rev.* 2017;38(2):103–122.
31. Alagoma I, Arthur O. Hypertensive encephalopathy as the initial manifestation of Cushing's syndrome. *J Med Res.* 2016;2(6):144–145.
32. Isidori AM, Sbardella E, Zatelli MC. Conventional and nuclear medicine imaging in ectopic Cushing's syndrome: a systematic review. *J Clin Endocrinol Metab.* 2015;100(9):3231–3244.
33. Nicolaus AWB, Ali B, Mouhammed AH, et al. Cushing syndrome: diagnostic workup and imaging features, with clinical and pathological correlation. *Am J Roentgenol.* 2017;209(1):19–32.
34. Dennedy MC, Annamalai AK, Prankerd-Smith O, et al. Low DHEAS: a sensitive and specific test for the detection of subclinical hypercortisolism in adrenal incidentalomas. *J Clin Endocrinol Metab.* 2017;102(3):786–792.
35. Yener S, Yilmaz H, Demir T, Secil M, Comlekci A. DHEAS for the prediction of subclinical Cushing's syndrome: perplexing or advantageous? *Endocrine.* 2015;48(2):669–676.

36. Susmeeta TS. An individualized approach to the evaluation of Cushing syndrome. *Endocr Pract.* 2017; 23(6):726–737.
37. Andre L, Richard AF, Constatine AS, Lynnette KN. Cushing's syndrome. *Lancet.* 2015;386(9996):913–927.
38. Marina SZ, Lynnette KN. Utility of various functional and anatomic imaging modalities for detection of ectopic adrenocorticotropin-secreting tumors. *J Clin Endocrinol Metab.* 2010;95(3):1207–1219.
39. Barbot M, Ceccato F, Scaroni C. The pathophysiology and treatment of hypertension in patient with Cushing's syndrome. *Front Endocrinol (Lausanne).* 2019;10:321.
40. Lenders JW, Duh QY, Eisenhofer G, et al. Pheochromocytoma and paraganglioma: an endocrine society clinical practice guideline. *J Clin Endocrinol Metab.* 2014;99:1915–1942.
41. Carroll Ty B, Peppard WJ, Hermann DJ, et al. Continuous etomidate infusion for management of severe Cushing syndrome: validation of a standard protocol. *J Endocr Soc.* 2019;3(1):1–12.

CHAPTER 13

Pheochromocytoma: Perioperative and Intraoperative Management

Maureen McCartney Anderson ■ Tara Corrigan ■ Alexander Shifrin

CHAPTER OUTLINE

Incidence, Clinical Significance, and Diagnosis

Pheochromocytoma is defined as a tumor arising from the chromaffin cells in the adrenal medulla that produces catecholamines: norepinephrine, epinephrine, and dopamine.[1] The incidence of pheochromocytoma in the hypertensive population is 0.1% to 0.6%.[2] It has been reported that approximately 5% of patients with an incidental finding of adrenal masses on imaging have a pheochromocytoma.[1] Pheochromocytomas can occur sporadically or can be inherited, and at least one-third of patients have an inheritable germline mutation.[1]

With a patient presenting with an incidental finding of adrenal nodule or with hypertension, it is prudent to confirm the presence and treat pheochromocytomas. The hypersecretion of catecholamines can lead to significant cardiovascular morbidity and mortality.[1] Hypertensive crisis as defined by systolic blood pressure greater than 180 mm Hg and diastolic pressure of greater than 120 mm Hg, with or without end organ failure, can be elicited through tumor manipulation from surgery, exercise, various medications such as beta blockers, corticosteroids, and intravenous contrast.[3,4] Recurrent episodes of catecholamine excess can result in myocyte necrosis and inflammation leading to cardiomyopathy.[4] In addition to the cardiovascular morbidity, at least 10% to 15% of pheochromocytomas are malignant.[1] Malignant is defined as the presence of metastasis at sites where chromaffin histology is not usually present.[1]

The classic symptoms of pheochromocytoma include headache, palpitations, or diaphoresis in hypertensive patients, although some patients present normotensive with the less common symptoms of fatigue, nausea, flushing, or orthostatic hypotension.[5] Patients may also present with signs of end organ failure from hypertensive crisis including myocardial infarction, arrythmia, or stroke.[5] As discussed earlier, up to a third of pheochromocytomas can be inheritable, so it is important to screen patients with the following diseases: multiple endocrine neoplasia type A/B, Von Hippel–Lindau disease, and neurofibromatosis type 1.[4]

Diagnosis of pheochromocytoma can be confirmed with biochemical testing (plasma and urine) as well as anatomic imaging. The Endocrine Society Clinical Practice Guidelines on Pheochromocytoma and Paraganglioma published in 2014 recommend taking measurements of plasma free metanephrines or urinary fractioned metanephrines.[1] This recommendation is echoed by the European Society of Endocrinology Clinical Practice Guidelines with measurements of plasma and urinary metanephrines as well as a chromogranin A.[6]

Measurements of plasma free metanephrines or urinary fractioned metanephrines are the initial testing for patients suspected of pheochromocytoma.[1] Plasma metanephrines have the highest sensitivity (99%) and specificity (89%) for diagnosis.[4] Levels greater than or equal to three times the upper reference value for either metanephrine or normetanephrine should be considered highly suspicious for pheochromocytoma.[2] Where values are not indicative of pheochromocytoma but are mildly elevated, tests should be repeated with prudence to evaluate if offending medications (i.e., levodopa, acetaminophen, certain beta blockers, or antidepressants) can be eliminated. Make sure the test is performed with the patient in a supine position for at least 30 minutes.[2]

Modalities for initial anatomic imaging include computed tomography (CT) and magnetic resonance imaging (MRI). Recommendation 2.2 from the Endocrine Society guidelines suggests CT instead of MRI as the first choice imaging due to its spatial resolution for the abdomen, pelvis, and thorax.[1] Sensitivity for localization on CT with contrast for pheochromocytomas is between 88% and 100%.[1] More than 85% of pheochromocytomas elicit a mean attenuation of more than 10 Hounsfield units on unenhanced CT.[1] On MRI scans, two-thirds of pheochromocytomas show increased signal intensity on T2-weighted images.[2] Functional imaging such as ^{123}I-metaiodobenzylguanidine (MIBG) and ^{18}F-fluorodihydroxy-phenylalanine (^{18}F-FDG) positron-emission tomography (PET)/CT scanning have been recommended for patients with metastatic disease.[1] The Endocrine Society guidelines suggest ^{18}F-FDG PET/CT as the preferred imaging modality for known metastatic disease.[1] The sensitivity of ^{18}F-FDG PET was reported to be between 74% and 100% for patients with metastatic disease.[1]

Once biochemical diagnosis and imaging confirm pheochromocytoma, the treatment of choice is surgical excision. Minimally invasive adrenalectomy is recommended for most pheochromocytomas.[1] Laparoscopic (lateral transabdominal/transperitoneal) or posterior retroperitoneoscopic approaches are the gold standard for pheochromocytomas, for masses less than 6 cm.[7] Open resection is reserved for large adrenal masses greater than 6 cm or invasive tumors to ensure complete tumor resection, prevent the rupture of the tumor capsule, and to prevent local recurrence.[1] A laparoscopic approach is associated with less blood loss, less pain, less hospital days, and less surgical morbidity than open adrenalectomy.[1]

Preoperative Management

CATECHOLAMINES AND ADRENORECEPTORS

An excess surge of catecholamines, both epinephrine and norepinephrine, produce different effects on the adrenoreceptors on the body's various organ systems. Both epinephrine and norepinephrine stimulate the alpha receptors that produce vasoconstriction, which leads to either paroxysmal or sustained hypertension. Beta 1 receptors located in the cardiovascular system stimulated by both epinephrine and norepinephrine result in increased heart rate and contractility, also contributing to hypertension. The epinephrine stimulation of beta 2 receptors located in the bronchioles of the lungs and the arteries of skeletal muscle cause vasodilation. In addition, epinephrine stimulates glycogenolysis and gluconeogenesis, resulting in hyperglycemia. Understanding the effects of catecholamine excess can help the clinician in the preoperative management of the pheochromocytoma patient with appropriate alpha blockade, as well as helping the clinician anticipate the possible postoperative complications following catecholamine withdrawal.

The Endocrine Society guidelines recommend that all patients with functional pheochromocytoma should have preoperative blockade to prevent perioperative complications.[1] Perioperative complications from induction of anesthesia to tumor manipulation may lead to severe hemodynamic instability leading to reduced cardiac output resulting in end organ ischemia.[7] Successful preoperative alpha blockade has reduced the number of perioperative complications to less than 3%.[5] α-Adrenergic blockers are the first-line drugs of choice, followed by the add on support of calcium channel blockers and beta blockers.[1] The length of blockade preoperatively is for 7 to 14 days to allow for control of hypertension and heart rate.[1] In our practice, we tend to increase the length of alpha blockade to about 3 to 4 weeks to assure an adequate and stable control of blood pressure. The goal of therapy is to have blood pressure less than 130/80 mm Hg while sitting and systolic pressure greater than 90 mm Hg and heart rate of 60 to 70 beats per minute when seated and 70 to 80 beats per minute when standing.[1,2] Although this is a good goal for older patients with preexisting hypertension, for younger and healthy patients we try to reach blood pressure goals of between 110/60 mm Hg to 120/70 mm Hg. In addition to the antihypertensive medications mentioned previously, a liberal high-sodium diet of 5000 mg for at least 3 to 5 days prior to the procedure, as well as increased fluid intake to counteract the catecholamine-induced volume contraction, is started.[1,8]

ALPHA ADRENERGIC BLOCKERS

Phenoxybenzamine is a noncompetitive, nonselective α-adrenergic blockade for both alpha 1 and 2 receptors.[9] It blocks postganglionic synapses in exocrine glands and smooth muscle.[10] Phenoxybenzamine onset of action is about 2 hours, its maximum effect is reached in 4 to 6 hours, and it has a half-life of 24 hours.[10] The recommended starting dose is 10 mg by mouth twice daily, with titration by increasing to 10 to 20 mg every 2 to 3 days until the blood pressure goal is reached, to a maximum of 1 mg/kg per day.[1,9] Common adverse side effects include reflex tachycardia, orthostatic hypotension, drowsiness, fatigue, miosis, and nasal congestion.[10] It has been reported that, due to its longer half-life, intraoperative hemodynamics are better controlled during tumor manipulation but the occurrence of postoperative hypotension is more frequent than the alpha 1 selective α-adrenergic blockers. It is of note and important to consider when prescribing to patients with limited medical insurance coverage that phenoxybenzamine is considerably more expensive than an alpha 1 selective blocker, costing over $100 per capsule compared with 0.50 cent to $1.

Selective α1-adrenergic blockers include prazosin, doxazosin, and terazosin. They competitively inhibit postsynaptic α1-adrenergic receptors, which in return vasodilate veins and arterioles to decrease total peripheral resistance and blood pressure.[10] Due to their shorter half-life than phenoxybenzamine, α1-selective blockers are associated with less postoperative hypotension.[8] The longest half-life of the selective α1-adrenergic blockers is doxazosin, which accounts for its once/day dosing, starting at 1 to 2 mg/day with dose titration to desired effects up to 16 mg/day.[1,2,10] Time to peak effect is approximately 2 to 3 hours, which may lead to a side effect of orthostatic hypotension; patients are urged to take it at night prior to going to bed.[3,10] Prazosin is administered in doses of 1 mg 2 to 3 times per day up to 15 mg/day in two to three divided doses, and terazosin is given in doses of 1 to 5 mg/day to a maximum of 20 mg/day.[2,3,10] Common adverse reactions of selective alpha 1 blockers include orthostatic hypotension, central nervous system depression, drowsiness, dizziness, fatigue, and weakness. Selective alpha blockers are associated with less reflex tachycardia than phenoxybenzamine.[8] This is due to the preferential alpha 1 blockade causing vasodilation to the lesser extent of binding to alpha 2 unlike phenoxybenzamine that causes the reflex tachycardia.[9] They are also less expensive, making them a more attractive choice for pheochromocytoma patients.

Calcium channel blockers are added as an adjunct to alpha blockage for patients when blood pressure goals are not achieved, or patients are intolerable to the side effects of alpha blockade, or for patients with intermittent hypertension.[3,9,11] Calcium channel blockers function through the inhibition of the norepinephrine-mediated calcium transit into vascular smooth muscle cells, which controls hypertension and tachyarrhythmias and is less likely to cause orthostatic hypotension.[3,7,9] This class of drug also prevents catecholamine induced vasospasm, which is useful in the subset of pheochromocytoma patients who present with coronary vasospasm or myocarditis.[3,7] Calcium channel blockers that are frequently used as add on therapy include: nifedipine, amlodipine, nicardipine, and verapamil. Common side effects are headache, peripheral edema, nausea, constipation, fatigue, flushing, and tachycardia.[2] The starting dose for amlodipine is 2.5 to 5 mg/day, titrating weekly to the desired effect to a maximum dose of 10 mg/day.[2] The starting dose for nicardipine is 20 mg orally three times daily, titrated every 3 days to the desired effect to a maximum dose of 120 mg/day.[2,9] The extended-release form of nifedipine has a starting dose of 30 mg/day, with titration every 7 days to the desired effect to a maximum dose of 90 mg/day.[1–3,9] Verapamil, the extended release starts at 180 mg/day with a maximum dose of 540 mg/day.[12]

β-Adrenergic receptor blockers are also an adjunct to alpha blockade for the preoperative management of pheochromocytoma patients. Beta blockers should only be added after the patient is on alpha blockade. The Endocrine Society guidelines published in 2014 stated that the addition of β-adrenergic blockers should only be added after at least 3 to 4 days of alpha blockade.[1] Adding prior to alpha blockade may lead to a hypertensive crisis due to the unopposed stimulation of α-adrenergic receptors by exacerbating the epinephrine-induced vasoconstriction through losing the vasodilator properties of beta receptors.[1,3] The preference for β1-selective adrenergic blockers over nonselective β-adrenergic blockers has not been validated.[1] Beta blockers help control the reflex tachycardia that is commonly seen with α-adrenergic receptor blockers, as well as assisting in achieving target blood pressure.[1] The side effects of β-adrenergic blockers include bradycardia, fatigue, dizziness, confusion, and exacerbation of asthma.[2] Beta blockers used as adjunct treatment in pheochromocytoma patients include atenolol, metoprolol, and propranolol. The starting dose of atenolol is 25 mg/day, with titration weekly to a maximum dose of 100 mg/day.[1,9] Propranolol has a starting dose of 20 mg orally three times daily, adjusted up to goal heart rate to a maximum of 120 mg/daily in three divided doses.[1,9] Metoprolol has a starting dose of 50 mg orally twice day, with titration weekly to a maximum dose of 400 mg/day in two divided doses.[2] β-Adrenergic receptor blockers not recommended in the treatment of pheochromocytoma include labetalol and carvedilol. Labetalol has both alpha and beta antagonistic activity; however, its fixed ratio of alpha to beta (1:7) can lead to paradoxical hypertension or crisis.[1,9] It is recommended to achieve a desired antihypertensive effect that the ratio of alpha to beta should be at least 4:1.[9] Carvedilol has effects similar to labetalol.[9]

Less commonly used as an adjunct to alpha blockade for patients with refractory hypertension is metyrosine. It may be beneficial for patients with significantly excessive amounts of catecholamines.[8,9] Predictors of intraoperative hemodynamic instability include larger mass size and higher preoperative metanephrine/catecholamine levels.[2] Metyrosine controls catecholamine production by inhibiting the enzyme tyrosine hydroxylase, which is involved in catecholamine synthesis, thus depleting adrenal catecholamine stores.[8] The maximum effect of significantly depleted stores occurs after 3 days of treatment.[9] Its depletion of stores is not entirely complete, thus alpha blockade is still recommended with the use of metyrosine.[8] It is recommended to initiate treatment approximately 1 to 3 weeks prior to surgery, with starting doses of 250 mg orally every 8 to 12 hours and titration of dose every 3 days by 250 to 500 mg/day to a total dose of 1.5 to 2 g/day.[3,9] Limitations to metyrosine use is due to its limited availability, cost, and side effects.[9] Metyrosine crosses the blood–brain barrier leading to both peripheral and central decreased catecholamine synthesis, which in turn causes side effects of sedation, depression, anxiety, diarrhea, tremors, and extrapyramidal signs.[3,8,9]

Treatment with α-adrenergic blocker alone will only restore the blood volume in 60% of patients.[3] Patients with pheochromocytoma have significant volume contraction and require preoperative intravascular fluid resuscitation. This will help minimize refractory postoperative hypotension after tumor resection.[8] The patient is instructed to start a high-sodium diet (greater than 5000 mg/day) about 3 days prior to surgery with adequate fluid intake to promote volume expansion.[9] Patients with multiple comorbidities may require admission to hospital 1 day prior to surgery to have an intravenous administration of isotonic fluids[1,2] to aid with volume expansion. Aggressive volume expansion may be contraindicated in patients with renal insufficiency or heart failure.

Anesthetic Preoperative Assessment and Optimization

The process to achieve patient optimization as described earlier can take from 5 to 15 days or longer in patients with cardiomyopathy or refractory hypertension.[12,13] Prior to undergoing anesthesia, the following objectives should be met to assure proper patient optimization[13]:

- arterial pressure control
- reversal of chronic circulating volume depletion
- heart and arrhythmia control
- assessment and optimization of myocardial function
- reversal of electrolyte and glucose disturbances.

ARTERIAL PRESSURE CONTROL

Severe preoperative and intraoperative hypertension can lead to stroke, arrhythmias, myocardial ischemia, left ventricular failure, and subsequent refractory hypotension following tumor resection. Preoperative alpha blockade is standard practice to provide preoperative blood pressure control. Successful alpha blockade is reflected by normalizing blood pressure with only mild orthostasis.[7] Adequacy of blockade is assessed using Roizen's criteria[14]:

1. Blood pressure less than 160/80 mm Hg
2. Orthostatic hypotension not less than 80/60 mm Hg
3. No more than one premature ventricular contraction (PVC) in 5 minutes
4. No new ST-T changes on the electrocardiogram (ECG) within the previous week.

Although these criteria were established in 1982, they have remained consistently reliable.[7]

VOLUME DEPLETION

A patient in a chronic hypertensive state is volume-depleted secondary to the intense vasoconstriction through the α-1 receptors. This vasoconstriction is ameliorated by initiation of alpha blockade as mentioned previously; however, this can result in severe orthostatic hypotension in the preoperative phase and during tumor removal.[14] In the patient with pheochromocytoma, the Endocrine Society guidelines recommend the patient increase fluid and salt intake. This can be achieved with 2 to 3 L of fluid orally, with 5 to 10 g of salt in the days prior to surgery. This volume expansion can be monitored and titrated with serial hematocrits.[1] Hematocrit levels can fall 5 % to 10% in a patient who has been well hydrated.[12]

HEART RATE AND ARRHYTHMIA CONTROL

Tachyarrhythmias can be the result of the epinephrine/dopamine secreting tumor or secondary to the alpha blockade treating the tumor. Selective β1-antagonists are the preferred treatment modality but must be started after complete alpha blockade. In doing so, unopposed alpha-mediated vasoconstriction that could occur after antagonism of β2-mediated dilation will be avoided. Should a selective β1-antagonist be started prior to proper and complete alpha blockade, a hypertensive crisis could occur, and the negative inotropic effect of the beta blockade will further compromise myocardial function.[13]

ASSESSMENT OF MYOCARDIAL FUNCTION

Patients with a pheochromocytoma need to be assessed for the effect of catecholamine excess on end organs. The end organ most commonly effected is the heart and it can present as dilated and/or catecholamine cardiomyopathy with varying degrees of heart failure.[7,12] All patients undergoing removal of pheochromocytoma need a complete cardiovascular evaluation. This will involve a 12-lead echocardiogram, which will show the presence and severity of left ventricular strain, hypertrophy, bundle branch blocks, and ischemia. Preoperative echocardiography is helpful to assess systolic and valve function as well as delineate the degree of diastolic dysfunction.[7] Left ventricular hypertrophy can correlate with the severity, duration, and degree of blood pressure control. Catecholamine induced cardiomyopathy can cause both cardiogenic and noncardiogenic pulmonary edema.[7] The impaired cardiac function associated with pheochromocytoma may improve once catecholamine levels return to normal.[13]

REVERSAL OF ELECTROLYTE AND GLUCOSE DISTURBANCES

Assessment of electrolytes can identify catecholamine-induced renal impairment. Hypercalcemia can occur secondary to a pheochromocytoma and is often associated with a parathyroid adenoma. Hyperglycemia can result from increased glycogenolysis, impaired insulin release, lipolysis, and increased glucagon release. This, coupled with peripheral insulin resistance, requires standard therapies of oral hyperglycemics and/or insulin.[13]

Anesthetic Preparation and Goals for the Operating Room

Preparation of hypotensive and vasoactive drugs should be prepared prior to the patient entering the operative suite. Commonly used hypotensive drugs are sodium nitroprusside (SNP), nitroglycerine (NTG), esmolol, vasopressin, phenylephrine, and norepinephrine. Vasoactive drugs commonly used include magnesium sulfate, labetalol, and nicardipine.[14] In patients with catecholamine cardiomyopathy, inotropes inclusive of epinephrine and dopamine may be necessary.[7] Fluids in the form of colloids, crystalloids, blood, and blood products should also be readily available. Preparing all infusions in a programed intravenous pump with tubing to a manifold allows for quick and ready administration.[7] Traditional general anesthesia set up is warranted with an endotracheal tube (ETT) and basic standards of monitoring as recommended by the American Society of Anesthesiologists. Invasive blood pressure monitoring with an arterial line is imperative in patients with pheochromocytoma.

Positioning of the patient can vary dependent on the surgical approach. Overall, the primary goal is to deliver an anesthetic that provides stable hemodynamics despite catecholamine surges during anesthetic induction, peritoneal insufflation, surgical stimulation, and tumor handling followed by the opposite with tumor ligation.[7] Careful planning and open communication with the surgical team is pivotal.

Anesthetic Induction and Monitoring

Preinduction relief from anxiety with a benzodiazepine will assist in keeping the patient calm. Apprehension and anxiety can predispose to catecholamine surges. The benzodiazepine of choice in the hospital setting and prior to entering the operative suite is intravenous midazolam. However, some patients may need lorazepam or diazepam the night before to assist in anxiety relief.[7,14]

One of the most critical portions of anesthetic delivery is the direct visual laryngoscopy (DVL) and endotracheal intubation, which is why a preinduction arterial line insertion is recommended. The allowance for continuous beat-to-beat monitoring and rapid pharmacologic intervention as needed during this critical time is necessary.[7] The anesthetic induction goal is to limit the hemodynamic stresses of DVL and ETT insertion.[7,14] Anesthetic induction agents often include propofol and etomidate. Propofol is preferred because it produces vasodilation and blunts the response to laryngoscopy and intubation, whereas etomidate is recommended for its cardiovascular stability.[14] Ketamine is avoided due to its sympathomimetic effects. All agents that cause histamine release should be avoided. Neuromuscular blockade is generally achieved with a nondepolarizing blocker such as rocuronium, vecuronium, or cisatracurium. The depolarizing neuromuscular blocker succinylcholine is avoided as research has shown the potential for catecholamine surges from the muscle fasciculations that it produces with administration. It is said that the muscle fasciculations in the abdominal compartment can mechanically compress the tumor, which can result in catecholamine surge. Succinylcholine can also stimulate the autonomic ganglia, which can result in cardiac arrhythmia.[7,14]

Central venous access is a consideration for guiding fluid therapy as well as providing access to the central venous compartment for administration of vasodilators and vasoconstrictors. Central venous access is not mandatory and surgical resection can be achieved without insertion but should be considered in particularly compromised patients.[12] If a central venous catheter is not utilized, two large-bore peripheral intravenous catheters should be initiated.

Anesthetic Maintenance

Maintenance of anesthesia can be maintained with inhalational agents or total intravenous anesthetics. Sevoflurane is preferred for its cardio stability and lack of arrhythmogenic potential. Isoflurane lowers peripheral vascular resistance and blood pressure, and therefore can also be used. Halothane and desflurane should be avoided secondary to their arrhythmia potential and sympathetic stimulation, respectively. Total intravenous anesthesia is often maintained with propofol and remifentanil or dexmedetomidine. Propofol is a short-acting drug that acts by increasing inhibitory γ-aminobutyric (GABA) synapses and inhibiting glutamate. This, coupled with the short-acting opioid remifentanil, acts by binding μ-receptors in the brain, spinal cord, and peripheral nerves. Synergistically the drugs can decrease the hemodynamic response during pheochromocytoma resection.[14]

Intraoperative transesophageal echo can be utilized for real-time monitoring of intravascular volume status, as well as early detection of myocardial wall motion abnormalities, suggesting myocardial ischemia. Noninvasive methods for cardiac output estimation and stroke volume variation to diagnose fluid deficit can also be utilized.[12] Fluid management and balance are critical, as underhydration can lead to severe hypotension following tumor resection, whereas overhydration can lead to pulmonary edema and congestive heart failure in a heart that is already compromised.[12]

Hyperglycemia is a common result of catecholamine excess, and insulin infusion therapy should be routine management in this patient population.[7]

Anesthetic Management of Intraoperative Hypertension and Hypotension

The main complication anticipated during surgery on a pheochromocytoma is the hemodynamic instability with hypertension prior to the tumor removal and hypotension after tumor isolation.[12] However, hypertension can also result from a multitude of sources prior to tumor manipulation, such as patient positioning, anesthetic induction, pneumoperitoneum, and surgical incision. In these situations, the catecholamine release is from excessive stores in nerve endings and is generally more transient and responsive to therapy.[7] Communication with the surgeon is critical prior to and during tumor manipulation. Risk factors for hemodynamic instability include large tumor, baseline mean arterial pressure more than 100 mm Hg, and a high plasma norepinephrine concentration.[14]

Tumor manipulation can cause a significant increase in plasma levels of norepinephrine and epinephrine. Management of hypertension should be with short-acting and potent vasodilators (Table 13.1). The secretion of norepinephrine will result in intense hypertension with either

TABLE 13.1 ■ **Commonly Used Drugs During Resection of Pheochromocytoma**

Drug	Class	Dosage	Considerations
Fenoldopam	Selective D1 receptor partial agonist	0.2 mg/kg per minute	Tachycardia, hypokalemia Caution in pts with CVA hx
Sodium nitroprusside	Vasodilator/ NO-releasing agent	0.5–1.5 μg/kg per minute up to 4 μg/kg per minute	Cyanide toxicity in prolonged use and higher dosages; reflex tachycardia, severe hypotension
Nitroglycerin	Nitrate	5–25 μg/minute	Reflex tachycardia, tachyphylaxis; methemoglobinemia, cerebral vasodilation
Nicardipine	Calcium channel blocker	3–5 mg/hour; bolus of 1–2 mg for crisis	Hypotension, bradycardia, heart failure
Phentolamine	Alpha-adrenergic blocker	1–5 mg	Minimal side effects
Esmolol	Selective beta-1-blocker	0.5–1 mg/kg bolus and 50 μg/kg per minute infusion	Caution in pts with conduction disturbances, and severe heart failure. Can cause bradycardia and postural hypotension. May potentiate effect of calcium channel blockers. Nonselective beta blocker should be used with caution or avoided in asthmatics
Metoprolol	Selective beta-1-blocker	2.5–5 mg	
Labetalol	Nonselective beta blocker; 7:1 beta to alpha alockade	5–10 mg	
Magnesium Sulfate	Antidysrhythmic; alectrolyte	1–3 g bolus dose with 1–4 mg/hour maintenance dose	Potentiates neuromuscular blockade; caution in heart block and with severe renal impairment

D1, Dopamine; *CVA*, cerebrovascular accident; *hx*, history; *NO*, nitric oxide; *pts*, patients.

bradycardia or tachycardia, with bradycardia being more common. Epinephrine secretion will result in severe tachycardia (paroxysmal supraventricular tachycardia and ventricular arrhythmias) and hypertension, but with less severity.[14] Immediate response to the hemodynamic change should occur with deepening of the anesthetic and rapidly administering SNP and/or nitroglycerin. SNP will have rapid onset of arterial dilation with the infusion started at 0.5 to 1.5 μg/kg per minute.[13] Both drugs have a rapid onset of action and can be easily titrated to achieve hemodynamic stability and preload reduction.[7] Esmolol (0.5 to 1 mg/kg intravenous bolus or infusion) is a short-acting beta-receptor antagonist and can be an adjunct for vasodilatation to combat intraoperative hypertension and tachycardia.[12] Labetalol (5 to 10 mg intravenously) can also be used to control these crises.[14] In resistant cases, nicardipine and/or fenoldopam can be used. Nicardipine, a dihydropyridine calcium channel antagonist, is a potent arterial vasodilator and can be used as a bolus or infusion. The half-life of 40 to 60 minutes for nicardipine can result in persistent hypotension.[13] Fenoldopam (dose of 0.2 mg/kg per minute) causes peripheral vasodilation while increasing renal blood flow.[14] Magnesium sulfate can be used as a potent arterial vasodilator inhibiting catecholamine release by directly inhibiting their receptors. It is generally used as an intravenous bolus in 1 to 3 g and is a strong calcium antagonist. Catecholamine excess will often result in hyperglycemia, and insulin infusion therapy, as indicated, should be considered.[1]

After the adrenal gland has been removed, severe hypotension can occur as a result of the residual action of vasodilators, bleeding/reduced circulating volume, catecholamine withdrawal, and adrenoceptor down regulation.[14] Initial treatment is with volume replacement of 2 to 4 L of crystalloid, which can be initiated just prior to tumor ligation.[7] If ineffective, the patient may require inotropes such as epinephrine, norepinephrine, phenylephrine, dopamine, and vasopressin.[14] Norepinephrine can be initially used to increase peripheral vascular resistance for refractory hypotension.[13] Vasopressin's action on the V1 receptors causes a systemic vasoconstriction and pulmonary vasodilation. The action on the V2 receptors in the distal convoluting tubule and collecting ducts of the kidney will increase water reabsorption[13] (Table 13.2).

TABLE 13.2 ■ **Commonly Used Drugs Immediate Post Adrenalectomy**

Drug	Class	Dose	Consideration
Epinephrine	α- and β-adrenergic agonist	1–20 μg/minute	Positive inotrope, chronotropic effect
Norepinephrine	α- and β-adrenergic agonist	1–30 μg/minute	Decreases organ blood flow; can compromise perfusion to extremities
Dopamine	α- and β-adrenergic agonist	5–20 μg/kg per minute	Dose-dependent agonist; increases cardiac output; may cause tachycardia. At <5 μg/kg per min will act as dopamine agonist
Vasopressin	V1 and V2 agonist; synthetic antidiuretic hormone (arginine vasopressin)	Bolus of 0.4–20 units Infusion 1–3 mU/kg per minute	May cause myocardial infarction and/or fluid retention
Phenylephrine	Alpha agonist	Bolus 40–200 μg; infusion 10–100 μg/minute	Increase preload and afterload; reflexive bradycardia

Postoperative Management

The most common complications postoperatively after an adrenalectomy include hypotension, hypertension, and rebound hypoglycemia.[1] It is recommended that blood pressure, heart rate, and plasma glucose values be monitored for 24 up to 48 hours in either the intensive care unit or a closely monitored unit.[1,9] For patients undergoing bilateral adrenalectomy, bilateral cortical sparing adrenalectomy, or unilateral cortical sparing adrenalectomy of a sole remaining adrenal gland, treatment to avoid adrenal insufficiency should be instituted such as glucocorticoid/mineralocorticoid replacement.[1]

The prevalence of postoperative hypotension after tumor resection is between 20% and 70%.[9] Postoperative hypotension is defined as blood pressure less than 90/60 mm Hg or any degree of hypotension leading to ischemia/end organ failure.[15] Causes of postoperative hypotension include prolonged preoperative α-adrenergic blockade half-life, decreased circulating plasma volume, abrupt decline of catecholamine release with down regulation of adrenoreceptors, and blood loss.[15] Treatment includes aggressive fluid resuscitation with isotonic intravenous fluids with or without the aid of intravenous vasopressor infusion. In the immediate postoperative period, it is important to gradually titrate preoperative antihypertensive medications to avoid further hypotension. The vasopressor infusions used to treat refractory hypotension despite adequate fluid resuscitation are norepinephrine, epinephrine, and vasopressin. Norepinephrine (Levophed, Pfizer Inc) is considered the first-line drug of choice after adequate fluid resuscitation. It is an α- and β-adrenergic agonist with higher affinity for alpha 1.[15] The starting dose is 8 to 12 μg/minute intravenously with titration to effect mean arterial pressure greater than 65 mm Hg.[15] Epinephrine (adrenalin) stimulates both α- and β-adrenergic receptors which increase mean arterial pressure by vasoconstriction, and increases cardiac output.[15] The starting dose is 0.05 to 2 μg/kg per minute with titration by 0.05 to 0.2 μg/kg per minute to target pressure. Vasopressin has no action on adrenoreceptors. It acts on vasopressin receptors in the kidney to reabsorb water, as well as on arterial smooth muscle to increase systemic vascular resistance to restore blood pressure and fluid balance.[15] The starting dose is 0.03 units/minute intravenously, titrated up to 0.04 units/minute.

Postoperative hypertension can be the result of inadequate tumor removal, metastasis, overzealous intravenaous fluid supplementation, excessive use of vasopressor agents, or underlying essential hypertension.[15] Hypertensive crisis (180/120 mm Hg) should be managed with intravenous antihypertensives. Phentolamine is a competitive α1- and 2-adrenoreceptor blocker recommended for postoperative hypertensive crisis following pheochromocytoma resection. It is given as an intravenaous bolus of 5 mg.[15] Its main side effect is reflex tachycardia and it is usually paired with a short-acting β1-adrenergic receptor blocker, esmolol, starting at 50 μg/kg intravenously with titration by 50 μg/kg per minute to a maximum dose of 200 μg/kg per min.[15] Calcium channel blockers are also recommended agents for hypertensive crisis post tumor resection; they promote arterial vasodilation by inhibiting norepinephrine-mediated calcium influx in vascular smooth muscle.[12] The most common calcium channel blocker used is nicardipine, given as a starting dose of 5 mg/hour intravenously with titration of 2.5 mg/hour every 5 to 15 minutes to a maximum of 15 mg/hour.[15] Other drugs recommended for treatment of hypertensive crisis following pheochromocytoma resections are clevidipine, labetalol, nitroglycerin, magnesium sulfate, and hydralazine.[15]

Postoperative hypoglycemia can occur in about 10 % to 15% of resected pheochromocytoma surgical cases.[4] Preoperative hyperglycemia is caused by catecholamine-stimulated glycolysis, increased peripheral insulin resistance, and inhibited insulin secretion from the pancreas.[15] With abrupt cessation of catecholamines, patients will have a rebound hyperinsulinemia leading to hypoglycemia. In our institution, blood glucose levels are monitored at regular intervals for the first 24 hours, hourly in the first 4 hours, then every 4 hours × 24 hours. Hypoglycemia is treated emergently with either IV ampule Dextrose 50% or glucagon and maintenance with dextrose 5% in intravenous fluids, with the goal of blood glucose of 100 mg/dL.[15]

Postoperative Follow-Up

The recommendations on postoperative surgical follow-up from the Endocrine Society to ensure adequate tumor removal include the measurement of plasma metanephrine levels approximately 2 to 4 weeks postoperatively.[1] The goal of postoperative testing is to document complete tumor resection; if levels are elevated, it is highly suspicious for persistent disease.[6] This should be followed by anatomic imaging to confirm the presence of residual or metastatic disease.[6]

The Endocrine Society guidelines recommend life-long annual biochemical testing to assess for recurrent or metastatic disease[1] as 5% of cases recur within 5 years of follow-up,[2] whereas the European Society of Endocrinology suggest follow-up for at least 10 years for all resected pheochromocytoma to monitor for local and metastatic recurrence or new tumors.[6] High-risk patients such as younger patients and those with an inheritable mutation should have life-long follow-up.[6]

Conclusion

The treatment of pheochromocytoma in the pre-, peri-, and postoperative course is a team approach with the patient actively involved. With the initiation of alpha blockade, open communication between provider and patient is essential for titration of doses and monitoring for side effects, as well as achieving the desired blood pressure and heart rate goals. Adequate preoperative alpha blockade will decrease the cardiovascular morbidity and mortality associated with surgical resection. The clinical team should be prepared to anticipate and treat common postoperative complications including hypo- and hypertension and hypoglycemia in the immediate postoperative course. Long-term follow-up is required to assess for metastases or recurrence of disease.

References

1. Lenders JW, Duh QY, Eisenhofer G, et al. Pheochromocytoma and paraganglioma: an Endocrine Society clinical practice guideline. *J Clin Endocrinol Metab*. 2014;99:1915–1942.
2. Pappachan JM, Tun NN, Arunagirinathan G, Sodi R, Hanna FW. Pheochromocytoma and hypertension. *Curr Hypertens Rep*. 2018;20:3.
3. Pacak K. Approach to the patient: preoperative management of the pheochromocytoma patient. *J Clin Endocrinol Metab*. 2007;92:4069–4079.
4. Pappachan JM, Raskauskiene D, Sriraman R, Edavalath M, Hanna FW. Diagnosis and management of pheochromocytoma: a practical guide to clinicians. *Curr Hypertens Rep*. 2014;16:442.
5. Chen H, Sippel RS, Pacak K. The NANETS consensus guideline for the diagnosis and management of neuroendocrine tumors: pheochromocytomas, paraganglioma and medullary thyroid cancer. *Pancreas*. 2010;39(6):775–783.
6. Plouin PF, Amar L, Dekkers OM, et al. European Society of Endocrinology clinical practice guideline for long term follow-up of patients operated on for a phaeochromocytoma or a paraganglioma. *Eur J Endocrinol*. 2016;174:G1–G10.
7. Ramakrishna H. Pheochromocytoma resection: current concepts in anesthetic management. *J Anaesthesiol Clin Pharmacol*. 2015;31(3):317–323.
8. Gregory SH, Yalamuri SM, McCartney SL, et al. Perioperative management of adrenalectomy and inferior vena cava reconstruction in a patient with a large, malignant pheochromocytoma with vena caval extension. *J Cardiothoracic Vascular Anesthesia*. 2017;31:365–377.
9. Garcia MIDO, Palasi R, Gomez RC, et al. Surgical and pharmacological management of functioning pheochromocytoma and paraganglioma. In: Mariani-Costantini R, ed. *Paraganglioma: A Multidisciplinary Approach* [Internet]. Brisbane, Australia: Codon Publications; 2019. doi:10.15586/paraganglioma.2019.ch4 Chapter 4.

10. *Lexicomp Online*. Hudson, OH: Wolters Kluwer Clinical Drug Information. Inc; 2020 January 24, 2020.
11. Mazza A, Armigliato M, Marzola MC, et al. Anti-hypertensive treatment in pheochromocytoma and paraganglioma: current management and therapeutic features. *Endocrine*. 2014;45:469–478.
12. Ramachandran R, Rewari V. Current perioperative management of pheochromocytomas. *J Urol*. 2017; 33(1):19–25.
13. Connor D, Boumphrey S. Perioperative care of phaeochromocytoma. *BJA Education*. 2016;16(5):153–158.
14. Gupta A, Garg R, Gupta N. Update in perioperative anesthetic management of pheochromocytoma. *World J Anesthesiol*. 2015;4(3):83–90.
15. Mamilla D, Araque KA, Brofferio A, et al. Postoperative management in patients with pheochromocytoma and paraganglioma. *Cancers*. 2019;11(7):936.

CHAPTER 14

Acute Adrenal Insufficiency

Ramya Punati ■ Raquel Kristin S. Ong ■ Stefan Bornstein

CHAPTER OUTLINE

Introduction

Adrenal crisis is the most severe manifestation of adrenal insufficiency (AI); it can be the first manifestation of AI or can occur in patients already established on glucocorticoid therapy. Adrenal crisis is a life-threatening medical emergency associated with high mortality unless it is promptly recognized and treatment is rendered immediately. In this chapter, we discuss the definition, epidemiology, clinical features, etiologies, and management of acute AI. The terms "adrenal crisis" and "acute AI" will be used interchangeably to refer to the same clinical entity.

DEFINITION AND PATHOPHYSIOLOGY

Adrenal crisis occurs when circulating adrenal steroid hormones are insufficient for physiologic requirements. This can arise due to an acute decrease in cortisol synthesis as a result of dysfunction or destruction of the adrenal glands themselves, or due to impaired pituitary secretion of adrenocorticotropic hormone (ACTH) that is responsible for signaling to the adrenal glands to produce cortisol. It can also occur if the body is unable to appropriately increase endogenous cortisol production during times of increased physiologic demand, such as during major surgery, injury, trauma, or infection. Adrenal crisis thus results in an acute deterioration in clinical status associated with absolute or relative hypotension; the hypotension and associated symptoms improve rapidly (within 1 to 2 hours) on parenteral glucocorticoid administration.[1]

EPIDEMIOLOGY

Adrenal crises have an estimated incidence of 5 to 10 cases per 100 patient years and are responsible for increased morbidity and mortality in patients with AI.[2] Each year, about 6% to 8% of patients with AI are reported to suffer an episode of adrenal crisis. About 40% of chronic AI patients have been reported to experience at least one adrenal crisis in their lifetime, and about 20% of chronic AI patients have experienced more than one adrenal crisis in their lifetime.[3] Adrenal crisis is slightly more common in patients with primary AI than in patients with secondary AI. Women make up about 60% of patients admitted with adrenal crisis, which reflects the increased prevalence of AI in women due to an increased predisposition to autoimmune disease.[4,5] A prospective study reported 0.5 deaths per 100 patient years from adrenal crisis.[5]

The most common causes of AI are outlined in Table 14.1.[1,6,7] Primary AI is most commonly due to autoimmune adrenalitis (Addison's disease) in the United States and other first-world countries. This can occur as isolated Addison's disease (in 40% of cases) or as part of an autoimmune polyglandular syndrome (in 60% of cases). In other parts of the world, infections (tuberculosis, HIV, cytomegalovirus [CMV], systemic fungal infections) remain the most common cause. Less frequent causes of primary AI include adrenal metastases, infiltrative diseases, hemorrhage, congenital adrenal hyperplasia, bilateral adrenalectomy, and drugs that impair glucocorticoid production and action. Of note, metastases and infiltrative diseases rarely cause AI because extensive damage to both adrenal glands is required to cause AI.

TABLE 14.1 ■ **Common Causes of Adrenal Insufficiency (AI)**

Type	Common Causes
Primary Causes of AI	

Autoimmune	• Adrenalitis/Addison's disease (40%)
	• Autoimmune polyglandular syndrome (60%)
	  • Type 1 (chronic cutaneous candidiasis + hypoparathyroidism)
	  • Type 2 (autoimmune thyroid disease + type 1 diabetes mellitus)

Infections	• Tuberculosis • Systemic fungal infections • AIDS
Metastasis	• Lung • Breast • Colon • Melanoma • Lymphoma
Adrenal hemorrhage	• Sepsis • Anticoagulants • Anticardiolipin/lupus anticoagulant syndrome
Infiltration	• Hemochromatosis • Primary amyloidosis
Bilateral adrenalectomy	• Cushing's syndrome • Bilateral pheochromocytoma
Congenital adrenal hyperplasia	• Most common etiology of AI in children (80%)

Drug induced	• Adrenal enzyme inhibitors
	  • Mitotane
	  • Ketoconazole
	  • Metyrapone
	  • Etomidate

Other	• Adrenomyeloneuropathy • Adrenoleukodystrophy

(continued)

TABLE 14.1 ■ **Common Causes of Adrenal Insufficiency (AI)–con't**

Type	Common Causes
Secondary Causes of AI	

Pituitary pathologies and insults	• Mass lesions
	  • Macroadenoma
	  • Craniopharyngioma
	  • Meningioma
	  • Metastasis
	• Surgery
	• Radiation
	• Infiltration
	  • Hemochromatosis
	  • Sarcoidosis
	  • Langerhans cell histiocytosis
	• Lymphocytic hypophysitis
	• Drug-induced hypophysitis (CTLA-4 inhibitors)
	• Apoplexy
	• Trauma
	• Empty sella syndrome

Suppression of HPA axis	• Chronic use of glucocorticoids or other specific steroids (e.g., megestrol acetate), opioids

HPA, Hypothalamic-pituitary-adrenal.

Secondary AI is more common than primary AI[8] and is caused by any process that leads to deficiency of ACTH. This is most frequently due to pituitary pathologies such as mass lesions, surgery, trauma, medications, and radiation-induced pituitary damage. Secondary AI can also be caused by the chronic use of glucocorticoids, opioids, or other drugs (e.g., checkpoint inhibitors). Exogenous glucocorticoid use by any route (oral, inhaled, topical, or injected) at supraphysiologic doses (prednisone 5 mg or higher per day, or its equivalent) for longer than 4 weeks is well known to suppress the hypothalamic-pituitary-adrenal axis.

Clinical Presentation

RECOGNIZING ACUTE ADRENAL INSUFFICIENCY

The cardinal manifestation of acute AI is absolute or relative hypotension, which ultimately leads to shock if untreated.[2,5,9] In addition to the defining feature of hypotension, patients with adrenal crisis frequently present with fever and acute abdominal pain. They may also exhibit milder symptoms of hypocortisolism such as fatigue, nausea, anorexia, myalgias, arthralgias, and postural dizziness. The clinical features of an adrenal crisis are compared and contrasted with those of chronic AI in Table 14.2.[1,6] Without hypotension or evidence of hemodynamic compromise, the presence of these other symptoms in a patient with a known diagnosis of AI should be considered distinct from, but a likely precursor to, an adrenal crisis.[10] Failure of hypotension to respond to vasopressor agents should be a clue to the possible presence of acute AI and an indication for the trial of glucocorticoid therapy. Prompt resolution of these features after parenteral glucocorticoid administration is a key feature of adrenal crisis. If the symptoms and hypotension attributed to

TABLE 14.2 ■ Clinical Features of Chronic Adrenal Insufficiency (AI) and Adrenal Crisis

	Chronic AI	Acute AI (Adrenal Crisis)
Symptoms	Fatigue, anorexia, weight loss, myalgias, arthralgias Dizziness Nausea, vomiting, diarrhea Salt craving (in primary AI only)	Severe weakness Acute abdominal pain Nausea, vomiting Syncope Confusion
Signs	Orthostatic hypotension Fever Hyperpigmentation of skin creases and buccal mucosa (in primary AI only)	Hypotension Fever Abdominal tenderness, guarding Reduced consciousness, delirium
Laboratory Findings	Hyponatremia Hyperkalemia (in primary AI only) Hypoglycemia Hypercalcemia	Hyponatremia Hyperkalemia (in primary AI only) Hypoglycemia Hypercalcemia

an adrenal crisis fail to improve within 1 to 2 hours of sufficient glucocorticoid administration, alternative or coexisting diagnoses such as sepsis should be considered.

Due to its presentation with hypotension and fever, an adrenal crisis can initially lead clinicians to suspect infection. Patients with fever should indeed be treated as though they have an infection until proven otherwise. Infections are commonly the precipitating events of adrenal crisis.[3–5,11] Bacterial infections are common precipitants of adrenal crisis in elderly patients.[11] Gastroenteritis is a frequently cited trigger that can cause a particularly severe presentation due to rapid dehydration and an inability to tolerate oral medications and fluids.[3,9,12] Furthermore, the combination of abdominal pain, tenderness, and fever may mimic "acute abdomen," and abdominal exploration in such patients can be catastrophic.

Several biochemical abnormalities can be seen in patients with acute AI, although none distinguish adrenal crisis from chronic AI, as summarized in Table 14.2. Hyponatremia is the most common biochemical abnormality, occurring in 70% to 80% of cases. Hyponatremia can be seen in patients with any etiology of AI due to increased vasopressin secretion resulting from cortisol deficiency, although it is more common in primary AI in which mineralocorticoid deficiency compounds the problem via natriuresis and volume depletion.[1,13] Patients with primary AI can have hyperkalemia due to mineralocorticoid deficiency. Hypoglycemia may be seen in AI of any etiology due to glucocorticoid deficiency causing impaired gluconeogenesis. Hypoglycemia is more commonly seen in children with adrenal crisis than in adults.[10] It is also more common in cases of secondary AI caused by isolated ACTH deficiency.[14,15] In a minority of cases of adrenal crisis, patients may have the additional laboratory abnormalities of hypercalcemia (thought to occur due to hypovolemia, acute kidney injury, and decreased renal excretion of calcium)[16] and normocytic anemia (cortisol is required for the maturation of blood progenitor cells and pernicious anemia may coexist in autoimmune polyglandular syndromes).[17]

PRIMARY ADRENAL INSUFFICIENCY

Certain features of a patient's presentation with acute AI vary according to etiology and can serve as clues to the etiology of AI (Table 14.3). As mentioned previously, hyponatremia and especially hyperkalemia indicate primary AI. Patients with chronic primary AI who present in crisis may

TABLE 14.3 ■ **Clinical Features Suggestive of Specific Etiologies of Adrenal Insufficiency (AI)**

	Clinical Feature	Potential Etiology
History	Personal or family history of autoimmune disease	Addison's disease (autoimmune adrenalitis) – classical primary AI
	Salt craving	Primary AI
	Recent induction of general anesthesia or rapid-sequence intubation	Primary AI due to etomidate
	On anticoagulant therapy	Bilateral adrenal hemorrhage
	Coagulopathy	Bilateral adrenal hemorrhage
	Abdominal or back trauma	Bilateral adrenal hemorrhage
	Post-partum hemorrhage	Sheehan syndrome
	Acute headache	Pituitary apoplexy
	On immune checkpoint inhibitor therapy, especially CTLA-4 inhibitor or combination therapy	Hypophysitis
Signs	Hyperpigmentation	Chronic primary AI
	Vitiligo	Addison's disease (autoimmune adrenalitis) – classical primary AI
	Petechial rash	Waterhouse-Friderichsen syndrome
	Nuchal rigidity, delirium	Meningococcal meningitis
	Abdominal tenderness, guarding	Bilateral adrenal hemorrhage
	Peripheral visual field deficit	Pituitary apoplexy
Laboratory Findings	Hyperkalemia	Primary AI
	Hypoglycemia	Secondary AI (more common) > Primary AI

have hyperpigmentation, which occurs due to the chronic hypersecretion of ACTH that is cosecreted with melanocyte-stimulating hormone (MSH). This hyperpigmentation is seen in 41% to 74% of cases, and is most noticeable in palmar creases and buccal mucosa, as demonstrated in Figs. 14.1 and 14.2.[6,13,18,19]

An important etiology of acute AI is bilateral adrenal hemorrhage and infarction. In contrast to patients with chronic primary AI, these patients do not have hyperpigmentation due to acuity of the changes (lack of prolonged elevation of ACTH and cosecreted MSH). The majority of patients with bilateral adrenal hemorrhage have abdominal, flank, back, or lower chest pain.[20] These patients can rapidly deteriorate to shock without preceding hypotension. Risk factors for adrenal hemorrhage include thromboembolic disease, anticoagulant therapy, underlying coagulopathy (such as antiphospholipid antibody syndrome or disseminated intravascular coagulation), blunt trauma, and postoperative state.[20] When a patient with such risk factors develops changes such as fever, hypotension, or abdominal pain, clinicians should promptly suspect adrenal crisis due to hemorrhage. A noncontrast computed tomography (CT) scan can confirm the diagnosis, with acute adrenal hemorrhage appearing as bilaterally enlarged, hyperdense adrenal glands, as shown in Fig. 14.3.[20–22]

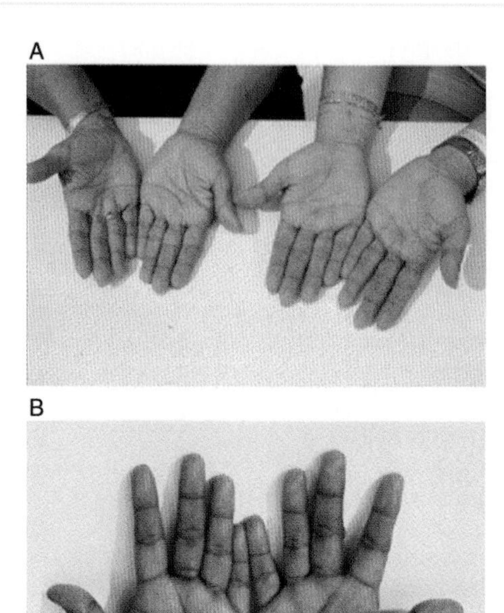

Fig. 14.1 (A, B) Hyperpigmentation of palmar creases in patients with Addison's disease. (From Nieman LK, Chanco Turner ML. Addison's disease. *Clin Dermatol.* 2006;24(4):276–280.)

Various infections have also been associated with acute hemorrhagic necrosis of the adrenal glands, which is known as Waterhouse–Friderichsen syndrome (WFS) and is more common in children than in adults. This may be typically caused by bacterial infection, and has classically been described in the context of meningococcemia in the prevaccine era. However, WFS has also been reported due to sepsis from other bacterial pathogens such as *Haemophilus influenzae*, *Pseudomonas aeruginosa*, *Escherichia coli*, *Mycoplasma pneumoniae*, *Streptococcus pneumoniae*, and *Staphylococcus aureus*.[23–26] Viral infections including CMV, parvovirus B19, varicella zoster, and Epstein–Barr virus have also been reported to cause WFS.[27] Physical findings in patients with WFS include petechial rash, purpura fulminans, and neurologic changes in meningitis, in addition to typical signs of infection.

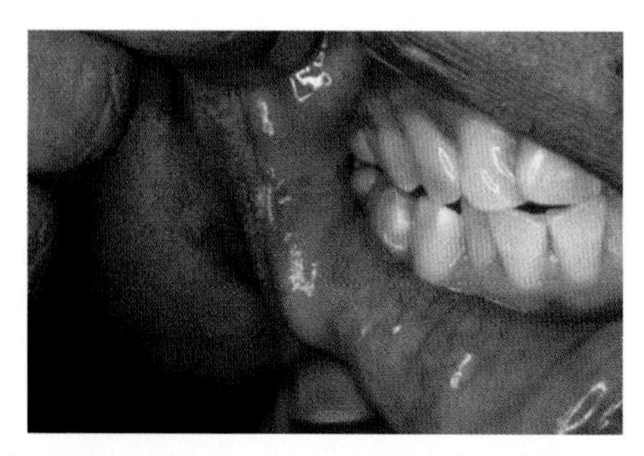

Fig. 14.2 Hyperpigmentation of buccal mucosa in a patient with Addison's disease. (From Nieman LK, Chanco Turner ML. Addison's disease. *Clin Dermatol.* 2006;24(4):276–280.)

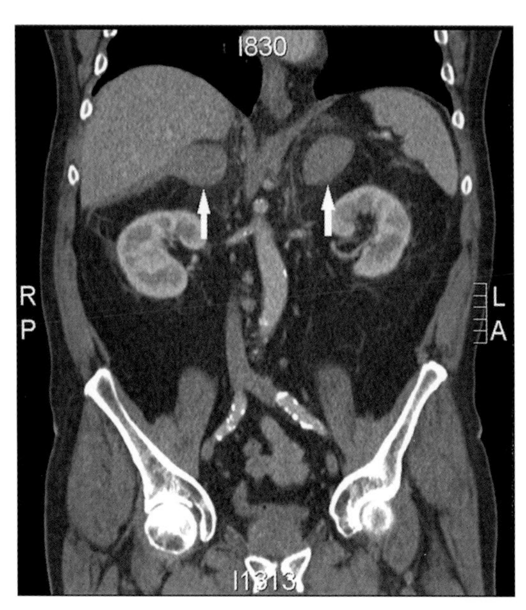

Fig. 14.3 Computed tomography of chest, abdomen, and pelvis, with *arrows* highlighting dense bilateral adrenal masses in a patient with bilateral adrenal hemorrhage leading to adrenal crisis. (From McGowan-Smyth S. Bilateral adrenal haemorrhage leading to adrenal crisis. *BMJ Case Reports.* 2014;2014.)

Finally, several drugs can precipitate adrenal crisis. Mechanisms of drug-induced primary AI include an inhibition of enzymes involved in cortisol biosynthesis (e.g., ketoconazole, metyrapone, etomidate) and an increase in glucocorticoid metabolism (e.g., carbamazepine, rifampin, phenytoin). Additionally, initiation of thyroxine therapy (thyroid hormone) in hypothyroid patients with undiagnosed AI may potentially precipitate acute AI, as thyroid hormone may increase the clearance of cortisol.[14,28,29] This is particularly important to consider because patients with AI often have concomitant hypothyroidism, either as part of autoimmune polyglandular syndrome type 2 (primary autoimmune AI and hypothyroidism) or due to pituitary disease (secondary/central AI and hypothyroidism).

SECONDARY ADRENAL INSUFFICIENCY

Acute AI is slightly less frequent in patients with secondary AI, likely because these patients have partial preservation of cortisol secretion, and because mineralocorticoid secretion is preserved. Still, adrenal crisis can occur when there is acute loss of pituitary function causing acute hypocortisolism, such as in cases of pituitary apoplexy (sudden hemorrhage, usually occurring into a pituitary macroadenoma), infarction of the pituitary gland after post-partum hemorrhage (Sheehan syndrome), during pituitary surgery, or head trauma. The majority of patients with pituitary apoplexy have headache and visual field deficit.[30] Other pituitary axes may be compromised as well.

Immune checkpoint inhibitor therapy, which is increasingly used in the treatment of melanoma and other cancers, can cause acute AI, either due to hypophysitis causing secondary AI or due to adrenalitis causing primary AI. In a large metaanalysis, the incidence of hypophysitis in patients on checkpoint inhibitor therapy was found to be 6.4% with combination therapy, 3.4% with CTLA-4 inhibitors, 0.4% with PD-1 inhibitors, and less than 0.1% with PD-L1 inhibitors.[31] A separate study found that in patients with hypophysitis due to checkpoint inhibitor therapy, secondary AI was the most common anterior pituitary deficiency, present in 83% of cases.[32] Primary AI is less frequently observed, with 4.2% incidence in patients receiving combination therapy and 0.7% with any checkpoint inhibitor.[31]

Patients with chronic exogenous glucocorticoid use can present with acute secondary AI when the glucocorticoid therapy is abruptly discontinued, either due to patient nonadherence or clinician error. Such patients may have physical signs of Cushing's syndrome such as wide violaceous striae, dorsocervical and supraclavicular fat pads, proximal muscle wasting, thin skin, ecchymoses, and central adiposity. However, one study in Australia found that adrenal crises were rare in patients with glucocorticoid-induced AI.[33]

Chronic opioid use is an increasingly important cause of secondary AI to recognize in the modern era of the opioid epidemic. Among patients treated with chronic opioids, the estimated prevalence of opioid-induced AI ranges from 9% to 29%.[34] Clinically significant adrenal crisis in patients with opioid-induced AI has been described in some case reports.[35,36]

Diagnosis

In the hemodynamically unstable patient in whom adrenal crisis is clinically suspected, therapy should be initiated promptly prior to biochemical confirmation of the diagnosis. Thus, having a high index of suspicion for this condition based on patient history and clinical presentation is of the utmost importance. When acute AI is suspected, blood should be drawn for serum cortisol and electrolyte testing, ideally just prior to giving the first dose of glucocorticoid. Some experts also recommend drawing and holding blood samples for ACTH, renin, and aldosterone, to be processed later if the diagnosis of AI is likely.[6]

A serum cortisol of less than 5 μg/dL during a period of acute stress or illness (regardless of time of day) strongly supports the diagnosis of AI. Conversely, a serum cortisol concentration greater than 20 μg/dL excludes the diagnosis. In cases in which the serum cortisol is indeterminate (5 to 20 μg/dL), glucocorticoid therapy should be continued until the patient has recovered, and further testing (which may include an ACTH stimulation test) can be conducted later to clarify the diagnosis. There is no role for ACTH stimulation testing during an acute hemodynamic decompensation that is suspected to be due to AI.

If the cortisol concentration is low, suggesting the diagnosis of AI, then the clinician should use additional laboratory tests to determine the level of the defect. Elevated ACTH concentration indicates primary AI, and in these cases, one would expect low aldosterone with elevated renin. Low or inappropriately normal ACTH concentrations indicate secondary AI; aldosterone and renin would be normal in these cases. Further testing, such as imaging of the adrenal glands (using CT) or pituitary (using magnetic resonance imaging), may be obtained as clinically indicated to determine the specific etiology of the AI.

A caveat to interpretation of cortisol concentrations in critically ill patients is that patients may have abnormalities of binding proteins (cortisol-binding globulin, albumin) that affect the total serum cortisol (which is routinely measured) but do not affect the free cortisol (which is biologically active). Testing the free cortisol concentration in saliva or serum has been suggested but is not routinely performed or recommended due to the lack of availability, expense, and lack of validity and established criteria for interpretation.[37] In lieu of testing the free cortisol concentration, clinicians should measure total cortisol and albumin, and consider conditions that may alter binding protein levels in a patient, such as liver cirrhosis, nephrotic syndrome, and estrogen use (e.g., in oral contraceptives). Also, physiologic states like pregnancy may result in elevated total cortisol levels due to increased cortisol-binding globulin.

In addition to suspecting and diagnosing acute AI, clinicians should perform a thorough evaluation for the precipitating cause, which usually includes reviewing the patient's medications, testing for infection, and obtaining imaging as indicated.

Management of Acute Adrenal Insufficiency

Treatment of patients with possible adrenal crisis should not be delayed while diagnostic tests are being completed. Prompt treatment includes immediate parenteral administration of hydrocortisone 100 mg; if intravenous access is not available, intramuscular injection can be given. Concurrently, it is necessary to administer aggressive fluid resuscitation of 1 L of isotonic saline with or without 5% or 10% glucose (depending on the presence of hypoglycemia) in the first hour. Then, hydrocortisone is given intravenously either via continuous infusion to equal 200 mg in a 24-hour period or 50 mg intravenously every 6 hours in 24 hours. Intravenous isotonic saline is continued based on the patient's hemodynamic stability, volume status, and urine output.[6,38]

If hydrocortisone is not available, prednisolone could be used. Dexamethasone is the least favorable steroid to use, especially in adrenal crisis due to primary AI, because it has no mineralocorticoid activity, whereas hydrocortisone 40 mg has an equivalent of 100 μg of fludrocortisone.[6]

Blood gas and glucose should be monitored hourly until acidosis and hypoglycemia resolve and then every 2 to 4 hours thereafter. Electrolytes should be monitored every 4 hours. Caution is recommended to not exceed correction of hyponatremia greater than 10 to 12 mEq/L in the first 24-hour period due to the risk of central pontine myelinolysis. Cortisol replacement can induce water diuresis, and in cases of secondary AI can also suppress antidiuretic hormone. In combination with isotonic fluid replacement, these changes can lead to overcorrection of hyponatremia and osmotic demyelination syndrome.[39] Hyperkalemia usually normalizes with fluid, electrolyte, and steroid replacement. Cardiac monitoring should be in place to assess for any ECG changes (peaked T waves, widened QRS complexes, and/or flattened P waves) due to hyperkalemia.

The identification and treatment of the illness or injury that precipitated the adrenal crisis is also important.

On day 2, if clinically improved, hydrocortisone could be decreased to 100 mg/24-hour period (i.e., 25 mg every 6 hours). As the patient continues to improve, the patient can be transitioned from parenteral to oral glucocorticoids.

Chronic Management of Adrenal Insufficiency and Prevention of Adrenal Crisis

The optimal glucocorticoid maintenance regimen is hydrocortisone 15 to 25 mg/day or cortisone acetate 20 to 35 mg/day. This should be divided into twice daily or three times daily doses with the highest dose in the morning and the lowest in the afternoon (not later than 4 to 6 hours before bedtime)[6] in order to mimic endogenous glucocorticoid pulsatile circadian release, which reaches its highest peak in the morning. Hydrocortisone and prednisolone are active glucocorticoids, whereas prednisone and cortisone acetate are prodrugs that require activation via 11β-hydroxysteroid dehydrogenase type 1 in the liver before exerting their activity.

Patients with primary AI need mineralocorticoid replacement to maintain water, electrolyte, and blood pressure homeostasis. Mineralocorticoid replacement is given in the form of fludrocortisone at initial doses of 50 to 100 μg in adults.[6] Patients are recommended to not restrict the salt in their diet.

Patient education, such as increasing dose of replacement therapy ("stress dosing") when sick or planned for a medical procedure/surgery, using parental hydrocortisone as necessary, and seeking medical assistance promptly, is the best approach to prevention of adrenal crisis.[6,38,40] Follow-up care with an endocrinologist is necessary to periodically reevaluate for symptoms of inadequate glucocorticoid replacement (symptoms of AI) or for signs of excessive glucocortocoid replacement (features of Cushing's syndrome). The endocrinologist should monitor for adverse metabolic effects of excessive glucocorticoid therapy, such as weight gain, hyperglycemia, dyslipidemia, and low bone density. The adequacy of mineralocorticoid replacement should be assessed by measuring orthostatic vital signs, serum potassium, and plasma renin activity. Additionally, the endocrinologist should counsel patients to wear a medical alert identification and reeducate patients at each visit about how to recognize adrenal crisis, when and how to increase glucocorticoid dosing during illness, how to self-administer parenteral glucocorticoid, and when to seek emergent medical care.[6,13]

References

1. Puar TH, Stikkelbroeck NM, Smans LC, Zelissen PM, Hermus AR. Adrenal crisis: still a deadly event in the 21st century. *Am J Med.* 2016;129:339e1–339e9.
2. Rushworth RL, Torpy DJ, Falhammar H. Adrenal crises: perspectives and research directions. *Endocrine.* 2017;55(2):336–345.
3. Hahner S, Loeffler M, Bleicken B, et al. Epidemiology of adrenal crisis in chronic adrenal insufficiency: the need for new prevention strategies. *Eur J Endocrinol.* 2010;162:597–602.
4. Smans LC, van der Valk ES, Hermus AR, Zelissen PM. Incidence of adrenal crisis in patients with adrenal insufficiency. *Clin Endocrinol* (Oxf). 2016;84:17–22.
5. Hahner S, Spinnler C, Fassnacht M, et al. High incidence of adrenal crisis in educated patients with chronic adrenal insufficiency: a prospective study. *J Clin Endocrinol Metab.* 2015;100:407–416.
6. Bornstein SR, Allolio B, Arlt W, et al. Diagnosis and treatment of primary adrenal insufficiency: an Endocrine Society clinical practice guideline. *J Clin Endocrinol Metab.* 2016;101(2):364–389.
7. Bornstein SR. Predisposing factors for adrenal insufficiency. *N Engl J Med.* 2009;360:2328–2339.
8. Arlt W, Allolio B. Adrenal insufficiency. *Lancet.* 2003;361:1881–1893.
9. Allolio B. Extensive expertise in endocrinology: adrenal crisis. *Eur J Endocrinol.* 2015;172:R115–R124.
10. Rushworth RL, Torpy DJ, Falhammar H. Adrenal crisis. *N Engl J Med.* 2019:852–861.
11. Rushworth RL, Torpy DJ. A descriptive study of adrenal crises in adults with adrenal insufficiency: increased risk with age and in those with bacterial infections. *BMC Endocr Disord.* 2014;14:79.
12. White K, Arlt W. Adrenal crisis in treated Addison's disease: a predictable but under-managed event. *Eur J Endocrinol.* 2010;162:115–120.
13. Bancos I, Habner S, Tomlinson J, Arlt W. Diagnosis and management of adrenal insufficiency. *Lancet Diabetes Endocrinol.* 2015;3(3):216–226.
14. Burke CW. Adrenocortical insufficiency. *Clin Endocrinol Metab.* 1985;14:947–976.
15. Stacpoole PW, Interlandi JW, Nicholson WE, Rabin D. Isolated ACTH deficiency: a heterogeneous disorder. Critical review and report of four new cases. *Medicine.* 1982;61:13–24.
16. Ahn SW, Kim TY, Lee S, et al. Adrenal insufficiency presenting as hypercalcemia and acute kidney injury. *Int Med Case Rep J.* 2016;9:223–226.
17. Arlt W. The approach to the adult with newly diagnosed adrenal insufficiency. *J Clin Endocrinol Metab.* 2009;94:1059–1067.
18. Lovas K, Husebye ES. Addison's disease. *Lancet.* 2005;365(9476):2058–2061.
19. Nieman LK, Chanco Turner ML. Addison's disease. *Clin Dermatol.* 2006;24(4):276–280.
20. Rao RH. Bilateral massive adrenal hemorrhage. *Med Clin North Am.* 1995;79:107–129.
21. McGowan-Smyth S. Bilateral adrenal haemorrhage leading to adrenal crisis. *BMJ Case Reports. 2014.* 2014.
22. Logaraj A, Tsang VH, Kabir S, Ip JC. Adrenal crisis secondary to bilateral adrenal hemorrhage after hemicolectomy. *Endocrinol Diabetes Metab Case Rep. 2016.* 2016:16–0048.
23. Khwaja J. Bilateral adrenal haemorrhage in the background of *Escherichia coli* sepsis: a case report. *J Med Case Rep.* 2017;11:72.
24. Adem PV, Montgomery CP, Husain AN, et al. *Staphylococcus aureus* sepsis and the Waterhouse-Friderichsen syndrome in children. *New Engl J Med.* 2005;353:1245–1251.
25. Tormos LM, Schandl CA. The significance of adrenal hemorrhage: undiagnosed Waterhouse-Friderichsen syndrome, a case series. *J Forensic Sci.* 2013;58:1071–1074.
26. Hamilton D, Harris MD, Foweraker J, Gresham GA. Waterhouse–Friderichsen syndrome as a result of non-meningococcal infection. *J Clin Pathol.* 2004;57:208–209.
27. Heitz AFN, Hofstee HMA, Gelinck LBS, et al. A rare case of Waterhouse-Friderichsen syndrome during primary varicella zoster infection. *Neth J Med.* 2017;75:351–353.

28. Kang MS, Sandhu CS, Singh N, et al. Initiation of levothyroxine in a patient with hypothyroidism inducing adrenal crisis requiring VA ECMO: a tale of preventable disaster. *BMJ Case Reports CP.* 2019; 12:e230601.
29. Shaikh MG, Lewis P, Kirk JM. Thyroxine unmasks Addison's disease. *Acta Paediatr.* 2004;93:1663–1665.
30. Randeva HS, Schoebel J, Byrne J, et al. Classical pituitary apoplexy: clinical features, management and outcome. *Clin. Endocrinol* (Oxf). 1999;51:181–188.
31. Barroso-Sousa R, Barry WT, Garrido Castro AC, et al. Incidence of endocrine dysfunction following the use of different immune checkpoint inhibitor regimens: a systematic review and meta-analysis. *JAMA Oncol.* 2018;4:173–182.
32. Tan MH, Iyengar R, Mizokami-Stout K, et al. Spectrum of immune checkpoint inhibitors-induced endocrinopathies in cancer patients: a scoping review of case reports. *Clin Diabetes Endocrinol.* 2019;5:1.
33. Rushworth RL, Chrisp GL, Torpy DJ. Glucocorticoid-induced adrenal insufficiency: a study of the incidence in hospital patients and a review of peri-operative management. *Endocr Pract.* 2018;24:437–445.
34. Donegan D, Bancos I. Opioid-induced adrenal insufficiency. *Mayo Clin Proc.* 2018;93(7):937–944.
35. Oltmanns KM, Fehm HL, Peters A. Chronic fentanyl application induces adrenocortical insufficiency. *J Intern Med.* 2005;257(5):478–480.
36. Flamarion E, Saada N, Khellaf M, et al. Insuffisancesurrénalesecondaire aux opioïdes: rapport de cas et synthèse de la littérature [Opioid-induced adrenal insufficiency: Case report and synthesis of the literature]. *Rev Med Interne.* 2019;40(11):758–763.
37. Hamrahian AH, Oseni TS, Arafah BM. Measurements of serum free cortisol in critically ill patients. *N Engl J Med.* 2004;350(16):1629–1638.
38. Dineen R, Thompson CJ, Sherlock M. Adrenal crisis: prevention and management in adult patients. *Ther Adv Endocrinol Metab.* 2019:10–20.
39. Verbalis JG, Goldsmith SR, Greenberg A, et al. Diagnosis, evaluation, and treatment of hyponatremia: expert panel recommendations. *Am J Med.* 2013;126:S1–S42.
40. Pazderska A, Pearce SH. Adrenal insufficiency—recognition and management. *Clin Med.* 2017;17(3): 258–262.

PART 5

Endocrine Pancreas and Pancreatic Neuroendocrine Tumors

CHAPTER 15

Diabetic Emergencies: Ketoacidosis, Hyperglycemic Hyperosmolar State, and Hypoglycemia

Heidi Guzman ■ David Wing-Hang Lam

CHAPTER OUTLINE

Diabetic Ketoacidosis

INTRODUCTION

Diabetic ketoacidosis (DKA) is an acute metabolic complication of diabetes characterized by an absolute or relative insulin deficiency resulting in hyperglycemia, hyperketonemia, and metabolic acidosis. DKA is an endocrine emergency that requires immediate treatment and close monitoring for metabolic derangements. It most commonly occurs in patients with a known history of type 1 diabetes; however, patients with type 2 diabetes are also at risk during states of acute illness. In some cases, DKA may be the first manifestation of diabetes, especially in developing countries.

DEFINITION

The diagnostic criteria for DKA include hyperglycemia with a blood glucose level greater than 250 mg/dL, the presence of serum ketones, an anion gap metabolic acidosis with a pH less than 7.3, a serum bicarbonate less than 18 mEq/L, and an anion gap greater than 12.[1]

Euglycemic Diabetic Ketoacidosis

Euglycemic DKA (euDKA) is characterized by an anion gap metabolic acidosis and hyperketonemia as in traditionally described DKA, but with the exception that patients present with a serum glucose level less than 200 mg/dL.

EPIDEMIOLOGY

DKA continues to be an important cause of morbidity and mortality among patients with diabetes. The prevalence of DKA hospitalizations has been on the rise in the United States with an increase in the rate from 19.5 to 30.2 per 1000 persons with diabetes between 2009 and 2014. This increase in prevalence was consistent across all age groups and sexes, with the highest rates seen in persons aged less than 45 years.[2] The reason for the rise in hospitalization rates for DKA is unknown. Possible explanations include the rising incidence of type 1 and type 2 diabetes in children and adolescents, suggesting that more patients are presenting with DKA at diagnosis. There is also an increase in provider awareness and identification of milder forms of DKA that may have previously gone unrecognized.[3] The rates of in-hospital case-fatalities have decreased from 1.1% to 0.4% during this same time period, with the highest case-fatality rates among the elderly and patients with concomitant life-threatening conditions.[2] Patients presenting with shock or coma on admission had a worse prognosis, with the main causes of death being infection, hypokalemia, and circulatory collapse. DKA also remains as the most common cause of death in children and adolescents with type 1 diabetes.[1]

DKA is more common among patients with type 1 diabetes, but it can also occur in patients with type 2 diabetes. Patients with poorly controlled type 2 diabetes with concurrent illnesses and patients with a history of ketosis-prone type 2 diabetes are at higher risk. Ethnic minorities, specifically patients of African-American or Hispanic descent, have a higher prevalence of ketosis-prone type 2 diabetes and typically have a strong family history of diabetes with associated negative autoimmune markers.[4] DKA as an initial presentation for diabetes is also common, but incidence rates vary drastically between countries, ranging from 13% to 80%, with the highest incidence rates seen in developing countries.[5]

EuDKA was first described in a case series in 1973 when 37 of 211 patients admitted for DKA were found to have mild hyperglycemia with metabolic acidosis. The majority of patients described in the case series had type 1 diabetes with associated recent carbohydrate reduction, vomiting, or decreased insulin doses.[6] Although previously rare, there is also a growing rise of euDKA in association with sodium-glucose cotransporter 2 (SGLT-2) inhibitors. In patients with type 1 diabetes and SGLT-2 inhibitor use, the incidence of DKA has been reported to be 9.4%, as compared with 0.2% in patients with type 2 diabetes on SGLT-2 inhibitors.[7,8] In summary, euDKA is more likely to occur in patients with type 1 diabetes but can also occur in patients with type 2 diabetes.

PATHOPHYSIOLOGY

DKA is triggered by an insulin-deficient state that leads to activation of counterregulatory hormones that promote lipolysis, glycogenolysis, and gluconeogenesis, and clinically manifests with hyperglycemia, ketosis, and metabolic acidosis with profound volume depletion.

Insulin Deficiency and Counterregulatory Hormones

DKA results from an absolute or relative insulin-deficient state. Patients may become insulin deficient in a variety of settings including new-onset diabetes, nonadherence to insulin treatment regimen, insulin pump failure, medication or illicit drug use interactions, or during acute physiologic states that require an increase in circulating insulin levels. Insulin deficiency leads to a perceived fasting or low glucose state at the cellular level activating insulin counterregulatory hormones including glucagon, cortisol, growth hormone, and catecholamines. The counterregulatory hormones antagonize the effects of insulin by increasing the blood glucose level through the activation of alternative mechanisms of energy production. Glucagon plays a key role by promoting glycogenolysis, gluconeogenesis, and lipolysis. Cortisol, catecholamines, and growth hormone also stimulate lipolysis by activating hormone-sensitive lipase in adipose tissue, leading to the release of free fatty acids and glycerol. Glycerol is then recycled in the liver as an important substrate in the gluconeogenesis pathway and further promotes the rise of blood glucose, leading to hyperglycemia.

Free Fatty Acids in Diabetic Ketoacidosis

The free fatty acids released from lipolysis are transported to the liver where they become the precursors to ketoacids and further suppress the production of insulin. Under the stimulation of glucagon, the enzyme malonyl-coenzyme A (CoA) becomes upregulated in the liver, facilitating the transport of free fatty acids into the mitochondria. Once in the mitochondria, free fatty acids are limited from entering the Krebs cycle, as the key substrate pyruvate is diverted from glycolysis to gluconeogenesis during the perceived cellular fasting state. This Krebs cycle roadblock gives rise to an accumulation of free fatty acids in the mitochondrial matrix that are then catabolized into acetyl-CoA and ketoacids B-hydroxybutyrate and acetoacetate, which can be used as energy in the body. The production of ketones leads to a ketonemia that is further maintained by reduced liver ketone clearance. At baseline, ketone bodies are acidic, but the body is able to produce extracellular and intracellular buffers to neutralize the acidity. However, in DKA, the body is unable to meet the buffering demand imposed by the ketone excess, leading to an anion gap metabolic acidosis. The metabolic acidosis is also worsened by further conversion of pyruvate into lactate in the cells.

Dehydration

The counterregulatory hormones work to promote glycogen breakdown and glucose synthesis, leading to hyperglycemia. When the glucose level in the blood reaches an approximate concentration of 225 mg/dL, glucose will start to leak into the renal tubules, creating an osmotic gradient and water diuresis. The diuresis can be quite significant and lead to volume depletion and dehydration if patients cannot sufficiently maintain their oral fluid intake.

Ketones also contributes to the diuresis. As the ketone concentration accumulates in the blood, it also collects in the urine where it is combined with sodium to form a buffer that can be excreted. The creation of the sodium gradient drives further movement of water that is excreted, leading to more dehydration.

The hyperglycemia-induced osmotic diuresis also promotes the loss of other electrolytes in the urine including potassium, calcium, phosphorous, and magnesium. The fluid loss also leads to a decrease in glomerular filtration in the kidneys, which then causes a decrease in glucosuria and worsens the hyperglycemia.

Pathophysiology of Euglycemic Diabetic Ketoacidosis

The pathophysiology of euDKA is not entirely known; possible causes could be as simple as recent insulin administration before presentation and therefore masking hyperglycemia, but can also be a result of significant carbohydrate restriction, excess alcohol consumption, chronic liver disease or liver cirrhosis, glycogen storage disorders, pancreatitis, or pregnancy.[9]

One possible mechanism in euDKA patients stems from decreased hepatic glucose production during a fasting state. Through fasting or perceived starvation, which can occur from decreased carbohydrate caloric intake, acute illness, pregnancy, or substance misuse, the body is depleted of glycogen. This leads to a milder hyperglycemia when triggered in DKA. Another proposed explanation is that some patients may have an enhanced excretion of urinary glucose caused by a surplus in counterregulatory hormones or SGLT-2 inhibitor use, leading to reduced serum glucose.[10]

In the United States, SGLT-2 inhibitors were Food and Drug Administration (FDA) approved in 2013 for the treatment of type 2 diabetes, and work by promoting glucose reabsorption from the proximal renal tubule leading to a decrease in serum glucose and an increase in glucosuria. If a patient was in DKA while on an SGLT-2 inhibitor, the SGLT-2 inhibition provides an insulin-independent mechanism for lowering glucose levels through urinary glucose excretion with the end result being euDKA.

The association of euDKA with the use of SGLT-2 inhibitor medications prompted an FDA drug safety warning about the associated risk.[11]

CLINICAL PRESENTATION

Clinical Findings

DKA is a rapidly evolving condition with symptoms typically presenting within a 24-hour period. Patients in DKA most commonly present with symptoms of hyperglycemia, including polyuria and polydipsia. EuDKA can pose a diagnostic challenge to providers given the presence of a milder hyperglycemia, which may lead to a delay in treatment and medical complications.

Patients may also have feelings of fatigue, weight loss, nausea, vomiting, and abdominal pain. Severe presentations of DKA may also include mental status changes that can vary from altered sensorium to lethargy and coma. On physical examination, patients may appear dehydrated with dry mucous membranes, poor skin turgor, tachycardia, and hypotension. The physical examination may also reveal a fruity breath odor as a result of elevated serum acetone levels and rapid and shallow Kussmaul breaths as a compensatory mechanism for metabolic acidosis. Features of the precipitating trigger for DKA may also be present.

Laboratory Findings

Once the clinical suspicion for DKA is established, the diagnosis must be confirmed with laboratory testing. This includes measurement of glucose, metabolic panel, pH, and serum ketones.

An immediate point-of-care fingerstick should be done to confirm hyperglycemia of greater than 250 mg/dL. It is important to note that in cases of euDKA, the blood glucose value will be less than 200 mg/dL, but the laboratory findings of an anion gap metabolic acidosis with positive serum ketones will still be present.

To assess for metabolic acidosis, an arterial sample to measure the pH along with a metabolic panel to calculate an anion gap should be obtained. If an arterial sample is not available, venous blood gas can be used to assess the pH and has a 97.8% sensitivity and 100% specificity in the diagnosis of DKA.[12] The anion gap is calculated by measuring the difference of cations (which is represented as corrected serum sodium) and anions (which is represented as the sum of serum chloride and bicarbonate).

For ketone analysis, the American Diabetes Association recommends serum ketone testing in favor of urinalysis ketone testing to allow for a more accurate diagnosis. Ketone urinalysis only measures acetone and acetoacetate, and not B-hydroxybutyrate, which is produced in a 20:1 ratio in DKA, making it the primary ketoacid. Serum B-hydroxybutyrate testing has a sensitivity of 98% and a specificity of 79%, compared with ketone urinalysis testing, which has a sensitivity of 98% and specificity of 35%.[13]

In addition to diagnostic testing, laboratory studies should include measurements of electrolytes potassium; magnesium, which may be low and require supplementation; and phosphate, which may be normal or initially elevated at presentation. Patients should also have a complete blood count, urinalysis, an electrocardiogram, and their hemoglobin A1c measured. Focused testing of precipitating triggers may also be indicated depending on the clinical presentation.

DIFFERENTIAL DIAGNOSIS

Many medical conditions share the individual components that together define DKA: hyperglycemia, anion gap metabolic acidosis, and ketosis. Hyperglycemia can be a marker of a variety of conditions including uncontrolled type 1 or type 2 diabetes, physiologic stress, infection, and, in severe cases, hyperosmolar hyperglycemic state (HHS). HHS presents with marked hyperglycemia, typically with blood glucose greater than 600 mg/dL. However, unlike DKA, patients with HHS will have minimal acidosis with pH greater than 7.3 and serum bicarbonate greater than 15 mmol/L, absent to mild ketosis, and elevations in serum osmolality to more than 320 mOsm/L.

Several conditions can also present with an anion gap metabolic acidosis. This list includes alcohol intoxication, uremia, rhabdomyolysis, and toxicity from salicylates, paraldehyde, methanol, or ethylene glycol ingestion. Lactic acidosis also leads to an anion gap metabolic acidosis and has its own differential including infection, pancreatitis, ischemia, and seizure.

Ketosis can occur in states of starvation. When the body is depleted of glucose, the liver will start to produce ketone bodies in order to generate ATP for the brain. Patients with a history of chronic alcoholism can also develop an alcoholic ketoacidosis. Ethanol can be metabolized to ketones but it can also suppress gluconeogenesis and lead to a perceived state of starvation.

Given this broad differential diagnosis which can have similar laboratory findings to DKA, it is important to consider the combination of laboratory diagnostics along with the clinical history and physical examination to accurately diagnose DKA.

DIABETIC KETOACIDOSIS PRECIPITANTS

DKA most commonly occurs among patients with a known history of diabetes who acutely run out of insulin or stop taking their insulin. In this scenario, it is important to investigate the barriers or causes contributing to insulin nonadherence. In addition to medication nonadherence, it is also important to consider that other precipitants and stressors which can activate an increase in the counterregulatory hormones cortisol, catecholamines, and glucagon can precipitate DKA.

Illness can be a major stressor, particularly if secondary to infection, myocardial infarction, and stroke. Illness associated with vomiting is also a common precipitant for DKA by promoting dehydration and may lead to patients omitting or decreasing the amount of insulin they are administering in order to avoid hypoglycemia.

Medications can also precipitate DKA. Corticosteroids, high doses of thiazide diuretics, atypical antipsychotics, and diazoxide have all been associated triggers for DKA. The use of SGLT-2 inhibitors has also been associated with precipitating euDKA. Illicit drug use and alcohol also increases the risk of DKA by interfering with medication adherence. More obscure precipitant causes of DKA include Cushing's syndrome, acromegaly, glucagonoma, pancreatic destruction caused by a virus or neoplasm, and pregnancy.

TREATMENT

The management aims in DKA are to restore fluid, electrolyte, and hormonal homeostasis while minimizing the risks for complications. Treatment requires close monitoring to assess the response and resolution of hyperglycemia and to correct laboratory abnormalities. Due to the need for close monitoring, patients with DKA are best managed in an intensive care unit (ICU) or step-down unit.

Fluid Replacement

The osmotic diuresis precipitated by hyperglycemia in DKA leads to volume depletion and dehydration. Fluid resuscitation will correct the intravascular volume depletion while enhancing renal perfusion and promoting further glucose diuresis. Additionally, fluid replacement helps to decrease the counterregulatory hormone response by restoring the intravascular volume and further decreasing glucose levels in the blood.[14]

Patients with DKA have an estimated water deficit of about 5 to 7 L, or 100 mL/kg, which represents a 10% to 15% loss in body weight. The initial goal in fluid repletion is to expand the intravascular volume and restore hemodynamic function. In the absence of heart failure, pulmonary edema, or end-stage renal disease, isotonic saline (0.9% sodium chloride) is infused at a general rate of 500 to 1000 mL/hour or 15 to 20 mL/kg per hour for the first 2 hours. If the patient is hypotensive and in hypovolemic shock from severe dehydration, 3 or 4 L of isotonic saline may be required to restore blood pressure. To assess for successful fluid replacement, patients should be hemodynamically monitored for improvements in blood pressure, heart rate, urine output, laboratory values, and physical examination.

After correcting the intravascular depletion, the remaining goal of fluid management is to replace half of the estimated fluid deficit over the course of 12 to 24 hours. If the corrected serum sodium remains low, the normal saline infusion can be continued but in general decreased to 250 to 500 mL/hour. If the corrected serum sodium level is normal or high, indicating a remaining free water deficit, then the infusion can be changed to half-normal saline and decreased to 250 to 500 mL/hour. Once the blood glucose level drops to 250 mg/dL or below, fluids should contain dextrose 5% to 10% to prevent hypoglycemia, whereas insulin therapy is still required to decrease ketones and correct acidosis.

Electrolyte Replacement

Potassium. At presentation, patients in DKA typically present with potassium abnormalities. Most commonly, patients will present with hyperkalemia despite a total-body potassium depletion. This paradox is due to the normal action of insulin to drive potassium intracellularly and out of the serum. The insulin deficiency characteristic of DKA causes a redistribution of potassium into the serum. In addition, the metabolic acidosis in DKA further causes potassium to move out of the cell as potassium is exchanged for hydrogen. As insulin therapy and fluids are administered during treatment, serum potassium levels begin to decrease. The insulin moves the potassium back into the cells, whereas the fluid repletion can cause a dilution of the serum potassium, increasing the risk for hypokalemia. Hypokalemia must be closely monitored, prevented, and treated. To prevent hypokalemia, potassium should be repleted after potassium levels fall below 5.2 mEq/L. Typically, 20 to 30 mEq of potassium is given with each liter of intravenous fluid for a goal potassium of 4 to 5 mEq/L; however, lower doses may be required in patients with decreased renal function.

In rare cases, patients in DKA may present with hypokalemia. The osmotic diuresis may lead to significant urinary losses of potassium. If the potassium level is less than 3.3 mEq/L, potassium repletion should be given with the initial fluid resuscitation and insulin treatment should be delayed to avoid cardiac arrhythmias. Once potassium levels are greater than 3.3 mEq/L, insulin therapy can be administered.

Phosphate. As with potassium, patients in DKA generally have a total body depletion in phosphate. However, most patients will have normal or increased levels of phosphate at initial presentation. The initial hyperphosphatemia is likely secondary to the concentrated levels in the setting of intravascular volume depletion and acute renal impairment.[15] Serum phosphate levels will decrease with insulin and fluid therapy. Studies have not shown any benefit of phosphate replacement in the management of DKA, but replacement is indicated in those with severe hypophosphatemia with serum phosphate levels less than 1 mg/dL.[16] In the event of severe hypophosphatemia, 20 to 30 mEq of potassium phosphate can be added to the fluids to prevent complications, which include cardiac arrhythmias and respiratory compromise.

Bicarbonate. Bicarbonate therapy is typically only given in DKA for patients with serum pH levels of 7 or below. There is controversy in this recommendation, as there is no current evidence that demonstrates improved DKA outcomes with bicarbonate administration. Proponents of bicarbonate advocate that bicarbonate may help patients with severe acidosis and therefore decrease risks for cardiac and vital organ dysfunction. Opponents to bicarbonate argue that bicarbonate administration can worsen outcomes by increasing the risk for pH shifts, fluid retention, and cerebellar edema.[17]

Insulin

Insulin is used to correct hyperglycemia by increasing peripheral glucose uptake into the cells and decreasing hepatic gluconeogenesis. Insulin therapy also directly inhibits ketoacid production and decreases the release of free fatty acids. Currently, there is no consensus on a single insulin protocol for the treatment of DKA; however, all protocols share the same goals of insulin therapy – to correct hyperglycemia and restore acid–base balance.

Intravenous insulin therapy has long been favored for the treatment of DKA due to its rapid onset of action and short half-life, giving the treating provider the ability to dynamically adjust doses based on glucose response to insulin. However, there is growing interest and use of subcutaneous insulin protocols that have the advantage of decreasing the intensity of care required and possibly avoiding the need for an ICU admission for relatively mild cases of DKA.

Insulin should only be started after initiating fluid resuscitation and correcting hypokalemia, if indicated, to avoid worsening cellular fluid and potassium shifts. When insulin therapy is started, it is important to closely monitor glucose levels every hour, in addition to monitoring serum electrolytes, glucose, magnesium, phosphorous, blood urea nitrogen, creatinine, and venous pH every 2 to 4 hours.

Most intravenous insulin protocols utilize a weight-based dose for the infusion rate (0.1 to 0.15 units/kg per hour) with titration based upon the change in glucose each hour and a goal of a decrease between 50 and 75 mg/dL per hour and a target blood glucose of less than 200 to 250 mg/dL. Some protocols may also utilize an intravenous bolus of insulin before starting an insulin infusion.

RESOLUTION OF DIABETIC KETOACIDOSIS

Resolution of ketoacidosis occurs when the blood glucose level is below 200 mg/dL, serum bicarbonate levels are greater than 18 mEq/L, venous pH is greater than 7.3, and the calculated anion gap is less than 12 mEq/L. Once these targets are reached, patients can be bridged to subcutaneous insulin therapy from intravenous insulin therapy. It is important for there to be a period of overlap during the transition to avoid iatrogenically causing an insulin-deficient state and the possibility of the patient re-developing DKA. To avoid this, the basal insulin dose should be administered and the intravenous insulin infusion can be discontinued 2 hours after the dose is given.

Patients with a known history of diabetes can typically be given their home dose of basal insulin. Patients with a new diagnosis of diabetes can be started on a weight-based insulin regimen or insulin doses can be estimated based on total insulin required during resolution of DKA.

COMPLICATIONS OF DIABETIC KETOACIDOSIS

Hypokalemia and Hypoglycemia

The most common complications in the management of DKA include hypoglycemia and hypokalemia. Hypoglycemia can occur from high insulin infusion rates without sufficient intravenous fluid dextrose administration. Although there is no universal protocol for insulin dosing, the need for treatment monitoring with monitoring of hourly glucose to both prevent and identify hypoglycemia is critical. Monitoring is especially important because some patients in DKA may not develop traditional symptoms of hypoglycemia due to a blunted adrenergic response. Hypokalemia is also a common complication that occurs from both insulin therapy and fluid repletion. Insulin administration drives extracellular potassium into cells, and fluid repletion can dilute the concentration of serum potassium. Levels of potassium should be monitored every 2 hours and repleted when potassium levels fall below 5.2 mEq/L.

Cerebral Edema

More rare but severe complications in DKA can also occur, the most worrisome of which is cerebral edema. Cerebral edema carries a high mortality rate of 21% to 90%.[18,19] Cerebral edema occurs from an elevated osmolar gradient caused by hyperglycemia, which leads to a water shift from the intracellular space to the extracellular space and cell volume contraction. Cerebral edema is more common in children and adolescents and typically presents with headache, vomiting, and decreased mental status followed by seizures, bradycardia, and respiratory arrest. Risk factors for cerebral edema include younger age, severe acidosis with low bicarbonate level on presentation, and hyponatremia with rapid hydration. Patients with cerebral edema need to be transferred to an intensive care setting and treated with intravenous mannitol.

Other Complications

Other complications in DKA management include pulmonary edema from volume repletion in patients with CKD or heart failure. Less commonly, patients may also experience rhabdomyolysis. The exact etiology of rhabdomyolysis in DKA is not known but presumed to be a combination of hyperosmolarity and hypophosphatemia. If left untreated, DKA can also lead to ischemic stroke, cerebral venous thrombosis, and hemorrhagic stroke from cerebral hypoperfusion.

PREVENTION OF DIABETIC KETOACIDOSIS

Hospitalizations for DKA have been on the rise, and preventing both the initial event as well as recurrent episodes is of utmost importance. Many patients admitted for DKA present with new-onset diabetes, most commonly in type 1 diabetes and ketosis-prone diabetes in ethnic minorities. Patients most at risk for developing type 1 diabetes include children and adolescents with a parent or sibling with type 1 diabetes and patients with other autoimmune conditions. Medical providers should be appropriately educated on these risk factors and should screen high-risk patients. If screened negative for diabetes, health care providers should continue to closely monitor their high-risk patients in addition to educating their patients and the patient's family members on the signs and symptoms of diabetes. Research has shown that educational prevention programs on early recognition of diabetes and DKA symptoms can significantly decrease the number of children admitted with DKA at diagnosis.[20]

Recurrent admissions for DKA must also be prevented to decrease both the morbidity and mortality associated with diabetes, as recurrent hospitalizations are associated with an increased mortality risk. Hospital readmissions are more likely to occur in patients with type 1 diabetes, but patients with type 2 diabetes can account for up to 35% of recurrent DKA cases.[21] It is important that all patients admitted for DKA be counseled on strategies for its prevention. This includes discussing the signs and symptoms of hyperglycemia, early recognition of DKA with use of home ketone monitoring systems, and reviewing sick-day management with patients and family members. During an acute illness, patients need to establish early contact with their health care providers. Patients and family should also be counseled on the importance of continuing insulin, monitoring blood sugars, hydration, and providing correctional doses of rapid-acting insulin for hyperglycemia during acute illness.

Prevention of recurrent DKA also requires assessing the precipitating factors that may have triggered prior DKA hospitalizations. This includes assessing for insulin nonadherence related to poor health literacy, financial difficulties, substance abuse, and psychological stressors.

Insulin nonadherence may be prevented through intensive patient education and outpatient follow-up with a diabetes health care provider. Patients should also be provided with the necessary diabetes medications and supplies on discharge.

Hyperglycemic Hyperosmolar State

INTRODUCTION

The HHS is a metabolic complication of diabetes mellitus that represents a separate hyperglycemic emergency to DKA despite many similarities. HHS is characterized by severe hyperglycemia, hyperosmolarity, and dehydration in the absence of significant ketoacidosis and is more commonly found in patients with type 2 diabetes.

DEFINITION

The diagnostic criteria for HHS include hyperglycemia with a blood glucose level often exceeding 600 mg/dL, serum osmolality greater than 320 mOsm/kg, and absence of significant ketoacidosis.[22]

PATHOPHYSIOLOGY

The pathophysiology of HHS is similar to that of DKA with some specific intricacies. At the cornerstone of both conditions is a deficiency in insulin. However, in HHS, the insulin deficiency is only relative, as the pancreas continues to make insulin but is unable to keep up with the demand needed to overcome peripheral tissue insulin resistance. In the setting of a relative insulin deficiency, the cells in the periphery enter a perceived "starvation" state leading to the release of the counterregulatory hormones glucagon, cortisol, growth hormone, and catecholamines. The counterregulatory hormones work to promote glycogenolysis and gluconeogenesis, leading to worsening hyperglycemia. The hyperglycemia then leads to a direct and indirect increase in serum osmolality. Serum osmolality is determined by the formula 2[serum sodium] + [serum glucose]/18 + BUN (i.e., blood urea nitrogen); therefore as the serum glucose levels rise, there will be a direct increase in the serum osmolality. Additionally, hyperglycemia triggers an osmotic diuresis, which leads to the loss of free water, glucose, and electrolytes through the urine, resulting in the indirect increase in serum osmolality concentration and worsening of dehydration.[23]

Combined, the hyperglycemia and dehydration lead to a mixed hyponatremia. The hyperglycemia results in a hyperosmolar hyponatremia that can be corrected by decreasing the serum sodium 1.6 mEq/L per 100 mg/dL glucose rise above 100 mg/dL. In addition, the concurrent dehydration produced from osmotic diuresis leads to a hypovolemic hyponatremia that must be corrected with intravenous hydration.

A key difference in the pathophysiology of HHS in comparison to DKA is the minimal to absent production of ketones. In HHS, the pancreas continues to produce insulin, and the amount of insulin produced is sufficient to inhibit lipolysis. In the absence of lipolysis, there is no fatty acid oxidation and therefore no production of ketone bodies and resultant acidemia.

CLINICAL PRESENTATION

Clinical Findings

HHS has a clinical presentation that commonly resembles the signs and symptoms seen in DKA. Patients in HHS may present with polyuria, polydipsia, severe dehydration, weight loss, blurred vision, and changes in mental status. However, a distinguishing feature is the timing of the symptoms. Patients in DKA will often present with more acute symptoms, whereas patients in HHS may have symptoms develop over several days to weeks. A careful history should be performed to assess for any precipitating factors such as infection, cardiovascular compromise, dietary indiscretions, changes in medications, and general compliance with prescribed diabetic regimen.

On physical examination, patients may appear dehydrated with dry mucous membranes, decreased skin turgor, tachycardia, and hypotension. Unlike DKA, patients in HHS typically do not develop gastrointestinal distress. Neurologic symptoms such as decreased alteration, stupor, delirium, seizure, and focal neurologic deficits such as transient hemiplegia may also be present.

Laboratory Findings

Serum glucose will typically be above 600 mg/dL, even exceeding 1000 mg/dL in some cases. On chemistry panel, most patients will be hyponatremic with normal to elevated potassium levels. Patients will often have an elevated BUN and creatinine reflecting a prerenal azotemia. Serum osmolality will also be elevated to above 320 mOsmol/kg. In contrast to DKA, there will be an absence of significant ketoacidosis with typically normal to mildly elevated ketones, a pH greater than 7.3, and no anion gap.

TREATMENT

HHS is an endocrine emergency that requires prompt recognition and treatment. All patients must be acutely stabilized and mental status should be closely evaluated. Patients presenting with severe lethargy or stupor should be evaluated for respiratory compromise and intubated if necessary, for airway protection. Patients should be admitted to the ICU for close monitoring and care, and any precipitating causes should be investigated and treated.

Fluid Replacement

Once stabilized, patients should be treated with aggressive intravenous hydration and electrolyte replacement as needed. Isotonic fluid is preferred to restore intravascular volume depletion and decrease counterregulatory hormone action and hyperglycemia. An initial isotonic fluid bolus of 15 to 20 mL/kg during the first 1 to 2 hours of presentation, followed by 250 to 500 mL/hour, is typically recommended until glucose levels reach 300 mg/dL.[24]

Electrolyte Replacement

Similar to DKA, patients may have depleted potassium stores from urinary losses, and potassium levels must be greater than 3.3mEq before starting an insulin drip. Potassium should also be repleted once potassium levels fall to less than 5.5 mEq/L.

Insulin

After the initial 1 to 2 hours of fluid resuscitation, an intravenous insulin drip can be started as per the preferred hospital protocol. At this time, there are no clear consensus guidelines regarding the preferred insulin drip titration protocol. Once serum glucose levels reach 300 mg/dL, isotonic fluid should be replaced by intravenous D5 ½ normal saline and continued until the patient's mental status is restored and the serum osmolarity normalizes to less than 310 mOsmol/kg in order to maintain blood glucoses between 250 to 300 mg/dL.

During the course of HHS management, the goal is to keep glucose levels between 250 to 300 mg/dL in order to minimize the risk for cerebral edema. In animal studies, rapid correction of plasma and brain osmolality has resulted in cerebral edema. Although this has not been seen in humans, the theoretical fear of cerebral edema from osmolality overcorrection supersedes the benefit of euglycemia during HHS treatment.[22,24]

Hypoglycemia

DEFINITION

Hypoglycemia is defined as a low blood glucose concentration below the normal range that is associated with autonomic and neuroglycopenic symptoms. Due to variable levels in which patients may exhibit symptoms of hypoglycemia, a joint American Diabetes Association and Endocrine Society work group concluded that no specific glucose threshold could be used to define hypoglycemia.[25] In patients with diabetes, an alert value of less than 70 mg/dL was suggested to prompt attention to the patient due to the increased risk of harm from hypoglycemia by the same work group. Although any episode of hypoglycemia could be life-threatening to a patient due to its impact on cognition, severe hypoglycemia, defined as a hypoglycemic event that requires external assistance to administer carbohydrates or glucagon, can be considered an endocrine emergency.

CLINICAL PRESENTATION

Symptoms associated with hypoglycemia can be classified by their underlying cause – activation of the adrenergic system or neuroglycopenia:

- Adrenergic symptoms
  - Heart palpitations and tachycardia
  - Diaphoresis
  - Tremor
  - Hunger
  - Nausea
  - Anxiety
- Neuroglycopenic symptoms
  - Weakness
  - Lethargy
  - Altered mental status
  - Dizziness
  - Seizure
  - Coma/loss of consciousness

DIFFERENTIAL DIAGNOSIS

The differential diagnosis of hypoglycemia is quite different when being considered in a patient with diabetes or without diabetes. In patients with diabetes, medications for diabetes are nearly always the cause for severe hypoglycemia. In a patient without diabetes, the differential diagnosis is broad, including accidental or intentional administration of antihyperglycemic agents, alcohol use, hepatic failure, renal failure, adrenal insufficiency, insulinoma, nesidioblastosis, bariatric surgery–related hypoglycemia, and insulin autoimmunity. For a patient with limited known history, it is appropriate to begin with a broader differential diagnosis in their initial evaluation.

EVALUATION

The first step in the evaluation of a patient is a detailed history to determine if they have the diagnosis of diabetes and, if so, a detailed history including medications. A detailed history may help in narrowing the differential diagnosis and focusing the evaluation of the patient. However, in some cases, a medical history may not be obtainable and a broader differential diagnosis and work up maybe required.

History

The history obtained for a patient with severe hypoglycemia should first focus on recent events and activities that could precipitate hypoglycemia, such as changes in food intake, physical activity, alcohol intake, and recent illnesses. A detailed list of antihyperglycemic medications, recent additions, and any dose adjustments should be reviewed. Insulin and insulin secretagogues such as sulfonylureas and meglitinides can cause a hyperinsulinemic state resulting in hypoglycemia. Other classes of medications including metformin, thiazolidinediones, SGLT-2 inhibitors, glucagon-like peptide-1 (GLP-1) receptor agonists, dipeptidyl peptidase-4 (DPP-4) inhibitors, and alpha-glucosidase inhibitors do not result in a hyperinsulinemic state; however, if used in combination with insulin or insulin secretagogues, they can increase the risk of hypoglycemia. Lastly, other risk factors that can increase the risk of hypoglycemia, such as older age, longer duration of diabetes, chronic kidney disease, and malnutrition, should be assessed.

Laboratory Evaluation

In most cases of severe hypoglycemia, a capillary point-of-care glucose reading is the first available data to identify the diagnosis. Depending on the known history of the patient and the context of presentation, confirmation of hypoglycemia with measurement of blood glucose may not be necessary and should not delay treatment. However, if there is a question regarding the diagnosis of hypoglycemia, a plasma or serum glucose measurement should be obtained. Due to glycolytic enzymes in red cells and leukocytes, it is important that either sodium fluoride is added to the blood sample or the sample must be rapidly separated to prevent glycolysis and a false lowering of the measured glucose.

In the context of a limited or no history, other lab tests may be helpful in diagnosing the etiology of severe hypoglycemia including:

- Insulin
- Pro-insulin
- C-peptide
- Beta-hydroxybutyrate
- Sulfonylurea and meglitinide screen
- Cortisol

TREATMENT

In patients with severe hypoglycemia who require external assistance, the mainstay of treatment is the administration of glucose. The mode of administration primarily depends on the patient's mental status and vascular access. In the inpatient hospital setting, for patients who are able to safely ingest by mouth, treatment with a rapidly absorbed carbohydrate such as glucose tablets or gel may be used. For patients who are not able to take treatment by mouth, intravenous dextrose can be administered. The typical dose is administered as an intravenous push of a 50% dextrose solution in 25-g aliquots. Patients without intravenous access can be given 1 mg of glucagon intramuscularly.

Subsequent monitoring of glucose levels following treatment is necessary after initial treatment of hypoglycemia. Glucose monitoring should immediately follow treatment of hypoglycemia, but a plan for further monitoring must also be established. The decision regarding duration and frequency for monitoring takes into account the severity of hypoglycemia, the patient's mental status and ability to communicate, which antihyperglycemic medications were used and their duration of action, and the trend of glucose levels.

For subsequent treatment of recurrent hypoglycemia, the same treatment options may be used: oral administration of rapidly absorbed carbohydrates, intravenous dextrose, or glucagon. In some cases, a continuous intravenous infusion with a 5% or 10% dextrose may be required to maintain euglycemia. If a continuous infusion is utilized, attention must be given to the volume and respiratory status of the patient, and if receiving large volumes of fluids, electrolytes should be also be monitored.

Special Considerations

The treatment and monitoring plan for hypoglycemia depends on the medications taken by the patient. If the patient has taken acarbose, an alpha-glucosidase inhibitor, it is essential that oral treatment of hypoglycemia is with dextrose as opposed to sucrose (e.g., table sugar and candy) due to the inhibition of alpha-glucosidase in the intestine. Patients treated with insulin therapy may require prolonged monitoring and treatment depending on how recently insulin was administered and the duration of action of the insulin used. In addition, patient-specific factors such as impaired renal function and liver dysfunction, which can affect the metabolism of medications, may prolong the duration of monitoring and treatment of hypoglycemia. This especially applies to patients treated with insulin or insulin secretagogues.

PREVENTION

Prevention of hypoglycemia in patients with diabetes centers around three major themes: management of diabetes medications, patient education, and patient self-management of diabetes with blood glucose monitoring.

Following a hypoglycemic event, careful attention should be paid to evaluating the diabetes medication regimen. Medications thought to be primarily responsible for hypoglycemia should either be adjusted or removed, with appropriate alternatives prescribed. Subsequent encounters with the patient should review recurrent hypoglycemic events and the patient's self-monitored blood glucose testing.

Patients should be educated on their diabetes medications and the potential risk for hypoglycemia. Following this education, a patient should be told which medications they should withhold or reduce doses of in the event of decreased oral intake or fasting, increased physical activity, and alcohol intake. Symptoms of hypoglycemia should be reviewed with the patient and appropriate hypoglycemia treatments prescribed, such as glucose tablets and glucagon.

Self-monitored blood glucose testing should be provided and taught to patients who are on medications with an increased risk for hypoglycemia. Patients should be instructed to test their blood glucose if they recognize signs or symptoms of hypoglycemia. However, in the event of an emergency, treatment should be administered prior to testing. In addition, depending on the medication regimen of the patient, testing their blood glucose level prior to physical activity and driving a vehicle may be recommended. For some patients, a continuous glucose monitor that is capable of alerting the patient or caregiver of hypoglycemia and impending hypoglycemia may also be effective in its prevention.

Conclusion

DKA, HHS, and severe hypoglycemia are all serious life-threatening complications of diabetes that require prompt diagnosis, treatment, and close monitoring. The diagnosis of hyperglycemic emergencies, DKA and HHS, is made based on the presence of hyperglycemia, an assessment of acid–base status, and the presence or absence of ketonemia. Treatment for both DKA and HHS include fluid resuscitation, insulin, and close monitoring of electrolytes along with treatment of any underlying precipitating factors. The diagnosis of hypoglycemia is typically made based on point-of-care glucose testing; however, it may often require laboratory confirmation and evaluation. Although the treatment of hypoglycemia is straightforward, attention must be invested in identifying the cause and any precipitating events in order to prevent its recurrence. In all diabetes emergencies, there is a strong role of patient education in the early diagnosis and prevention of each.

References

1. Umpierrez G, Korytkowski M. Diabetic emergencies—ketoacidosis, hyperglycaemic hyperosmolar state and hypoglycaemia. *Nat Rev Endocrinol.* 2016;12(4):222–232.
2. Benoit Sr ZY, Geiss LS, Gregg EW, Albright A. Trends in diabetic ketoacidosis hospitalizations and in-hospital mortality—United States, 2000–2014. *MMWR Morb Mortal Wkly Rep.* 2018:362–365.
3. Vellanki P, Umpierrez GE. Increasing hospitalizations for DKA: a need for prevention programs. *Diabetes Care.* 2018;41(9):1839–1841.
4. Vellanki P, Umpierrez GE. Diabetic ketoacidosis: a common debut of diabetes among African Americans with type 2 diabetes. *Endocr Pract.* 2017;23(8):971–978.
5. Jefferies CA, Nakhla M, Derraik JG, Gunn AJ, Daneman D, Cutfield WS. Preventing diabetic ketoacidosis. *Pediatr Clin North Am.* 2015;62(4):857–871.
6. Munro JF, Campbell IW, McCuish AC, Duncan LJ. Euglycaemic diabetic ketoacidosis. *Br Med J.* 1973;2(5866):578–580.
7. Erondu N, Desai M, Ways K, Meininger G. Diabetic ketoacidosis and related events in the canagliflozin type 2 diabetes clinical program. *Diabetes Care.* 2015;38(9):1680–1686.
8. Henry RR, Thakkar P, Tong C, Polidori D, Alba M. Efficacy and safety of canagliflozin, a sodium-glucose cotransporter 2 inhibitor, as add-on to insulin in patients with type 1 diabetes. *Diabetes Care.* 2015;38(12):2258–2265.
9. Modi A, Agrawal A, Morgan F. Euglycemic diabetic ketoacidosis: a review. *Curr Diabetes Rev.* 2017; 13(3):315–321.
10. Rawla P, Vellipuram AR, Bandaru SS, Pradeep Raj J. Euglycemic diabetic ketoacidosis: a diagnostic and therapeutic dilemma. *Endocrinol Diabetes Metab Case Rep. 2017.* 2017:17–0081.
11. Gajjar K, Luthra P. Euglycemic diabetic ketoacidosis in the setting of SGLT2 inhibitor use and hypertriglyceridemia: a case report and review of literature. *Cureus.* 2019;11(4):e4384.
12. Menchine M, Probst MA, Agy C, Bach D, Arora S. Diagnostic accuracy of venous blood gas electrolytes for identifying diabetic ketoacidosis in the emergency department. *Acad Emerg Med.* 2011;18(10):1105–1108.
13. Arora S, Henderson SO, Long T, Menchine M. Diagnostic accuracy of point-of-care testing for diabetic ketoacidosis at emergency-department triage: β-hydroxybutyrate versus the urine dipstick. *Diabetes Care.* 2011;34(4):852–854.
14. Waldhausl W, Kleinberger G, Korn A, Dudczak R, Bratusch-Marrain P, Nowotny P. Severe hyperglycemia: effects of rehydration on endocrine derangements and blood glucose concentration. *Diabetes.* 1979;28(6):577–584.
15. Shen T, Braude S. Changes in serum phosphate during treatment of diabetic ketoacidosis: predictive significance of severity of acidosis on presentation. *Intern Med J.* 2012;42(12):1347–1350.
16. Fisher JN, Kitabchi AE. A randomized study of phosphate therapy in the treatment of diabetic ketoacidosis. *J Clin Endocrinol Metab.* 1983;57(1):177–180.
17. Chua HR, Schneider A, Bellomo R. Bicarbonate in diabetic ketoacidosis—a systematic review. *Ann Intensive Care.* 2011;1(1):23.
18. Umpierrez GE, Kelly JP, Navarrete JE, Casals MM, Kitabchi AE. Hyperglycemic crises in urban blacks. *Arch Intern Med.* 1997;157(6):669–675.
19. Wolfsdorf J, Craig ME, Daneman D, et al. Diabetic ketoacidosis in children and adolescents with diabetes. *Pediatr Diabetes.* 2009;10(Suppl 12):118–133.

20. Vanelli M, Chiari G, Ghizzoni L, Costi G, Giacalone T, Chiarelli F. Effectiveness of a prevention program for diabetic ketoacidosis in children. An 8-year study in schools and private practices. *Diabetes Care.* 1999;22(1):7–9.
21. Zhong VW, Juhaeri J, Mayer-Davis EJ. Trends in hospital admission for diabetic ketoacidosis in adults with type 1 and type 2 diabetes in England, 1998-2013: a retrospective cohort study. *Diabetes Care.* 2018;41(9):1870–1877.
22. Kitabchi AE, Umpierrez GE, Miles JM, Fisher JN. Hyperglycemic crises in adult patients with diabetes. *Diabetes Care.* 2009;32(7):1335–1343.
23. Adeyinka A, Kondamudi NP. Hyperosmolar hyperglycemic nonketotic coma. *StatPearls [Internet].* Treasure Island, FL: StatPearls Publishing; 2020.
24. Pasquel FJ, Umpierrez GE. Hyperosmolar hyperglycemic state: a historic review of the clinical presentation, diagnosis, and treatment. *Diabetes Care.* 2014;37(11):3124–3131.
25. Seaquist ER, Anderson J, Childs B, et al. Hypoglycemia and diabetes: a report of a workgroup of the American Diabetes Association and the Endocrine Society. *Diabetes Care.* 2013;36(5):1384–1395.

CHAPTER 16

Pancreatic Neuroendocrine Emergencies in the Adult (Gastrinoma, Insulinoma, Glucagonoma, VIPoma, Somatostatinoma, and PPoma/ Nonfunctional Tumors)

Vince Gemma ■ Jason D. Prescott

CHAPTER OUTLINE

Overview

The neuroendocrine component of the pancreas comprises highly specialized and tightly regulated cells responsible for the synthesis and secretion of specific peptide hormones. These cells are situated together within discreet, encapsulated and highly vascularized clusters called the islets of Langerhans, which are distributed throughout the pancreatic parenchyma. Approximately 3 million islets are present in the adult pancreas. The peptide hormones produced by specific islet cells include gastrin (G cells), insulin (beta cells), glucagon (alpha cells), vasoactive intestinal peptide (VIP, parasympathetic nerve cells), somatostatin (delta cells), and pancreatic polypeptide (PP, gamma/F cells), all of which are secreted directly into the associated islet blood supply. Under normal circumstances, the synthesis and secretion of each pancreatic neuroendocrine hormone are tightly regulated by intricate feedback mechanisms, so as to maintain normal physiology. However, overproduction of these hormones, often the result of tumor development from corresponding pancreatic neuroendocrine cells, can result in acute, potentially life-threatening morbidity. In general, emergent/life-threatening sequelae of excessive pancreatic neuroendocrine hormone production are not specific to the underlying hypersecretory tumor. Acute management therefore rarely involves direct diagnosis/treatment of the associated tumor but rather focuses on stabilization of the acutely ill patient.

Gastrinoma

Unlike most other pancreatic islet cells, G cells are not primarily pancreatic under normal circumstances, localizing also to the stomach antrum and duodenum. G cells are parasympathetic (vagal) neuroendocrine cells that function primarily to stimulate release of hydrochloric acid (HCl) from parietal cells of the stomach during digestion, which they mediate via gastrin secretion. The synthesis and secretion of gastrin, a 6–71-amino acid peptide (depending on the extent of posttranslational cleavage), are tightly regulated under normal circumstances: G cells secrete gastrin in response to vagal stimulation, stomach distention, increased blood calcium levels, and the presence of amino acids in the stomach. Gastrin secretion is normally inhibited by increasing stomach acidity, as well as by the regulatory hormones somatostatin, gastroinhibitory peptide, VIP, calcitonin, glucagon, and secretin.

Hypergastrinemia may result from inappropriate stimulation/loss of inhibition of otherwise normal G cells or, less commonly, from neoplastic G cell proliferation (gastrinoma). Approximately 25% of gastrinomas will develop from pancreatic G cells, with the incidence of pancreatic gastrinoma ranging between 0.1 and 0.4 per million individuals per year. Nonpancreatic gastrinomas may arise from the duodenum, stomach, liver, bile ducts, ovary, heart, or lung and the majority of gastrinomas are sporadic (approximately 80%), with most nonsporadic disease being associated with multiple endocrine neoplasia type 1 (MEN1). Gastrinomas develop disproportionately in men and diagnosis is most common between the ages of 20 and 50 years.[1]

The clinical manifestations of gastrinoma are collectively known as Zollinger–Ellison syndrome (ZES) and are the result of hypergastrinemia. Among the etiologies potentially responsible for gastrin hypersecretion, gastrinoma and pernicious anemia produce the highest blood gastrin levels and, correspondingly, the most potentially severe associated symptoms. In general, these are related to peptic ulcer disease (which develops in over 90% of ZES cases), and/or malabsorption, and include abdominal/esophageal/thoracic pain (75% prevalence), diarrhea (73% prevalence), and nausea. Potential associated signs include gastrointestinal (GI) hemorrhage (25% prevalence), weight loss/malnourishment (17% prevalence), steatorrhea, GI obstruction, GI perforation, and anorexia/food intolerance.

ACUTE/EMERGENT DISEASE: PRESENTATION, MANAGEMENT, AND OUTCOMES

In most cases, development of gastrinoma-related signs/symptoms is gradual, characterized by increasingly symptomatic and medically refractory peptic ulcer disease. Gastrinoma is rarely diagnosed in the acute setting and emergent manifestations are generally the result of unrecognized/neglected progressive disease. These include life-threatening GI hemorrhage, GI perforation, and GI obstruction (Table 16.1). It is important to note that management of these life-threatening disease manifestations is not specific to gastrinoma, but rather focuses on emergent stabilization of the acutely ill patient through resuscitative, supportive, and often surgical/procedural techniques. Such management usually occurs in the setting of an emergency department and always involves intravenous (IV) fluid resuscitation, basic biochemical (blood) testing, and diagnostic imaging, most commonly computed tomography (CT) scanning. The underlying diagnosis of gastrinoma, if not already known, is usually established and addressed well after urgent management is completed.

TABLE 16.1 ■ **Manifestations, Diagnostic Features, and Management of Gastrinoma (Hypergastrinemia)**

Emergent Manifestations	Critical Positive Diagnostic Features	Emergent Management: General Principles
1. Massive upper GI hemorrhage	**Vital signs:** Shock **PE/symptoms:** Cognitive impairment related to severe volume depletion **Biochemistry:** Anemia **Imaging:** Upper GI bleeding, bleeding ulcer (EGD)	1. +/− intubation, IV resuscitation, blood transfusion 2. IV proton pump inhibitor administration 3. Interventional EGD with thermal coagulation, mechanical clipping, hemostatic spray/powder application and/or epinephrine injection 4. Transarterial embolization or surgical management, if persistent bleeding
2. Upper GI perforation	**Vital signs:** Developing/frank shock **PE/symptoms:** Epigastric pain, peritonitis, nausea **Biochemistry:** Leukocytosis **Imaging:** Intraabdominal free air, intraabdominal free fluid/fluid collection, oral contrast extravasation	1. Intubation if frank shock, IV resuscitation 2. Empiric IV antibiotic and proton pump inhibitor administration 3. Surgical management for intraabdominal soilage clearance and ulcer repair
3. Gastric outlet obstruction	**Vital signs:** Tachycardia, hypotension **PE/symptoms:** Intractable vomiting **Biochemistry:** Hypochlorremic, hypokalemic metabolic alkalosis **Imaging:** Gastric distention, restriction/failure of oral contrast progression at gastric outlet, bowel edema at gastric outlet	1. IV resuscitation, nasogastric decompression, serum electrolyte correction 2. IV proton pump inhibitor administration 3. Balloon dilation

Hemorrhage

GI hemorrhage, in this case from duodenal and/or gastric ulceration, is the most common emergent complication of peptic ulcer disease, accounting for 73% of cases. Acute presentation is characterized by signs/symptoms of significant blood loss/hemorrhagic shock. Biochemical testing reveals marked anemia and, potentially, thrombocytopenia. If associated end organ ischemic time is short, hypokalemic, hypochloremic alkalosis may be incidentally noted. This finding is suggestive of underlying hypergastrinemia and may help guide resuscitation strategy.

The management of shock is not unique to hypergastrinemia-mediated GI hemorrhage. All patients presenting in shock should be treated emergently using a basic resuscitative algorithm designed to abrogate progressive life-threatening multiorgan failure. Such algorithms have been thoroughly described in the critical care/trauma literature and include airway stabilization, ventilatory support, resuscitation, and transfusion, in the context of frequent/real time vital sign monitoring.[2] Following successful resuscitative treatment, the underlying source(s) of bleeding must be identified. This requires diagnostic imaging, which may include CT arteriography, upper and lower endoscopy, catheter angiography and, potentially, tagged red cell scintigraphy and/or capsule endoscopy. For bleeding peptic ulcer disease, these imaging techniques, when positive, will reveal evidence of upper GI hemorrhage. In addition, CT scanning may identify one or more incidental abdominal soft tissue masses (gastrinomas) when ZES is present.

Endoscopy is always indicated when upper GI bleeding is suspected or is identified by nonendoscopic imaging. Associated sensitivity and specificity for bleeding ulcer identification exceed those of all other imaging modalities, approaching 98% and 100%, respectively. In addition, endoscopic intervention for active ulcer hemorrhage is generally employed simultaneously, including thermal coagulation, mechanical clipping, hemostatic spray/powder application, and/or epinephrine injection, thus making upper endoscopy both diagnostic and therapeutic. ZES is most commonly characterized by a solitary ulcer, usually less than 1 cm in diameter, localizing to the first portion of the duodenum (75% of cases). Nonetheless, a thorough upper endoscopic assessment is required, as multiple ulcers may be present and may localize to other portions of the upper GI tract, including the stomach, other domains of the duodenum, and/or the proximal jejunum.

Following emergent resuscitation, endoscopic intervention, as above, is the first-line treatment for bleeding peptic ulcers, achieving hemorrhage control in over 90% of cases. In the acute setting, ulcer discovery in general should also prompt IV treatment with a proton pump inhibitor and, if at all possible, any baseline anticoagulation should be reversed. Should endoscopic management fail to control ulcer bleeding, either during initial assessment or in the context of recurrence, surgical or endovascular approaches are indicated. These second-line options are generally considered equally effective, relative to one another. Catheter angiography with transarterial embolization is less invasive than surgery and success rates for initial bleeding control range between 52% and 98%. Surgical interventions include laparotomy, with enterectomy to oversew the ulcer and tamponade associated bleeding vessel(s), or ulcer resection with appropriate GI tract reconstruction, if the patient is stable. In each case, vagotomy and pyloroplasty should also be performed.[3]

Perforation

GI perforation is a second life-threating manifestation of ZES (Table 16.1). Like GI hemorrhage, perforation in this context is the result of advanced ulcer disease. These ulcers eventually erode through the full thickness of the stomach/bowel wall, ultimately allowing spillage of GI contents (including GI flora) into the peritoneal space. As such, acute presentation is the result of peritoneal irritation and, potentially, septic shock. Patients most often complain of sudden onset severe abdominal pain, with physical examination findings generally consistent with peritonitis, including rebound pain, focal epigastric tenderness, and guarding. Biochemical testing may reveal leukocytosis.

Immediate management focuses on resuscitation, especially if hemodynamic instability is present. Subsequent diagnostic imaging will reveal evidence of GI perforation. Upright abdominal plain film radiography may show subdiaphragmatic free air. More commonly, abdominal CT scanning is the initial diagnostic imaging performed, revealing free air and extraluminal fluid in the vicinity of the perforation. If oral contrast is used, this may be seen extravasating into the adjacent peritoneal space. Evidence of gastric/duodenal GI perforation requires prompt broad-spectrum IV antibiotic and proton pump inhibitor administration, as well as ongoing fluid resuscitation. In general, emergent surgery to address the perforation and remove the associated peritoneal soilage is then indicated, although nonoperative management, with or without percutaneous drainage, is an option for elderly patients having small, sealed perforations and who are poor surgical candidates.

Operative management most commonly involves laparotomy, although laparoscopic approaches have been described. Surgical options for perforated gastric ulcers include total gastrectomy (if underlying gastric malignancy cannot be excluded and the patient is stable, without significant peritoneal soilage), as well as gastric wedge resection or omental (Graham) patch repair, with vagotomy and pyloroplasty in both cases. Perforated duodenal ulcers may be managed with patching, especially in hemodynamically unstable patients, or by pyloroplasty (with perforation incorporation) and vagotomy. More complex procedures/resections are generally not required but may be necessary if a large perforation is present in a hemodynamically stable patient.[4]

Gastric Outlet Obstruction

Inflammation and edema associated with progressive peptic ulcer disease involving the distal stomach and/or duodenum may cause gastric outlet obstruction (Table 16.1). In the emergent setting, presenting signs and symptoms include intractable nonbilious vomiting, epigastric pain, abdominal distention, and dehydration. Biochemical testing may reveal hypochloremic, hypokalemic alkalosis, in the setting of prolonged vomiting and gastrinemia-mediated chronic HCl secretion. Diagnostic plain film imaging may demonstrate gastric distention (if the stomach has not been decompressed by nasogastric tube suctioning or excessive vomiting) and CT scanning with oral contrast will identify severe restriction/failure of contrast progression at the gastroduodenal junction, with bowel edema involving the gastric outlet.

Initial management focuses on fluid resuscitation, IV proton pump inhibitor administration, and basic biochemical testing, with correction of identified electrolyte abnormalities. Nasogastric tube placement with gastric decompression should be employed if abdominal distention is noted or when imaging reveals gastric outlet obstruction. Following resuscitation, upper endoscopy should be performed to delineate the cause of obstruction. For underlying peptic ulcer disease, an endoscopic balloon dilation is generally attempted. This requires advancement of the endoscope beyond the obstruction and is associated with a low rate of perforation, depending on the size of the balloon used. Recurrence rates in the context of ZES are unacceptably high, however, and successful initial balloon dilation is thus considered a temporizing measure in this context. Surgical management is therefore often required to definitively relieve the obstruction and treat the underlying ulcer disease. Options include open or laparoscopic distal gastrectomy/antrectomy with vagotomy, or bypass drainage with vagotomy.

Outcomes

Management outcomes for emergent manifestations of gastrinoma depend on specific presentation (upper GI hemorrhage, GI perforation, or gastric outlet obstruction), as well as on the extent of patient comorbidity. Mortality rates in the acute setting may be as high as 18% for peptic ulcer hemorrhage and 20% for peptic ulcer perforation, whereas these rates are exceedingly low in cases of peptic ulcer-related (benign) gastric outlet obstruction. Regardless, formal workup for gastrinoma is vitally important following successful acute management in these patients, as failure to establish this underlying diagnosis will increase the probability of recurrence in each case and may allow disease progression if malignant gastrinoma is present. Diagnosis is based on marked elevation in serum gastrin level (greater than 1000 pg/mL) or, in cases with less marked hypergastrinemia, on positive secretin stimulation testing.[5]

Insulinoma

The insulin producing beta islet cells account for 60% to 85% of the endocrine pancreas. Insulin functions in glucose homeostasis by driving glucose uptake in skeletal muscle, liver, and adipose tissue, and by inhibiting both glycogenolysis and gluconeogenesis. Insulin synthesis and secretion are tightly regulated under normal circumstances, so as to maintain euglycemia. Excess insulin/hyperinsulinemia produces hypoglycemia, which results in end organ energy deprivation, the most severe manifestations of which are irreversible brain injury and death.

Insulinoma is the most common functional pancreatic neuroendocrine tumor, with an incidence of 4 cases per 1 million person years. Characteristically, these tumors secrete excess insulin, producing symptomatic hypoglycemia between meals in effected individuals. Approximately 90% of insulinomas are less than 2 cm in maximal diameter and tumors may localize at any site within the pancreas. Insulinomas are most commonly benign (90%) and are generally discreetly localized/noninvasive. Given the small nature of most insulinomas, symptoms related to associated mass/mechanical effects are rare.

ACUTE/EMERGENT DISEASE: PRESENTATION, MANAGEMENT, AND OUTCOMES

Emergent/life threatening manifestations of insulinoma are the result of severe hypoglycemia, which, if left untreated, can result in irreversible brain injury or death (Table 16.2). A nondiabetic hypoglycemic patient presenting with symptoms of sympathoadrenal activation, such as tremors, sweating, and palpitations, should raise concern for a diagnosis of insulinoma. Regardless of underlying diagnosis, however, expeditious management of hypoglycemia is the most critical component of emergent care in these patients.

Undifferentiated Hypoglycemia

Severe hypoglycemia can produce disrupted mentation, including behavioral changes, fatigue, confusion and seizure, or loss of consciousness/coma, which should trigger a general emergency management algorithm used for any poorly responsive or unresponsive patient. This includes evaluation of airway (with intubation, if indicated), breathing, and circulation. Vital sign assessment may reveal signs of central/autonomic nervous system disruption, including tachycardia/dysrhythmia, hypertension/hypotension, and tachypnea. Basic emergency biochemical testing will reveal profound hypoglycemia, with plasma glucose levels generally less than 55 mg/dL. In this setting, IV blood sugar replacement should be initiated promptly, most commonly using a 50% dextrose solution, to provide 12.5 to 25 g of sugar. In general, this should lead to rapid clinical improvement. Glucagon, administered in 1 mg doses, can be given via a subcutaneous or intramuscular route if immediate IV access cannot be obtained. Serial blood sugar monitoring should be performed every 5 to 10 minutes until plasma glucose levels exceed 70 mg/dL. The restoration of euglycemia may be brief in this setting, depending on the level of underlying hyperinsulinemia, and, as such, a continuous infusion of 5% dextrose should be maintained following initial blood sugar stabilization.

TABLE 16.2 ■ **Manifestations, Diagnostic Features, and Management of Insulinoma (Hyperinsulinermia)**

Emergent Manifestations	Critical Positive Diagnostic Features	Emergent Management: General Principles
Hypoglycemic crisis	**Vital signs:** Tachycardia, hypotension **PE/symptoms:** Altered mentation, seizures, coma **Imaging:** Nonspecific	1. IV dextrose, 50% solution, to provide 12.5-25 g sugar 2. Glucagon, 1 mg subcutaneous or intramuscular 3. Blood glucose level monitoring every 5-10 minutes 4. Continuous infusion of 5% dextrose solution to maintain blood glucose >70 mg/dL 5. For known underlying insulinoma: diazoxide or octreotide

Refractory Hypoglycemia With Known Insulinoma

Patients having a known diagnosis of insulinoma may present with recurrent, refractory episodes of severe hypoglycemia. In addition to the general emergent management strategy described above, treatment in this setting also focuses on optimizing glucose homeostasis. The most common initial measure in such cases is diazoxide administration, which inhibits insulin secretion. Secondary agents include octreotide, or other somatostatin analogs, which must be used with caution as administration may lead to paradoxical worsening of hypoglycemia in the context of concomitant inhibition of glucagon secretion, which is also mediated by these agents.

Outcomes

Outcomes related to emergent insulinoma-mediated hypoglycemia depend on presenting severity, timing, and degree of treatment responsiveness. In the acute setting, prompt treatment of severe hypoglycemia will have good outcomes, without long-term sequelae. For patients with generalized prolonged hypoglycemic encephalopathy (which is not specific to insulinoma), outcomes are poor, with 60% of patients suffering from permanent disability or death. Following emergent management, all patients must undergo a hypoglycemia workup, including assessment for insulinoma and nesidioblastosis. Endogenous hyperinsulinemia in the context of hypoglycemia is diagnostic of insulinoma. Long-term outcomes for resectable insulinoma are excellent, whereas palliative management of unresectable malignant disease may be challenging. In general, however, aggressive surgical tumor debulking in the setting of metastatic or locally invasive disease improves long-term survival.[6]

Glucagonoma

Alpha cells account for approximately 20% of pancreatic islet volume and are responsible for the synthesis and secretion of glucagon. Glucagon is a 29-amino-acid peptide hormone that functions to regulate energy homeostasis by increasing blood sugar concentration, primarily though stimulation of hepatic glycogenolysis and gluconeogenesis. As is the case for all pancreatic neuroendocrine hormones, the synthesis and secretion of glucagon are normally regulated by intricate feedback mechanisms, with hypoglycemia being the most important driver of glucagon secretion.

Glucagonomas are rare functional neuroendocrine tumors derived from alpha cells. The annual incidence in the United States ranges between 0.01 and 0.1 cases per 100,000 people and most glucagonomas are diagnosed in the fifth or sixth decade of life. Gender distribution is equal among effected individuals and the majority of cases are characterized by the sporadic (greater than 80%) development of a solitary tumor, typically arising in the distal pancreas. Like other pancreatic neuroendocrine tumors, familial/syndromic glucagonomas are most frequently associated with MEN1 syndrome, which accounts for approximately 20% of cases. Up to 80% of glucagonomas will be metastatic at the time of initial diagnosis.

The constellation of signs and symptoms characterizing glucagonoma are together known as the glucagonoma/4D syndrome and are the product of hyperglucagonemia. Classically, this includes weight loss (prevalence 90%), rash/mucosal inflammation (necrolytic migratory erythema, prevalence up to 90%), diabetes (prevalence approximately 40%), diarrhea (prevalence 30%), neuropsychiatric disturbance (depression, psychosis, agitation, delusions, ataxia, and/or hyperreflexia, prevalence over 50%), and deep venous thrombosis/pulmonary embolism (DVT/PE, prevalence 50%). The 4D designation refers to dermatitis, depression, DVT, and diabetes. Among these signs/symptoms, glucagon-mediated hyperglycemia is responsible for the development of associated diabetes, although the mechanism(s) whereby hyperglucagonemia produces the remaining features of this syndrome are not well understood.

ACUTE/EMERGENT DISEASE: PRESENTATION, MANAGEMENT, AND OUTCOMES

Glucagonoma-related signs/symptoms tend to develop gradually, and these tumors are rarely diagnosed in an emergent setting. Nonetheless, unrecognized and/or neglected disease may eventually produce emergent/life-threatening morbidity. The most important emergent manifestation is acute PE, which is a responsible for most glucagonoma syndrome-related mortality (Table 16.3). Rare cases of glucagonoma-related dilated cardiomyopathy have been described, as have very uncommon cases of associated diabetic ketoacidosis. In addition, stroke, in the context of a patent foramen ovale, is a theoretical manifestation of embolic disease in patients diagnosed with glucagonoma, although no specific instances have been formally reported.

Pulmonary Embolism

The presentation of acute PE is not specific to glucagonoma, when present, and is prototypically characterized by shortness of breath/dyspnea, tachycardia/palpitations, cough, pleuritic chest pain, and, rarely, hemoptysis. Vital sign assessment will confirm tachycardia and, potentially, hypoxia and/or hypotension. Evidence of DVT may be identified during the physical examination, including unilateral distal extremity swelling/edema, with skin warmth, erythema and tenderness, an associated palpable cord (representing an area of thrombosis), and/or pain with foot dorsiflexion while the knee is extended (positive Homan's sign). An electrocardiogram (ECG) may demonstrate evidence of right heart strain. Biochemical testing will reveal an elevated D-dimer level, which is sensitive, but not specific, for DVT/PE, and an atrial blood gas assessment may identify hypoxemia and hypocapnia. Concomitant findings of hyperglycemia, hypoproteinemia/hypoalbuminemia, and mild anemia are suggestive of, but not specific for, underlying glucagonoma.

Clinical suspicion for PE should prompt diagnostic imaging, either by CT angiogram or, less commonly, ventilation-perfusion (VQ) scanning. In addition to embolus identification, CT scanning may identify infarction involving lung parenchyma distal to the point of vascular obstruction and, in cases of underlying glucagonoma, evidence of soft tissue pancreatic mass(es) and/or metastatic disease. Right ventricular dilation may also be noted in severe cases. Bedsides echocardiography should be performed to assess for pulmonary hypertension and right heart failure, if hemodynamic instability is present. Once a diagnosis of PE is made, the coexistent presence of

TABLE 16.3 ■ **Manifestations, Diagnostic Features, and Management of Glucagonoma (Hyperglucagonemia)**

Emergent Manifestations	Critical Positive Diagnostic Features	Emergent Management: General Principles
Pulmonary embolism	**Vital signs:** Tachycardia, tachypnea, hypoxia **PE/symptoms:** Shortness of breath, cough, pleuritic chest pain, rash (necrolytic migratory erythema), diarrhea, depression **Biochemistry:** Positive D-dimer, hyperglycemia, hypoxemia, hypoproteinemia **Imaging:** Pulmonary thrombosis (CT angiography), positive VQ scan, +/– right heart strain noted by echocardiogram/EKG	1. Supplemental oxygen 2. IV therapeutic anticoagulation 3. +/– endovascular thrombolysis or thrombectomy

rash (necrolytic migratory erythema), especially if distributed to the face, perineum, lower abdomen, and/or distal extremities, should immediately alert the clinician to the possibility of associated glucagonoma.

Acute management of PE in this context is not specific to the underlying glucagonoma. All cases of acute PE require supplemental oxygen administration, which may include intubation and ventilatory support in severe cases. Therapeutic anticoagulation should be initiated expeditiously, most commonly by continuous heparin (or equivalent agent) infusion. Severe cases with associated hemodynamic instability, right heart strain/pulmonary hypertension, and/or ineffective oxygenation despite maximal ventilatory support, require procedural intervention, either by endovascular thrombolysis or embolectomy.

Outcomes

Management outcomes for acute PE are not specific to those cases associated with glucagonoma. Overall, mortality rates depend on the extent of embolic disease and, in particular, on the presence or absence of associated hemodynamic instability/shock, which, when present, confers a 30% to 50% risk of mortality. In addition, untreated PE is associated with an overall mortality rate of 30%, illustrating the criticality of early diagnosis and treatment.

A careful assessment for signs and symptoms of glucagonoma is crucial in all patients following successful management of acute PE, as thromboembolism recurrence rates in this context are high, especially if therapeutic anticoagulation is eventually discontinued. Moreover, subsequent nonemergent surgical, ablative, and medical treatment(s) for associated glucagonoma will decrease or abrogate thromboembolism recurrence risk, effectively treat other manifestations of the glucagonoma/4D syndrome present, and potentially prevent/delay tumor progression, if a malignant glucagonoma is present. A 10-fold (or greater) elevation in serum glucagon level is diagnostic of underlying glucagonoma.[7]

VIPoma

VIP is a 28-amino-acid peptide hormone and neurotransmitter synthesized and secreted by parasympathetic nerve cells. VIP is produced in many different tissues, and its function depends on the specific cell type/organ targeted, although the net effect of this hormone on the human GI tract is to increase motility and overall luminal secretion. VIP synthesis and secretion are tightly regulated under normal circumstances. The specific mechanisms of this regulation, however, are generally not well understood and may differ between involved organ systems.

VIP-secreting tumors (VIPomas) are rare neuroendocrine neoplasms, with an annual incidence rate of approximately 1 per million individuals. In adults, 95% of these tumors will develop in the pancreas, with the remaining 5% potentially arising from multiple different tissues, including the lung, colon, nervous system, adrenal glands, or liver. The majority of pancreatic VIPomas will be solitary, less than 3 cm in maximal diameter, and will localize to the tail of the pancreas (~75%). The most common age range for diagnosis in the adult is between 30 and 50 years, and up to 80% will be metastatic at the time of initial detection. Most VIPomas are sporadic (~95%), although familial/genetic predisposition to VIPoma development is associated with MEN1 syndrome (as is the case for other pancreatic neuroendocrine tumor types).

Most VIPomas overproduce VIP, which results in a secretory diarrheal syndrome termed Verner–Morrison syndrome, pancreatic cholera, or **W**atery **D**iarrhea, **H**ypokalemia, and hypochlorhydria or **A**chlorhydria (WDHA) syndrome. Like other pancreatic neuroendocrine hormone-mediated syndromes, symptomatic development of WDHA is usually gradual, depending on a progressive increase in VIP blood levels as tumor growth proceeds over time. VIPomas can produce emergent/life-threatening morbidity, however, if progressive disease is neglected or undiagnosed (Table 16.4).

TABLE 16.4 ■ **Manifestations, Diagnostic Features, and Management of VIPoma (VIPemia)**

Emergent Manifestations	Critical Positive Diagnostic Features	Emergent Management: General Principles
Severe dehydration, serum electrolyte abnormalities	**Vital signs:** hypothermia, tachycardia, tachypnea, hypotension **PE/symptoms:** Fatigue/altered mental status, palpitations, vomiting, muscle weakness/cramps, dry mucous membranes, loss of skin turgor, watery diarrhea **Biochemistry:** Hemoconcentration, hypokalemia, hyperalbuminemia, hypercalcemia, hyperglycemia, elevated blood creatinine **Imaging:** Nonspecific	1. Aggressive IV resuscitation with normal saline or lactated ringers 2. Serum electrolyte correction (IV) 3. Serial monitoring of serum electrolyte and creatinine levels 4. Short acting octreotide administration, if known diagnosis of VIPoma

ACUTE/EMERGENT DISEASE: PRESENTATION, MANAGEMENT, AND OUTCOMES

Emergent sequelae of VIP hypersecretion are the result of severe secretory diarrhea and include life-threatening dehydration and marked electrolyte imbalances. Presenting signs/symptoms in this context include fatigue/lethargy, dizziness/lightheadedness, irritability, heart racing/palpitations, vomiting, muscle weakness, and muscle spasms/cramps. Patients will describe a progressive history of chronic watery diarrhea, generally exceeding 1 L in daily volume. Abdominal pain/cramping is generally absent, and patients will often endorse decreased urine output/anuria in the acute setting. Vital sign assessment may identify relative hypothermia, hypotension, tachycardia, and tachypnea. Physical examination findings will be consistent with dehydration and may include altered mentation, loss of skin turgor, impaired capillary refill, dry mucous membranes, tachycardia, and tachypnea. Biochemical testing may demonstrate hemoconcentration, hypokalemia, hyperalbuminemia (with associated increased blood total calcium levels), hyperglycemia, and elevated blood creatinine levels. Osmotic gap assessment will reveal a value of less than 50 mOsm/kg, consistent with secretory diarrhea. Stool guaiac testing will be negative. An ECG may identify findings related to hypokalemia, including flattening or inversion of T waves, Q-T interval prolongation, U waves, and tachycardia. Radiologic assessment will be nonspecific, although abdominal imaging is likely to identify soft tissue pancreatic masse(s) representing the underlying VIPoma, with possible associated metastatic foci (most commonly hepatic). Endoscopic assessment will generally be unremarkable.

Acute treatment of severe dehydration is not specific to underlying VIP hypersecretion. As for all acutely ill patients, initial evaluation begins with assessment and management of airway, ventilation, and circulation. In cases of severe altered mentation/lethargy, intubation may be temporarily required to protect the airway. Aggressive IV resuscitation with normal saline or lactated ringers should be promptly initiated, with concomitant administration of IV potassium chloride if hypokalemia is present. These measures generally bring about rapid improvement in presenting signs and symptoms. A Foley catheter should be placed to facilitate urine output monitoring, which serves as an important gauge of fluid status in patients having intact kidney function. Nephrotoxic agents should be avoided in the context of acute prerenal kidney injury, including IV contrast and nonsteroidal antiinflammatory agents. Serial biochemical monitoring is required to verify and track blood electrolyte and creatinine level improvement. Copious watery diarrhea will persist, and may actually increase in volume/frequency, during acute resuscitation given persistent underlying VIPemia, and hospital admission to establish the underlying diagnosis (for which the differential is broad) will be required. If the underlying diagnosis of VIPoma has already been established, subcutaneous short-acting octreotide should also be administered in the acute setting, as somatostatin analogs can inhibit VIP secretion and thus decrease the severity of associated secretory diarrhea.

Outcomes

Outcomes following emergent treatment for single episodes of acute, severe secretory diarrhea are generally excellent, with associated mortality and long-term morbidity being uncommon. Secretory diarrhea resulting from VIPoma will be chronic, however, especially when untreated. In this setting, associated chronic/recurrent dehydration and electrolyte abnormalities eventually lead to renal and cardiac failure, which are primarily responsible for VIPoma-related mortality. Thus, although an initial acute episode of severe secretory diarrhea-induced dehydration is readily managed in the context of VIPoma, subsequent/concomitant diagnosis and treatment of this tumor are critically important to preventing/minimizing associated life-threatening chronic diarrhea. For this reason, recurrent severe watery diarrhea should prompt serum VIP level testing in all cases. A value greater than 75 pg/mL confirms an underlying diagnostic of VIPoma.[8]

Somatostatinoma

Somatostatin is an inhibitory peptide hormone produced in many different organ systems, including the pancreas/GI tract, nervous system, heart, thymus, thyroid, eye, and skin. In the pancreas, somatostatin is synthesized by islet delta cells, and, in this context, its function is to inhibit the secretion of the other GI hormones. Thus, the overall effect of somatostatin in the GI tract is to decrease motility and secretion.

Somatostatinomas are rare neoplasms that account for less than 5% of functional neuroendocrine tumors, with a reported annual incidence of 1 in 40 million individuals. These tumors are malignant in approximately 70% of cases and up to 70% will arise from the pancreas, most commonly within the pancreatic head. Somatostatin hypersecretion produces the triad of diabetes, cholelithiasis, and diarrhea, referred to as inhibitory syndrome. Diabetes manifests in 60% of cases and is the result of somatostatin-mediated inhibition of insulin secretion, whereas cholelithiasis, present in 70% of effected individuals, results from inhibition of cholecystokinin release. Somatostatin-induced inhibition of gastrin and of pancreatic enzyme secretion produces hypochlorhydria and steatorrhea, respectively. Nonfunctional/nonsecreting somatostatinomas have been described and may eventually enlarge/metastasize, ultimately producing mechanical/obstructive-based symptoms, including abdominal pain, nausea, and jaundice.

ACUTE/EMERGENT DISEASE: PRESENTATION, MANAGEMENT, AND OUTCOMES

Inhibitory syndrome (glucose intolerance, cholelithiasis or cholestasis, diarrhea with or without steatorrhea, and hypochlorhydria) will manifest in up to 66% of pancreatic somatostatinomas. Like other hypersecretory pancreatic neuroendocrine syndromes, the development of somatostatinoma-related symptoms is incremental. As tumor growth proceeds, blood somatostatin levels gradually rise, resulting in progressive symptom development. Ultimately, these symptoms can be life-threatening, especially if the tumor remains undetected.

Symptomatic somatostatinomas most commonly manifest with mild to moderate hyperglycemia. A small number of cases presenting with hyperglycemic crisis (diabetic ketoacidosis[DKA] or hyperosmolar hyperglycemic state[HHS]) have been reported, however (Table 16.5). Morbidity in this context is not specific to somatostatin hypersecretion and associated signs/symptoms are

TABLE 16.5 ■ **Manifestations, Diagnostic Features, and Management of Somatostatinoma (Somatostatinemia)**

Emergent Manifestations	Critical Positive Diagnostic Features	Emergent Management: General Principles
Hyperglycemia crisis (diabetic ketoacidosis or hyperosmolar hyperglycemic state)	**Vital signs:** Hypothermia, tachycardia, tachypnea, hypotension **PE/symptoms:** Polyuria, polydipsia, progressive neurologic deterioration, nausea, vomiting, abdominal pain, dry mucous membranes, loss of skin turgor, 'fruity' smelling breath (DKA) **Biochemistry:** Hyperglycemia (>350 mg/dL DKA/>600 mg/dL HHS), anion gap metabolic acidosis, plasma osmolality >320 mOsmol/kg, hypo or hyperkalemia, elevated urine/blood ketone levels (DKA) **Imaging:** Nonspecific, rare cerebral edema	1. Aggressive IV resuscitation with normal saline 2. IV regular insulin: 0.15 units/kg bolus, 0.1 units/kg/hour infusion, hourly blood glucome monitoring (goal 150–200 mg/dL) 3. Serum electrolyte abnormality correction (IV), with monitoring of levels every 2 hours 4. Blood pH correction if <6.9 with IV bicarbonate, target blood pH 7.2

typical of DKA/HHS in general. Patients present with rapidly progressive polyuria, polydipsia, and neurologic deterioration, including fatigue, confusion, lethargy, focal dysfunction (hemiparesis or hemianopsia), seizures, or coma. Associated nausea, vomiting, and abdominal pain may also be present. Vital sign assessment may reveal hypothermia, tachypnea, tachycardia, and hypotension. A physical examination will demonstrate neurologic findings, as above, as well as signs of severe dehydration, including loss of skin turgor, impaired capillary refill, and dry mucous membranes. The patient's breath may take on a fruity quality (akin to acetone) resulting from high ketone content, if DKA is present. Blood testing will reveal hyperglycemia, with blood glucose levels exceeding 350 mg/dL in most cases of DKA and greater than 600 mg/dL for HHS, an anion gap metabolic acidosis, and elevated plasma osmolality, usually greater than 320 mOsmol/kg. Other findings may include hyperkalemia or hypokalemia, elevated creatinine (prerenal acute kidney injury), and noninfectious leukocytosis. Arterial blood gas testing may reveal metabolic acidosis (DKA). Urinalysis will show elevated glucose and, for DKA, elevated ketone levels, the latter of which will also be elevated in the blood. Imaging studies will generally be nonspecific, although axial abdominal imaging in this context may identify the underlying somatostatinoma/associated metastatic disease. Rarely, axial imaging of the head may demonstrate cerebral edema.

Management begins with assessment of airway, breathing, and circulation. Severe neurologic dysfunction will require airway protection by intubation. Aggressive volume resuscitation with IV fluid, initially normal saline, should be initiated promptly. Control of hyperglycemia with IV insulin (0.15 units/kg bolus, followed by 0.1 units/kg per hour infusion) is undertaken to achieve stable blood glucose levels between 150 and 200 mg/dL. Careful serial monitoring of blood glucose (hourly) and urine output is required. Serum electrolyte level monitoring (every 2 hours), with correction of abnormalities, is also critical. In particular, hypokalemia must be promptly corrected, if present, with a serum target range between 3.3 and 5.5 mEq/L. Metabolic acidosis with blood pH less than 6.9 should prompt treatment with IV bicarbonate, with a blood pH target of 7.2. The majority of patients will experience rapid clinical improvement as glucose levels, electrolyte levels, blood osmolality, and volume status normalize.

While cholelithiasis and abdominal pain are common manifestations of somatostatinoma, associated emergent cholecystitis has not been reported. As such, cholelithiasis is generally managed with cholecystectomy at the time of somatostatinoma resection. Patients suffering from somatostatinoma-related diarrhea, with or without steatorrhea, may present semi-urgently for management of associated dehydration, although the related symptoms tend to be mild and are readily managed with IV fluid resuscitation and serum electrolyte level correction.

Outcomes

Management of hyperglycemic emergency is generally highly successful and, in patients having an underlying diagnosis of somatostatinoma, outcomes in the acute setting are not tumor specific. Recurrent/persistent hyperglycemia, in the presence of low blood insulin levels, cholelithiasis, and recurrent diarrhea, should prompt specific work-up for associated somatostatinoma, however, as recognition and management of the underlying tumor is critical to overall outcome. When inhibitory syndrome is present, blood somatostatin levels exceeding 30 pg/mL will be diagnostic of underlying somatostatinoma. Ultimately, long-term prognosis depends on tumor resectability.[9]

PPoma/Nonfunctional Neuroendocrine Tumors

Secretory neuroendocrine tumors that do not produce associated symptoms and nonsecretory tumor variants account for 60% to 90% of pancreatic neuroendocrine neoplasms and are termed nonfunctional (NF). Secretory tumors in this category produce clinically quiescent molecules/hormones, such as PP and/or chromogranin A. PP is a 36-amino acid cholecystokinin antagonist that plays a role in satiety signaling, inhibits pancreatic exocrine secretion, and may inhibit gastric emptying. Interestingly, PP hypersecretion does not produce symptomatic disease.

ACUTE/EMERGENT DISEASE: PRESENTATION, MANAGEMENT, AND OUTCOMES

Given the absence of attributable hypersecretory symptoms, NF pancreatic neuroendocrine tumors are usually discovered incidentally during unrelated axial imaging or during workup for associated nonspecific symptoms related to tumor growth and/or metastasis (e.g., abdominal pain, weight loss, and/or obstructive jaundice). Thus, these tumors generally do not produce emergent life-threatening morbidity. Rather, symptomatic disease generally results from gradual tumor progression, with compressive-type symptoms related to the primary tumor slowly developing in approximately 21% of patients, while symptoms resulting from distant metastasis will manifest in approximately 60% of cases. As such, patients do not generally present in extremis.

Management for NF pancreatic tumors is individualized, depending on presentation. In cases of associated nonspecific abdominal pain, with or without anorexia/oral nutrition intolerance, in an otherwise hemodynamically normal and stable patient, evaluation should include basic laboratory testing and CT imaging with IV contrast. Dehydration and electrolyte abnormalities should be addressed with IV fluid resuscitation/replacement. Associated evidence of bowel obstruction should prompt decompression by nasogastric tube placement. Evidence of jaundice on presentation should trigger liver function testing, fractionated bilirubin level assessment, and abdominal ultrasound for inspection of biliary anatomy. Associated fever and abdominal pain/peritonitis are suggestive of underlying cholangitis, which is very rare among patients presenting with NF pancreatic neuroendocrine tumors. Treatment of cholangitis in this context is not specific to the underlying tumor. As for cholangitis in general, prompt empiric antibiotic therapy and endoscopic biliary assessment, with decompression, are required.

Outcomes

Given that the nonspecific symptoms produced by NF pancreatic neuroendocrine tumors are generally related to advanced disease stage, associated prognosis is generally poor, relative to that of functional tumors. The overall 5-year survival for NF tumors is 31.1%, compared to 47.6% for their functional counterparts. The lower overall survival rate for NF disease reflects the general difference in extent of disease progression at the time of diagnosis between the two tumor categories, highlighting the fact that symptoms related to pancreatic hormone hypersecretion facilitate relative early detection in pancreatic neuroendocrine tumor development.[10]

References

1. Epelboym I, Mazeh H. Zollinger-Ellison syndrome: classical considerations and current controversies. *The Oncologist.* 2013;19(1):44–50.
2. Krausz MM. Initial resuscitation of hemorrhagic shock. *World J Emerg Surg.* 2006;27:1–14.
3. Kaminskis A, Ivanova P, Kratovska A, et al. Endoscopic hemostasis followed by preventive transarterial embolization in high-risk patients with bleeding peptic ulcer: 5-year experience. *World J Emerg Surg.* 2019;14:45.
4. Søreide K, Thorsen K, Harrison EM, et al. Perforated peptic ulcer. *Lancet.* 2015;386(10000):1288–1298.
5. Storm AC, Ryou M. Advances in the endoscopic management of gastric outflow disorders. *Curr Opin Gastroenterol.* 2017;33(6):455–460.
6. Veltroni A, Cosaro E, Spada F, et al. Clinico-pathological features, treatments and survival of malignant insulinomas: a multicenter study. *Eur J Endocrinol.* 2020;182(4):439–446.
7. Wei J, Song X, Liu X, et al. Glucagonoma and Glucagonoma syndrome: one center's experience of six cases. *J Pancreat Cancer.* 2018;4(1):11–16.
8. Angelousi A, Koffas A, Grozinsky-Glasberg S, et al. Diagnostic and management challenges in vasoactive intestinal peptide secreting tumors: a series of 15 patients. *Pancreas.* 2019;48(7):934–942.
9. Nesi G, Marcucci T, Rubio CA, Brandi ML, Tonelli F. Somatostatinoma: clinico-pathological features of three cases and literature reviewed. *J Gastroenterol Hepatol.* 2008;23(4):521–526.
10. Watley DC, Ly QP, Talmon G, Are C, Sasson AR. Clinical presentation and outcome of nonfunctional pancreatic neuroendocrine tumors in a modern cohort. *Am J Surg.* 2015;210(6):1192–1195; discussion 1195–1196.

PART 6

Neuroendocrine Tumors: Gastrointestinal Neuroendocrine Tumors

CHAPTER 17

Carcinoid Syndrome and Carcinoid Crisis

Sarah M. Wonn ■ Rodney F. Pommier

CHAPTER OUTLINE

Introduction

Neuroendocrine tumors (NETs) are a rare malignancy arising throughout the aerodigestive tract. These tumors have recently been recognized to be increasing in incidence, reaching 6.98 per 100,000 per year.[1–3] The term *carcinoid* was first coined in 1907 as "karzinoide" and describes a multitude of primary locations of NETs. These tumors have the unique property of production of an array of neurotransmitters such as serotonin and histamine, peptides such as those in the kinin-kallikrein system, and catecholamines, among others.

Carcinoid syndrome is a constellation of symptoms (classically flushing, diarrhea, and bronchospasm) thought to be mediated by the various hormones secreted by NETs. Carcinoid syndrome is present in 19% of patients with NETs of any primary tumor type, and 40% of those with duodenal, jejunal, or ileal primary NETs.[4] The mechanism of carcinoid syndrome is incompletely understood, and in spite of this incomplete understanding, carcinoid crisis is hypothesized to be an extension of carcinoid syndrome. Carcinoid crisis has no universal accepted definition, but is frequently defined as a life-threatening form of carcinoid syndrome with marked hemodynamic instability.[5] Historically, carcinoid crisis has also been hypothesized to be caused by a massive release of hormones as described above due to their vasoactive effects.

The literature on carcinoid crisis is very limited given the rarity of these tumors and the spontaneity of crisis occurrence. To date, only seven single-center retrospective reviews and one prospective single-center review have been published. This leaves clinicians with the challenge of accepting expert opinion. More recently, studies have begun to challenge the paradigm that carcinoid crisis is caused by a massive release of hormones as an extension of carcinoid syndrome, which will be discussed within the chapter. Given the variety of origins of NETs and the differences in intraabdominal and cardiac operations, this chapter will not cover cardiac operations but will attempt to focus specifically on abdominal operations, though this may be challenging in the setting of small retrospective studies being the only available literature.

As expected from the lack of consensus definition and the recent questioning of the paradigm of carcinoid crisis, controversy exists over the management of carcinoid crisis. Two areas of disagreement exist: first, the use of somatostatin analogues (i.e., octreotide) as prophylaxis and treatment, and second, the use of β-adrenergic agonists. Much has changed about our understanding of carcinoid crisis in recent years and much remains to be learned about this unique endocrine emergency's pathophysiology and treatment strategies.

Definition

Carcinoid syndrome was first described in 1954 in a case series of 16 patients. In this series, the principal findings were described as a malignant carcinoid tumor with metastases to the liver having dependent edema, diarrhea, borborygmi, abdominal pain, generalized widening of the small vessels of the skin, peculiar patchy flushing, right-sided heart valvular disease, and attacks of bronchial asthma. In this work, serotonin is attributed as the major mediator for many of these symptoms.[6] Crisis was first described in a 1964 case report of a patient with peripheral vascular collapse, leading to the beginnings of the definition as "profound hypotension in patients with the malignant carcinoid syndrome has been noted during anesthesia, palpation of the tumor at operation, or spontaneous bouts of flushing." The cause of the crisis was unknown and was postulated once again to be due to serotonin, as the patient had no response to norepinephrine and did respond to cyproheptadine, an antiserotonergic agent.[7]

Currently, there is no strict definition of carcinoid crisis. Most studies define carcinoid crisis as an acute change with profound, life-threatening hemodynamic instability, though the degree of symptomatology and duration of crisis varies. Consensus guidelines, such as those published by the North American Neuroendocrine Tumor Society (NANETS) in 2017, defined crisis as "the sudden onset of hemodynamic instability that can occur during anesthesia, operations, or other invasive procedures."[5] There have been seven retrospective reviews and one prospective study of patients with NETs undergoing operation; the definitions of carcinoid crisis by each study are summarized in Table 17.1. Not having an accepted definition of carcinoid crisis has created two major challenges. First, studies on carcinoid crisis are difficult to compare directly, as different authors define carcinoid crisis in different ways. Second, there is a wealth of individual case reports on carcinoid crisis, but these must be interpreted with caution, as no accepted definition of crisis exists.

In addition, defining carcinoid crisis has been challenged by its unknown pathophysiology. Historically, carcinoid crisis was thought of as an extreme of carcinoid syndrome with a massive release of vasoactive substances, and some authors still define carcinoid crisis as an extreme of carcinoid syndrome.[8] More recently, other studies have begun to systemically disprove this theory with the fact that octreotide (a somatostatin analogue that causes inhibition of hormonal synthesis and release) does not help prevent or treat carcinoid crisis.[9,10] In addition, a prospective trial from 2019, which collected intraoperative levels of hormones and data on pulmonary vasculature via a pulmonary artery catheter and cardiac function via a transesophageal echocardiogram, found that carcinoid crisis is most consistent with distributive shock, and intraoperative hormone levels were not elevated with crisis.[11]

There is also an ethical consideration in defining carcinoid crisis—it is not ethical to subject a patient to 10 minutes of sustained, life-threatening hemodynamic instability in the interest of fulfilling a definition of carcinoid crisis. In addition, a study published in 2013 found higher rates of postoperative complications occur in those with intraoperative crises, and a follow-up study in 2016 demonstrated that those who have hypotension in excess of 10 minutes are more likely to have postoperative complications, and those with prompt treatment of crisis are less likely to have carcinoid crisis.[9] We implore specialty societies to define carcinoid crisis with a clinically relevant definition that allows for patient safety while also allowing studies on the incidence and risk factors, prevention, and treatment of carcinoid crisis to occur.

TABLE 17.1 ■ **Definitions of Carcinoid Crisis and Incidence Rates and Risk Factors**

Study	Definition	Incidence
Kinney et al. 2001[17]	"Flushing, urticaria, ventricular dysrhythmia, bronchospasm, ... total duration of SBP <80 mm Hg to the nearest 5 min, and treatment with vasopressor(s) (SBP <80 mm Hg for >10 min), and total duration of sustained tachycardia (defined as pulse >120 beats min^{-1}) to the nearest 5 min."	15/119 (12%) with intraoperative complications
Massimino et al. 2013[9]	"Intraoperative complications were defined as prolonged hypotension (...SBP ≤80 mmHg for ≥10 min) or report of hemodynamic instability (including hypotension, sustained hypertension, or tachycardia) not attributed to acute blood loss or other obvious causes by the attending anesthesiologist or attending surgeon." Carcinoid crisis was declared whenever attending anesthesiologist or attending surgeon declared a crisis.	23/97 (24%) with intraoperative complications 5/98 (5%) with carcinoid crisis
Woltering et al. 2016[42]	"Prolonged hypotension ([SBP] <80 for >10 minutes). In addition, patient records that had anesthesia or surgical staff notation of intra-operative hemodynamic instability (HTN, hypotension, or tachycardia), or if the term "crisis" was reported."	6/179 (3.4%)
Condron et al. 2016[10]	"Significant hemodynamic instability not attributed to other factors (such as compression of the inferior vena cava or significant blood loss). Hemodynamic instability was considered significant if SBP was <80 or >180 mm Hg, if the heart rate was greater than 120 beats per minute, or if the patient was displaying physiology that, if sustained, would be expected to cause end organ dysfunction (such as ventricular arrhythmias or bronchospasm causing difficulty with ventilation). The attending surgeon and anesthesiologist had to be in agreement to declare a crisis."	45/150 (30%)
Kinney et al. 2018[43]	"Sudden or abrupt onset of at least two of the following: flushing or urticaria that is not explained by an allergic reaction, bronchospasm or bronchodilator administration, hypotension ([SBP] <80 for >10 mins and treated with pressors) not explained by volume status or hemorrhage, dysrhythmia not explained by volume status or hemorrhage, tachycardia of 120 bpm or greater."	0/169 (0%)
Fouché et al. 2018[8]	Intraoperative carcinoid syndrome was defined as "rapid (onset period ≤5 min) hemodynamic changes (heart rate (HR) or blood pressure (BP) ≥40%, not explained by surgical or anaesthetic management and regressive ≥20% within 5 min after the octreotide bolus injection." Carcinoid crisis was defined as "a life-threatening intra-operative carcinoid syndrome refractory to octreotide boluses. Carcinoid crisis includes cardiogenic shock, severe cardiac dysrhythmias, cardiac arrest or bronchospasm refractory to bronchodilators and compromising mechanical ventilation."	139 episodes of intraoperative carcinoid syndrome was observed in 45/81 patients (55.6%); 0 intraoperative carcinoid crises

(continued)

TABLE 17.1 ■ **Definitions of Carcinoid Crisis and Incidence Rates and Risk Factors—cont.**

Study	Definition	Incidence
Kwon et al. 2019[18]	"CC [carcinoid crisis] was defined subjectively by clinical documentation of occurrence by any treating physician, including the anesthesiologist, surgeon, or interventional radiologist. The HDI [hemodynamic instability]... required at least 1 of following events sustained for a period of more than 10 minutes during the procedure: (1) hypotension (systolic blood pressure, <0 mmHg), (2) hypertension (systolic blood pressure, >180 mmHg), (3) tachycardia (heart rate, >120 beats per minute). If any of the above events could be attributable to causes other than CC, such as blood loss, inferior vena cava manipulation, or pain on anesthesia record review, the HDI episode was excluded."	24/75 (32%) with carcinoid crisis/ hemodynamic instability; 3/75 (4%) with carcinoid crisis
Condron et al. 2019[11]	"Clinically important hemodynamic instability not attributable to other factors, such as substantial blood loss or compression of the inferior vena cava. Hemodynamic instability was considered clinically important if the SBP was <80 or >180 mmHg, if the heart rate was greater than 120 beats per min, or if the patients was displaying physiology that, if sustained, would be expected to cause end organ dysfunction, such as ventricular arrhythmias or bronchospasm causing difficulty with ventilation. Consensus of the surgeon and attending anesthesiologist was necessary to declare a crisis."	16/46 (35%)

bpm, Beats per minute; *HTN,* hypertension; *SBP,* systolic blood pressure.

Incidence

A literature search on carcinoid crises reveals a surprising number of case reports of carcinoid crises during anesthesia and operations, physical examinations, or diagnostic procedures or examinations (such as echocardiograms, mammograms, biopsies, or endoscopic procedures).[12–15] As these case reports often do not include any definition of carcinoid crisis and no denominator is given for the number for patients undergoing these events, the incidence cannot be determined from these. In addition, as there is no accepted definition of carcinoid crisis, individual case reports must be interpreted with caution as being true carcinoid crises.

A summary of incidence rates of carcinoid crisis found in retrospective and prospective studies cited in the literature are summarized in Table 17.1. These vary between 0% and 35% but are difficult to generalize, as these studies classify things such as intraoperative complications (which in definition appear similar to carcinoid crisis), hemodynamic instability (in definition appears as a surrogate for intraoperative complication or crisis), intraoperative carcinoid syndrome (as reported by a single study), or carcinoid crisis (defined differently by each study).

Risk Factors

Historically, carcinoid crisis was considered an extension of carcinoid syndrome, so logically patients with functional tumors (i.e., patients who experience carcinoid syndrome) would be at risk of carcinoid crisis. In addition, it has long been thought that patients with hepatic metastases, metastases or primary tumors in locations that drain systemically, or high tumor burden were considered at risk. There are several hypotheses about the pathogenesis of carcinoid syndrome and crisis. First, tumors with hepatic metastases are hypothesized to bypass liver enzyme breakdown, leading to higher risk of carcinoid syndrome and crisis.[16] Second, tumors that develop from or spread to sites with systemic drainage (i.e., lungs or ovaries) are hypothesized to bypass portal circulation and breakdown, thus leading to higher risk of carcinoid syndrome and crisis.[16] Third, it is hypothesized that tumor burden can become so large that enzymatic breakdown systems are overwhelmed, leading to higher risk of carcinoid syndrome and crisis.[16] However, cases of carcinoid crisis have been documented in patients without functional tumors, systemically drained metastases or primary tumors, or hepatic metastases.[9,10]

Regarding the hypothesis that functional tumors are more likely to have carcinoid crisis, several investigators have looked at the correlation between 24-hour levels of urinary 5-hydroxyindoleacetic acid (5-HIAA), a breakdown product of serotonin, and rates of carcinoid crisis. In a series of 119 patients in 2001, it was found that most patients (94%) had a high preoperative 24-hour level of urinary 5-HIAA, and the median 5-HIAA was significantly higher in those who experienced complications.[17] In contrast, a series of 97 cases found 21% of patients with functioning tumors had intraoperative complications compared to 28% of patients with nonfunctioning tumors, although the authors did not define what made the diagnosis of functional versus nonfunctional tumors and no serum chromogranin A (CgA) or 5-HIAA levels were reported.[9] A later series of 127 patients who underwent 150 operations found that neither preoperative CgA nor 5-HIAA levels correlated with intraoperative crisis.[10] In a series of 75 patients published in 2019, there were no clinicopathologic characteristics that was associated with the development of carcinoid crisis or hemodynamic instability, including preprocedure 24-hour level of urinary 5-HIAA levels greater than twice the upper limit of normal.[18] With only one author documenting a high 5-HIAA level as a significant risk,[17] others documenting no correlation,[10,18] and one inconclusive, review articles are mixed in the recommendation to include a high 5-HIAA level as a risk factor for carcinoid crisis.[19,20] Regarding hepatic metastases as a risk factor for carcinoid crisis, this was confirmed in two studies.[9,10] The theory of systemic drainage primary tumors or metastatic tumors has not been reported in these studies as a risk factor. Interestingly, the single prospective study found only preincisional serotonin levels to be related to carcinoid crisis.[11]

With the only prospective study showing preincisional serotonin level to correlate with carcinoid crisis, the variability in the risk factors for carcinoid crisis as described above, and the observation that crisis occurred even in patients without the associated risk factors of hepatic metastases or carcinoid syndrome,[9,10] we are left to conclude that all patients with NETs are at risk for developing crisis.

Many of these articles were written on patients undergoing large operations under general anesthesia, but in light of case reports of carcinoid crisis with smaller procedures for which patients may not be under sedation at all (i.e., percutaneous biopsy or mammogram), questions remain regarding when these patients are at risk and when to provide prophylactic treatment for carcinoid crisis. A review article published in 2014 identified 28 articles with 53 unique patients identified who had carcinoid crisis.[21] In this review, triggering factors included anesthesia/operation in 63.5%, interventional therapy in 11.5%, radionuclide therapy in 9.6%, physical examination in 7.7%, medication in 3.8%, biopsy in 2%, and spontaneous in 2%.[21]

With an inability to know who is most at risk or when carcinoid crisis will occur, and given its obvious life-threatening possibility, clinicians are attempting to develop appropriate preventative and therapeutic measures for these patients. There have been several review articles published on the anesthetic management of patients with neuroendocrine tumors,[19,20,22–24] but we caution against accepting these as dogma when they are expert review and published before many of the articles cited previously were published. The 2017 NANETS guidelines state, "physicians should be prepared to manage carcinoid crisis events in patients with SBNETs [small bowel neuroendocrine tumors] who undergo operations or invasive procedures," and give no firm criteria for risk factors.

Current Understanding of Pathophysiology

The mechanism of carcinoid syndrome and crisis is incompletely understood, and several theories exist regarding their pathogenesis as discussed in the "Risk Factors" section. Many theories of the mechanism of carcinoid crisis are based in biochemical studies in the mid-1950s, starting with isolation of serotonin from carcinoid tumors in 1953 and increased levels of histamine in the blood of a patient with a carcinoid tumor in 1956.[25] A later publication in 1964 that reported a case of carcinoid crisis being successfully treated with cyproheptadine (an antiserotonin and antihistamine compound) while having no response to norepinephrine supported this theory.[7] Subsequent studies began to propose that serotonin may not be the sole mediator or a mediator at all for the following reasons. First, a breakdown product of serotonin, 24-hour urinary 5-HIAA, was not elevated in all patients with carcinoid syndrome.[24] Second, it became apparent that other hormones and peptides were produced by carcinoid tumors. The first of these was published in 1966 when bradykinin was demonstrated to be high in patients with carcinoid syndrome.[26] This finding was echoed in a publication from 2008, which found that tachykinin was independently correlated with carcinoid diarrhea.[27] In 1980, another publication showed substantial amounts of dopamine and norepinephrine were present in the mesenteric mass of an ileal carcinoid tumor.[28] This finding was confirmed in a 1994 publication that demonstrated 38% of patients with midgut carcinoids had elevated urinary dopamine metabolites (3-methoxytyramine) and 33% of patients with midgut NETs had elevated norepinephrine and epinephrine urinary metabolites (normetanephrine and metanephrine).[29] Each of these products, upon being isolated in patients with NETs, have been postulated to have a different role in the symptomatology of carcinoid syndrome. Additionally, each tumor likely has its own unique secretory pattern, making every patient's experience of carcinoid syndrome different.[30]

The theory that these hormones are the cause of carcinoid crisis should be questioned because, first only one of the published seven retrospective reviews have shown 5-HIAA levels are related. In addition, the single prospective study of 46 patients with liver metastases from NETs undergoing operation published in 2019 had fascinating results from their hormone assays. The investigators measured plasma levels of serotonin, histamine, kallikrein, and bradykinin at preincision, mid-crisis, and closing. The authors report that only preincision serotonin levels were significantly elevated for those who had a carcinoid crisis versus those who did not. Remarkably, the other measured hormones did not have any other significant increase in patients with carcinoid crises. The investigators concluded that without an increase in these measured hormones during a crisis, these hormones cannot be the direct cause for triggering a crisis.[11]

These studies are the basis on which we question the paradigm of carcinoid crisis being a massive release of hormones in functional tumors only. Acceptance of this paradigm would limit prophylaxis and treatment to only those with functional tumors and crises have been observed in those without the classically cited risk factors of carcinoid syndrome and hepatic metastases.[9,10] In addition, specialty societies recommend being ready to treat crisis in all NET patients.[5] These modern-era studies will need to be validated in future studies, although this does have several challenges: the rarity of NETs and spontaneity of carcinoid crises making it difficult for a single center to gather enough cases to power a study; the ethics of allowing a crisis to proceed for 10 minutes in order to fulfill a definition; and the life-threatening hemodynamic instability that mandates urgent treatment.

Treatment With Somatostatin Analogues (Octreotide)

The paradigm that carcinoid crisis was precipitated by a massive release of hormones was perpetuated by case reports showing the effectiveness of somatostatin (a 14-amino acid inhibitory hormone) for both carcinoid syndrome and carcinoid crisis. Carcinoid tumors are known to express somatostatin receptors, which are G-protein–coupled receptors with five subtypes.[31] The mechanism of somatostatin is a reduction of hormone synthesis (see previous section on pathophysiology—these tumors have been demonstrated to secrete an array of serotonin, histamine, tachykinins, dopamine, and catecholamines) and inhibition of the release of these hormones.[31,32] As somatostatin has very rapid breakdown in circulation and would have to be given as a continuous infusion to be effective, a somatostatin analogue (i.e., octreotide) was developed later, which had a longer duration of action, allowing for bolus doses intravenously (IV) or subcutaneously (SQ). Octreotide is known to bind to somatostatin receptor subtypes 2, 3, and 5 with high, low, and moderate affinity, causing the previously described effects—inhibition of hormone synthesis and release.[33] Somatostatin analogues were used to treat patients with carcinoid syndrome, and it has been shown that patients treated with octreotide had decreased 5-HIAA levels, proving its inhibition of serotonin release.[34] In addition, somatostatin and octreotide also cause reduced splanchnic blood flow via visceral vasoconstriction.[32]

Regarding carcinoid syndrome and crisis treatment, publications in 1978 began to demonstrate inhibition of carcinoid flush by somatostatin[35] and the use of somatostatin for the treatment of intraoperative hypotension, though the term "carcinoid crisis" was not used by the authors.[36] Thus the credit for the first use of a somatostatin analogue for the treatment of carcinoid crisis is generally given to Larry Kvols who published a letter to the editor in 1985 with a case report of a patient with an intraoperative carcinoid crisis that resolved with a somatostatin analogue, with a full publication following in 1987.[37,38] In addition to its treatment of carcinoid crisis, publications in the late 1980s also began to report the use of pretreatment with somatostatin analogues for its prevention.[39,40] Because of these case reports, many anesthesia reviews recommend the use of octreotide to prevent and treat carcinoid crises.[19,20,22–24] Recommendations on preoperative and intraoperative regimen dosage, timing/duration, and routes (IV or SQ) vary widely between these sources. In more recent years several retrospective reviews and one prospective study were published, which comment on the use of octreotide prophylactically or therapeutically for carcinoid crisis, which lend a higher level of evidence than the previously discussed individual case reports and review articles.

The first of these studies was a retrospective review published by Kinney et al. in 2001. In this review of 119 patients with metastatic carcinoids undergoing abdominal operation, 15 (12.6%) had perioperative complications (see Table 17.1 for definition of complication) or death.[17] The overall rate of intraoperative complications was 7%, with events occurring in seven (10%) of 67 patients who received no octreotide preoperatively or intraoperatively and one (17%) of six patients who received only a preoperative dose (median dose 300 μg IV or SQ, range 50 to 1000 μg). In the 45 patients who received intraoperative octreotide (median dose 350 μg, range 30 to 4000 μg), either alone or with a preoperative dose, no intraoperative complications occurred. In the results section, it is stated the authors have "no evidence that preoperative administration of octreotide is associated with a reduced frequency of intraoperative complications or that intraoperative administration is associated with a reduced frequency of postoperative complications." However, their conclusion hints heavily that "no intraoperative complications occurred in those who received octreotide intraoperatively," and many subsequent anesthesia review articles cite this paper as a reason to give intraoperative octreotide.[19,20,22]

As this article was unable to provide specific recommendations on optimal dosage, a systematic review was published in 2013 of 18 articles on the dosage of octreotide.[41] The authors found that doses of 25 to 500 μg given IV effectively managed carcinoid crises. These authors were unable to describe any secondary outcomes of deaths, length of stay in an intensive care unit or the hospital. However, they note that a small sample size, the inconsistent use of the term "carcinoid crisis," and the paucity of outcomes were limitations to their study.

Massimino et al. published a retrospective review in 2013 of 97 cases of patients with carcinoid tumors undergoing abdominal operations in which 90% were given preoperative prophylactic octreotide (median dose 500 μg, range 100 to 1100 μg) and 70% of patients were on outpatient octreotide.[9] Five of the 97 (5%) had life-threatening carcinoid crisis and 23 (24%) had an intraoperative complication (see Table 17.1 for definitions). In this series, it was found that significant intraoperative complications occur frequently in patients with hepatic metastases regardless of the presence of carcinoid syndrome, even though events were observed in those without hepatic metastases. The authors found no correlation between long-acting octreotide preoperatively or single-dose prophylactic octreotide with intraoperative complications. Fifty-six patients also received intraoperative boluses of octreotide (250 to 500 μg), and 46% of these patients still had a subsequent event. The authors of this study concluded that neither preoperative octreotide (whether long-acting dosage or prophylactic dosage as described earlier) nor intraoperative boluses of octreotide are sufficient to prevent carcinoid crises.

Further support that octreotide is not an effective prophylaxis for carcinoid crisis was demonstrated in a publication of a metaanalysis of 28 articles with 53 unique patients identified who had carcinoid crises, which was published in 2014.[21] This group found the overall pooled risk of perioperative carcinoid crisis was similar despite the prophylactic administration of octreotide. These authors concluded that the prophylactic use of somatostatin analogues was not effective in the prevention of carcinoid crisis.

A third retrospective review was published in 2016 by Woltering et al. of 150 patients with small bowel NETs who underwent 179 cytoreductive operations.[42] Their standard practice is a 500-μg/hour infusion preoperatively, intraoperatively, and postoperatively. They identified six cases (3.4%) who experienced a carcinoid crisis (see Table 17.1 for authors' definition of crisis for this particular study). Given their low rates of carcinoid crisis, the authors recommend clinicians give a high-dose continuous infusion of octreotide during surgical intervention, commenting specifically that a bolus dose without a continuous infusion will defeat the purpose of the bolus dose because of its short half-life.

In direct contradiction to the Woltering study is a fourth retrospective review published by Condron et al. in 2016 of 127 patients with carcinoid tumors who underwent 150 operations. All patients received a 500-μg/hour continuous infusion, but carcinoid crisis (see definition of crisis for this study in Table 17.1) occurred in 30% of cases.[10] In addition, they did find that with an earlier initiation of treatment for hypotension, the carcinoid crises events were no longer associated with complications, except when hypotension persisted for more than 10 minutes. The authors concluded that intraoperative continuous infusions of octreotide do not prevent crisis but prompt treatment was important to reduce postoperative complications. These two studies were not commented upon by the opposing author, as one was accepted but not published for a year, and during this time the other study was under review.

To continue to attempt to answer the question of octreotide prophylaxis and treatment for carcinoid crisis, a fifth retrospective review published in 2018 by Kinney et al. included 169 patients with metastatic NETs who underwent 196 procedures.[13] Of these 169 patients, 77% received prophylactic octreotide SQ and 23% were given additional intraoperative octreotide. No episodes of carcinoid crisis were observed (see Table 17.1 for definition according to this author). As no crises were observed, these authors are unable to comment on octreotide's efficacy.

A sixth retrospective review was published by Fouché et al. in 2018 of 81 patients undergoing operation for small bowel NETs.[8] The perioperative octreotide regimen is a continuous intravenous infusion of 40 μg/hour to 80 μg/hour for 12 to 48 hours prior to operation. In addition, an observation of intraoperative carcinoid syndromes (see Table 17.1 for the authors' definition) initiated treatment with additional octreotide boluses of 0.5 to 2 μg/kg. The authors observed 139 episodes of intraoperative carcinoid syndrome and no episodes of carcinoid crisis. These authors suggest that with no patients having a carcinoid crisis in their series, there is clinical relevance of a standardized octreotide prophylactic protocol.

The last retrospective review was published by Kwon et al. in 2019 of 75 patients with hepatic metastases from NETs undergoing hepatic resection, ablation, or embolotherapy. The authors found that 24 (32%) experienced carcinoid crisis or hemodynamic instability (see Table 17.1 for authors' definition). They found that periprocedural octreotide use was not associated with lower carcinoid crisis/hemodynamic instability occurrence. This supported the previous findings of Condron in 2016 and Massimino in 2013. These authors hypothesized that carcinoid crisis may be a phenomenon different from carcinoid syndrome.

In summary of these seven retrospective reviews, three of these articles[8,17,42] have little statistical support for the use of octreotide as a preventative or therapeutic strategy for carcinoid crisis, with three articles[9,10,18] showing that it has no efficacy, and one[43] is inconclusive. The only single prospective study was published in 2019 by Condron et al.[11] In this study, 46 patients with hepatic metastases from NETs undergoing operation were studied between 2015 and 2017 and 16 (35%) experienced intraoperative hypotensive crisis. In this series, the preoperative bolus of octreotide (500 μg) and continuous infusion (500 μg/hour) were given to eliminate the variable of not having octreotide from their results. These patients had invasive monitoring intraoperatively with pulmonary artery catheters, transesophageal echocardiographs, and arterial lines placed, as well as hormonal measurements of serotonin, histamine, kallikrein, and bradykinin at three time points (preincision, mid-crisis, and at case conclusion). The fascinating results of this study showed none of the hormone levels changed during a carcinoid crisis, which questions the theory that carcinoid crisis is a massive release of hormones. However, as all these patients received a preoperative bolus and continuous infusion of octreotide, we may be seeing that octreotide does effectively block the hormone release but does not block the physiologic changes of carcinoid crisis, questioning the theory that carcinoid crisis is due to the massive release of hormones. To expand upon this further, on the invasive monitoring equipment described earlier the authors observed a decrease in pulmonary vascular resistance, consistent cardiac hypovolemia on echocardiography, and a decrease in systemic vascular resistance. From this the authors concluded that carcinoid crisis is a distributive shock. Last, as all patients were receiving continuous octreotide infusions but a crisis incidence rate of 35% was still observed, these authors also concluded octreotide was not a preventative agent.

The most recent NANETs guidelines published in 2017 have discussed that recent literature does not support the notion that routine administration of octreotide prevents carcinoid crisis though it does not appear to increase complication rates and is generally safe.[5] As we have now found that the pathophysiology of carcinoid crisis is fundamentally different and several authors have proven octreotide's ineffectiveness at prevention of crises,[9–11,18] future studies in the pathophysiology of crisis and different treatment strategies are advised. We question if the known effect of splanchnic vasoconstriction causes the improvements in blood pressure, which is why there are so many reports of carcinoid crisis improving with octreotide administration.

Treatment With Vasopressors, Including β-Adrenergic Agonists

The use of vasopressors, including β-adrenergic agonists in patients with carcinoid syndrome and crisis, is historically controversial. The basis of this argument are physiology studies from the 1960s, starting with a publication of 10 normal subjects compared to 8 patients with carcinoid tumors, which implicated bradykinin in the understanding of carcinoid flushing. They found that bradykinin resulted in venoconstriction during a phase of arteriolar hypotension, followed by venodilation.[44] In addition, this study found that epinephrine caused flushing in carcinoid patients as well as a marked decline in forearm resistance that was significantly longer than normal subjects, which the authors interpreted as that "a substantial portion of the vascular phenomena might be the result of an indirect effect of epinephrine." In addition, they found a few of the carcinoid patients showed obvious venodilatation instead of venoconstriction with the administration of epinephrine.

Later physiology studies done in the 1980s began to show adrenergic control of serotonin release, particularly β-adrenergic receptors.[45–47] This was perpetuated by anesthetic review articles that recommended against the use of these drugs, as they could cause a canonical process of crisis.[22,24] However, outside of these physiology studies from the 1960s and 1980s, data to support the avoidance of β-adrenergic agonists are limited. In addition, some tertiary referral centers have also demonstrated β-adrenergic agonist safety when other traditionally used agents (phenylephrine and vasopressin) were insufficient.[8–10,17]

To investigate this area further, a retrospective review of 293 operations that identified 58 operations on 56 patients with carcinoid tumors, with 161 crisis events, was published in 2019.[48] Of these patients, 36 were treated with phenylephrine or vasopressin only and 22 were treated with β-adrenergic agonists as well. There was no significant difference in the incidence of paradoxical hypotension between patients treated with β-adrenergic agonists compared with non–β-adrenergic agonists. In addition, the dose-response curve for the administration of ephedrine or epinephrine showed no significant linear association in the percent decrease in mean arterial pressure (MAP). There were also no differences in crises duration or postoperative complications. Based on the results of this study, the authors conclude that β-adrenergic agonists may be considered to treat refractory hypotension in patients with carcinoid if phenylephrine and vasopressin are proven insufficient.[48]

The fact that β-adrenergic receptors can safely be given without precipitation of secondary crises supports the theory that there is a different mechanism at play as β-adrenergic agents would otherwise cause a canonical process of crises.

Conclusion

We implore specialty societies to decide upon a strict definition of carcinoid crisis in order to give generalizability to on-going research efforts. This will also help clinicians determine the true incidence and risk factors of carcinoid crisis. There is much to be learned about the unique pathophysiologic process of carcinoid crisis and its treatment. The unpredictability and urgency of these crises make research very difficult, especially in light of the ethical considerations of leaving a crisis untreated for greater than 10 minutes to fulfill a definition and a demonstrated higher complication rate if hypotension exceeds this threshold. Current recommendations would be not to rely on octreotide, as it has been demonstrated to not prevent or treat carcinoid crises. For the treatment of carcinoid crisis, we recommend intravenous fluids and vasopressors in the following order: vasopressin, phenylephrine, and finally β-adrenergic agents. β-Adrenergic agents are considered third-line agents, as the data are emerging that these are safe and do not provoke secondary crises. With these emerging studies showing that octreotide is not helpful and challenging the paradigm that the crisis is triggered by a massive release of hormones, much remains to be learned about the pathophysiology of crisis, and this should be investigated further in multicenter, prospective trials.

References

1. Modlin IM, Oberg K, Chung DC, et al. Gastroenteropancreatic neuroendocrine tumors. *Lancet Oncol.* 2008;9:61–72. doi:10.1017/CBO9781107415324.004.
2. Yao JC, Hassan M, Phan A, et al. One hundred years after "carcinoid": epidemiology of and prognostic factors for neuroendocrine tumors in 35,825 cases in the United States. *J Clin Oncol.* 2008;26(18):3063–3072. doi:10.1200/JCO.2007.15.4377.
3. Dasari A, Shen C, Halperin D, et al. Trends in the incidence, prevalence, and survival outcomes in patients with neuroendocrine tumors in the United States. *JAMA Oncol.* 2017;3(10):1335. doi:10.1001/jamaoncol.2017.0589.

4. Halperin DM, Shen C, Dasari A, et al. Frequency of carcinoid syndrome at neuroendocrine tumour diagnosis: a population-based study. *Lancet Oncol.* 2017;18(4):525–534. doi:10.1016/S1470-2045(17)30110-9.
5. Howe JR, Cardona K, Fraker DL, et al. The surgical management of small bowel neuroendocrine tumors. *Pancreas.* 2017;46(6):715–731. doi:10.1097/MPA.0000000000000846.
6. Thorson Å, Biörck G, Björkman G, Waldenström J. Malignant carcinoid of the small intestine with metastases to the liver, valvular disease of the right side of the heart (pulmonary stenosis and tricuspid regurgitation without septal defects), peripheral vasomotor symptoms, broncho-constriction, and an unusual type of cyanosis; a clinical and pathologic syndrome. *Am Heart J.* 1954;47(6):795–817. doi:10.1016/0002-8703(54)90152-0.
7. Kahil ME, Brown H, Fred HL. The carcinoid crisis. *Arch Intern Med.* 1964;114(1):26–28. doi:10.1001/archinte.1964.03860070072004.
8. Fouché M, Bouffard Y, Le Goff MC, et al. Intraoperative carcinoid syndrome during small-bowel neuroendocrine tumour surgery. *Endocr Connect.* 2018;7(12):1245–1250. doi:10.1530/EC-18-0324.
9. Massimino K, Harrskog O, Pommier S, Pommier R. Octreotide LAR and bolus octreotide are insufficient for preventing intraoperative complications in carcinoid patients. *J Surg Oncol.* 2013;107(8):842–846. doi:10.1002/jso.23323.
10. Condron ME, Pommier SJ, Pommier RF. Continuous infusion of octreotide combined with perioperative octreotide bolus does not prevent intraoperative carcinoid crisis. *Surg (United States).* 2016;159(1):358–367. doi:10.1016/j.surg.2015.05.036.
11. Condron ME, Jameson NE, Limbach KE, et al. A prospective study of the pathophysiology of carcinoid crisis. *Surg (United States).* 2019;165(1):158–165. doi:10.1016/j.surg.2018.04.093.
12. Bissonnette T, Gibney G, Berry R, Buckley R. Fatal carcinoid crisis after percutaneous fine-needle biopsy of hepatic metastasis: case report and literature case. 2005:1-2. papers2://publication/uuid/C7062069-8440-4B58-80DA-2D698879A585.
13. Salm EF, Janssen M, Breburda CS, et al. Carcinoid crisis during transesophageal echocardiography. *Intensive Care Med.* 2000;26(2):254. doi:10.1007/s001340050060.
14. Ozgen A, Demirkazik FB, Arat A, Arat AR. Carcinoid crisis provoked by mammographic compression of metastatic carcinoid tumour of the breast. *Clin Radiol.* 2001;56(3):250–251. doi:10.1053/crad.1999.0167.
15. Morrisroe K, Sim I-W, McLachlan K, Inder WJ. Carcinoid crisis induced by repeated abdominal examination. *Intern Med J.* 2012;42(3):341–342. doi:10.1111/j.1445-5994.2012.02720.x.
16. Rubin de Celis Ferrari AC, Glasberg J, Riechelmann RP. Carcinoid syndrome: update on the pathophysiology and treatment. *Clinics.* 2018;73:1–9. doi:10.6061/clinics/2018/e490s.
17. Kinney MAO, Warner ME, Nagorney DM, et al. Perianaesthetic risks and outcomes of abdominal surgery for metastatic carcinoid tumours. *Br J Anaesth.* 2001;87(3):447–452. doi:10.1093/bja/87.3.447.
18. Kwon DH, Paciorek A, Mulvey CK, et al. Periprocedural management of patients undergoing liver resection or embolotherapy for neuroendocrine tumor metastases. *Pancreas.* 2019;48(4):496–503. doi:10.1097/MPA.0000000000001271.
19. Dierdorf S. Carcinoid tumor and carcinoid syndrome. *Curr Opin Anaesthesiol.* 2003;16:343–347. doi:10.1097/01.aco.0000073233.10825.46.
20. Mancuso K, Kaye AD, Boudreaux JP, et al. Carcinoid syndrome and perioperative anesthetic considerations. *J Clin Anesth.* 2011;23(4):329–341. doi:10.1016/j.jclinane.2010.12.009.
21. Guo LJ, Tang CW. Somatostatin analogues do not prevent carcinoid crisis. *Asian Pacific J Cancer Prev.* 2014;15(16):6679–6683. doi:10.7314/APJCP.2014.15.16.6679.
22. Powell B, Al Mukhtar A, Mills GH. Carcinoid: the disease and its implications for anaesthesia. *Contin Educ Anaesthesia, Crit Care Pain..* 2011;11(1):9–13. doi:10.1093/bjaceaccp/mkq045.
23. Veall GRQ, Peacock JE, Bax NDS, Reilly CS. Review of the anaesthetic management of 21 patients undergoing laparotomy for carcinoid syndrome. *Br J Anaesth.* 1994;72(3):335–341. doi:10.1093/bja/72.3.335.
24. Vaughan DJA, Brunner MD. Anesthesia for patients with carcinoid syndrome. *Int Anesthesiol Clin.* 1997;35(4):129–142. doi:10.1097/00004311-199703540-00009.
25. Gustafsen J, Boesby S, Man WK. Histamine in carcinoid syndrome. *Agents Actions.* 1988;25(1-2):1–3. doi:10.1017/CBO9781107415324.004.
26. Oates JA, Pettinger WA, Doctor RB. Evidence for the release of bradykinin in carcinoid syndrome. *J Clin Invest.* 1966;45(2):173–178. doi:10.1172/JCI105329.

27. Cunningham JL, Janson ET, Agarwal S, Grimelius L, Stridsberg M. Tachykinins in endocrine tumors and the carcinoid syndrome. *Eur J Endocrinol.* 2008;159(3):275–282. doi:10.1530/EJE-08-0196.
28. Goedert M, Otten U, Suda K, et al. Dopamine, norepinephrine and serotonin production by an intestinal carcinoid tumor. *Cancer.* 1980;45(1):104–107. doi:10.1002/1097-0142(19800101)45:1<104::AID-CNCR2820450119>3.0.CO;2-I.
29. Kema IP, De Vries EGE, Slooff MJH, Biesma B, Muskiet FAJ. Serotonin, catecholamines, histamine, and their metabolites in urine, platelets, and tumor tissue of patients with carcinoid tumors. *Clin Chem.* 1994;40(1):86–95.
30. Lips CJM, Lentjes EGWM, Höppener JWM. The spectrum of carcinoid tumours and carcinoid syndromes. *Ann Clin Biochem.* 2003;40(6):612–627. doi:10.1258/000456303770367207.
31. Reubi JC, Kvols L, Krenning E, Lamberts SWJ. In vitro and in vivo detection of somatostatin receptors in human malignant tissues. *Acta Oncol (Madr).* 1991;30(4):463–468. doi:10.3109/02841869109092402.
32. Harris AG. Somatostatin and somatostatin analogues: pharmacokinetics and pharmacodynamic effects. *Gut.* 1994;35(3 SUPPL):4–7. doi:10.1136/gut.35.3_Suppl.S1.
33. Borna RM, Jahr JS, Kmiecik S, Mancuso KF, Kaye AD. Pharmacology of octreotide: clinical implications for anesthesiologists and associated risks. *Anesthesiol Clin.* 2017;35(2):327–339. doi:10.1016/j.anclin.2017.01.021.
34. Oberg K, Norheim I, Theodorsson E, Ahlman H, Lundqvist G, Wide L. The effects of octreotide on basal and stimulated hormone levels in patients with carcinoid syndrome. *J Clin Endocrinol Metab.* 1989;68(4):796–800. doi:10.1210/jcem-68-4-796.
35. Frolich JC, Bloomgarden ZT, Oates JA, McGuigan JE, Rabinowitz D. The carcinoid flush: provocation by pentagastrin and inhibition by somatostatin. *N Engl J Med.* 1978;299(19):1055–1057.
36. Thulin L, Samnegård H, Tydén G, Long DH, Efendić S. Efficacy of somatostatin in a patient with carcinoid syndrome. *Lancet.* 1978;312(8079):43. doi:10.1016/S0140-6736(78)91348-X.
37. Kvols LK, Martin JK, Marsh HM, Moertel CG. Rapid reversal of carcinoid crisis with a somatostatin analogue. *N Engl J Med.* 1985;313(19):1229–1230.
38. Marsh HM, Martin Jr JK, Kvols LK, et al. Carcinoid crisis during anesthesia: successful treatment wtih a somatostatin analogue. *Anesthesiology.* 1987;66:89–91.
39. Ahlman H, Ahlund L, Dahlstrom A, Martner J, Stenqvist O, Tylen U. SMS 201-995 and provocation trests in preparation of patients with carcinoids for surgery or hepatic arterial embolization. *Anesth Analg.* 1988;67(12):1142–1148. doi:10.1213/00000539-198812000-00003.
40. Parris WCV, Oates JA, Kambam J, Shmerling R, Sawyers JF. Pre-treatment with somatostatin in the anaesthetic management of a patient with carcinoid syndrome. *Can J Anaesth.* 1988;35(4):413–416. doi:10.1007/BF03010865.
41. Seymour N, Sawh SC. Mega-dose intravenous octreotide for the treatment of carcinoid crisis: a systematic review. *Can J Anesth.* 2013;60(5):492–499. doi:10.1007/s12630-012-9879-1.
42. Woltering EA, Wright AE, Stevens MA, et al. Development of effective prophylaxis against intraoperative carcinoid crisis. *J Clin Anesth.* 2016;32:189–193. doi:10.1016/j.jclinane.2016.03.008.
43. Kinney MAO, Nagorney DM, Clark DF, et al. Partial hepatic resections for metastatic neuroendocrine tumors: perioperative outcomes. *J Clin Anesth.* 2018;51(May):93–96. doi:10.1016/j.jclinane.2018.08.005.
44. Mason DT, Melmon KL. Abnormal forearm vascular responses in the carcinoid syndrome: the role of kinisns and kinin-generating system. *J Clin Invest.* 1966;45(11):1685–1699. doi:10.1172/JCI105475.
45. Nilsson O, Grönstad KO, Goldstein M, Skolnik G, Dahlstrom A, Ahlman H. Adrenergic control of serotonin release from a midgut carcinoid tumour. *Int J Cancer.* 1985;36(3):307–312. doi:10.1017/CBO9781107415324.004.
46. Grönstad KO, Nilsson O, Dahlström A, Skolnik G, Ahlman H. Adrenergic control of serotonin release from carcinoid tumor cells *in vitro* and *in vivo*. *J Surg Res.* 1987;42(2):141–146. doi:10.1016/0022-4804(87)90111-9.
47. Grönstad KO, Zinner MJ, Nilsson O, Dahlström A, Jaffe BM, Ahlman H. Vagal release of serotonin into gut lumen and portal circulation via separate control mechanisms. *J Surg Res.* 1988;44(2):146–151. doi:10.1016/0022-4804(88)90042-X.
48. Limbach KE, Condron ME, Bingham AE, Pommier SEJ, Pommier RF. B-Adrenergic agonist administration is not associated with secondary carcinoid crisis in patients with carcinoid tumor. *Am J Surg.* 2019;217(5):932–936. doi:10.1016/j.amjsurg.2018.12.070.

PART 7

Pituitary

CHAPTER 18

Postsurgical and Posttraumatic Hyponatremia

Ansha Goel ■ Joseph G. Verbalis

CHAPTER OUTLINE

Introduction

Hyponatremia, defined as a serum sodium concentration ([Na$^+$]) less than 135 mEq/L, represents a relative excess of body water relative to body sodium content. The reported prevalence of hyponatremia varies with different patient populations and health care settings.[1] Regardless, hyponatremia is still the most common electrolyte disorder seen in clinical practice and can significantly complicate a patient's hospital course. The strong association between hyponatremia and in-hospital mortality has been demonstrated in numerous studies.[2] Due to declining renal function, the presence of comorbidities, and high frequency of drug prescriptions, older patients are known to have a higher prevalence of hyponatremia. Data from the National Health and Nutrition Examination Survey (NHANES) also reveals that hyponatremia is more common in patients who have hypertension, diabetes, coronary artery disease, stroke, chronic obstructive pulmonary disease, cancer, and psychiatric disorders.[3] Chronic hyponatremia, despite less severe symptoms than acute hyponatremia, is also associated with increased morbidity and mortality. A study involving more than 50,000 hospitalizations at a teaching academic medical center showed that even mild hyponatremia was associated with an increased in-hospital mortality, and that the risk of death was increased by 2.3% for each 1 mEq/L decline of serum [Na$^+$].[4] With an estimated annual cost ranging between $1.6 billion and $3.6 billion, hyponatremia has a substantial financial burden on the United States' health care system.[5] Among hospitalized patients, the presence of hyponatremia is associated with prolonged length of stay by 3.2 days and a 32% increased risk of hospital admission compared with patients without hyponatremia.[4] Both the prolonged length of stay and increased hospitalization costs (including readmissions) account for approximately 70% of the total cost of the illness.[6]

The central nervous system (CNS) plays a crucial role in the regulation of sodium and water homeostasis. The neurohypophysis consists of the vasopressin neurons in the hypothalamus that project via the pituitary stalk to the posterior pituitary, where arginine vasopressin (AVP) is secreted from the axon terminals. Disruption of neurohypophyseal regulation can result in conditions of salt and water imbalance, such as the syndrome of inappropriate antidiuretic hormone secretion (SIADH) and diabetes insipidus (DI). These two phenomena have been well studied in the literature as potential risks after intracranial surgery; however, both can also occur after traumatic brain injury (TBI) as well.[7]

Elderly patients and those with comorbidities are more at risk for developing electrolyte derangements, particularly hyponatremia. Hyponatremia predisposes patients to gait instability, which can lead to more frequent falls and increased fracture rates.[8,9] A study showed that a 5-mmol/L decrease in serum $[Na^+]$ had about the same effect on falls as aging 13 years.[10] Increased fracture rates are also due to chronic hyponatremia-induced deterioration of bone mass and strength, and increased fragility. Evidence has shown that even patients with mild hyponatremia (serum $[Na^+]$ = 130 to 134 mEq/L) have an increased prevalence of osteoporosis. Epidemiologic analysis of the NHANES III database suggested that osteoporosis occurred at a significantly increased 2.5-fold odds ratio (OR) in hyponatremic subjects over age 50 compared with participants with a normal serum $[Na^+]$.[11] A more recent epidemiologic study of 2.9 million electronic health records indicated that chronic hyponatremia was significantly associated with both osteoporosis and bone fractures at OR of 3.97 and 4.61, respectively.[12] As chronic hyponatremia may not cause overt symptoms, it frequently remains undiagnosed and untreated until complications manifest. These complications can compromise postoperative rehabilitation, particularly in elderly patients.

Postoperative surgical patients and patients with TBI are also especially prone to the development of hyponatremia. Hyponatremia in the postoperative period is associated with worse surgical outcomes, including increased mortality.[13] Hyponatremia has traditionally been managed by internists, intensivists, endocrinologists, nephrologists, and geriatricians. However, with the increased incidence of preoperative, postoperative, and posttraumatic hyponatremia and its known adverse consequences, timely recognition and management by other providers such as surgeons is crucial for optimal management of their patients. This chapter will specifically focus on the recognition, evaluation, and treatment of patients with postoperative and posttraumatic hyponatremia.

Definition and Classification of Hyponatremia

As a brief overview, hyponatremia is defined as a serum $[Na^+]$ less than 135 mEq/L. Hyponatremia can be categorized by symptoms, serum $[Na^+]$, and duration. The most useful categorization from the point of view of treatment is by symptoms: mild, moderate, and severe. Mild hyponatremia is serum $[Na^+]$ less than 135 mEq/L with neurologic manifestations that can include headache, irritability, difficulty concentrating, altered mood, and depression. Usually mild hyponatremias are chronic (several days to many weeks/months), but these symptoms are also seen with early stages of more acute hyponatremias. Moderate hyponatremia includes symptoms of nausea, confusion, disorientation, altered mental status, and unstable gait with or without falls. Usually, the serum $[Na^+]$ is less than 130 mEq/L with a duration of more than 48 hours. Lastly, severe hyponatremia has more advanced neurologic symptoms, including vomiting, seizures, obtundation, respiratory distress, and coma. This usually occurs with acute hyponatremia of less than 24- to 48-hour duration with serum $[Na^+]$ less than 125 mEq/L (Table 18.1).[14] Of note, children are at a higher risk of developing symptomatic hyponatremia because of their larger brain-to-skull size ratio.

The etiology of underlying hyponatremia is usually classified based on three different components: the patient's plasma tonicity, extracellular fluid (ECF) volume status, and the severity of hyponatremia in terms of the serum $[Na^+]$ level.[14] Plasma tonicity is further delineated into

TABLE 18.1 ■ **Classification of Hyponatremia According to Severity of Presenting Symptoms**

	Serum Sodium	Neurologic Symptoms	Typical Duration of Hyponatremia
Severe	<125 mmol/L	Vomiting; seizures; obtundation; respiratory distress; coma	Acute (<24–48 h)
Moderate	<130 mmol/L	Nausea; confusion; disorientation; altered mental status; unstable gait/falls	Intermediate or chronic (>24–48 h)
Mild	<135 mmol/L	Headache; irritability; difficulty concentrating; altered mood; depression	Chronic (several days or to many weeks/ months

From Verbalis, JG. Emergency management of acute and chronic hyponatremia. In: Matfin G, ed. *Endocrine and Metabolic Emergencies.* Washington, DC: Endocrine Press; 2018.

hypotonic, isotonic, or hypertonic, which is characterized by the relationship of the plasma osmolality to the serum [Na^+]. As hypotonic hyponatremia causes a shift of water from the ECF into cells due to osmotic gradients, only patients with hypotonic hyponatremia should further be differentiated based on ECF volume status (hypovolemic, euvolemic, and hypervolemic). Hypovolemic hyponatremia can occur in patients who have had gastrointestinal, renal, or fluid losses, diuretic therapy, and renal salt wasting. Euvolemic hyponatremia can be due to SIADH, hypothyroidism, exercise-associated hyponatremia, low solute intake, polydipsia, or the use of nonsteroidal antiinflammatory drugs (NSAIDS).[15] Adrenal insufficiency can cause hyponatremia as a result of multiple factors, including renal salt wasting in primary adrenal insufficiency and impaired water excretion in secondary adrenal insufficiency. As a result, primary adrenal insufficiency causes hypovolemic hyponatremia, whereas secondary adrenal insufficiency causes euvolemic hyponatremia.[16] Lastly, hypervolemic hyponatremia can occur in volume overload states such as congestive heart failure, cirrhosis, renal failure, and nephrotic syndrome. In these conditions, there is increased activity of AVP via baroreceptor-mediated nonosmotic stimulation caused by reduced effective circulating arterial volume.[17]

Arginine Vasopressin

Arginine vasopressin (AVP), also known as antidiuretic hormone (ADH), is an essential peptide hormone that is synthesized in the hypothalamus and stored in the posterior pituitary gland, from which it is released into the circulation. AVP plays a major role in the regulation of water and sodium homeostasis by virtue of its antidiuretic action in the kidney. AVP secretion occurs either due to increased plasma osmolality or decreased arterial blood pressure and/or blood volume. Osmoreceptors are sensory receptors in the anterior hypothalamus that detect changes in osmotic pressure and contribute to maintaining fluid balance in the body. Changes that deviate by as little as ~3 mOsm/kg from the set point (280 to 285 mOsm/kg H_2O) trigger specific homeostatic responses to restore water balance.[18] Baroreceptors, on the other hand, are mechanoreceptor sensory receptors that detect changes in blood pressure. A decrease in blood pressure greater than 10% to 15% is detected by baroreceptors in the cardiac atria, aorta, and carotid sinus, leading to a decrease in tonic inhibition of AVP release, which ultimately leads to AVP release from the posterior pituitary gland.[19] AVP binding to AVP V2 receptors on the kidney collecting duct principal cells activates a signal transduction cascade that inserts aquaporin-2 (AQP2) water channels into the apical membrane of the collecting ducts, leading to reabsorption of water back into the circulation.[20] This results in what is known as antidiuresis: decreased renal free water clearance, increased urinary concentration, and reduced urinary volume. Along with osmoreceptor-stimulated thirst, this process promotes normalization of plasma osmolality. The function of AVP is especially important during periods of severe blood loss, such as hemorrhagic shock, or systemic infection, such as sepsis, when there is a lack of responsiveness to other vasoconstrictors (which is where AVP gets its name *vasopressin*).[19] By binding to the V1a receptors, which are expressed on vascular smooth muscle, AVP also produces vasoconstriction and increased peripheral vascular resistance, thus promoting increases in blood pressure.

Either a deficiency or excess of AVP can result in clinical disease. Conditions such as SIADH result in secretion of AVP that is inappropriate for the plasma osmolality, which results in water retention, hyponatremia, and oliguria. SIADH is suspected when the diagnostic evaluation reveals euvolemia on clinical examination, plasma osmolality less than 275 mOsm/kg H_2O, inappropriate urinary concentration (urine osmolality greater than 100 mOsm/kg H_2O), and elevated urinary [Na^+] (greater than 30 mmol/L). SIADH is a diagnosis of exclusion, after other causes of euvolemic hypoosmolality (hypothyroidism and hypocortisolism) have been ruled out. SIADH is largely a clinical diagnosis that is supported by biochemical parameters.[15] SIADH can be caused by underlying medical conditions such as CNS disturbances (e.g., stroke, hemorrhage, infection, trauma, and psychosis), malignancies (small cell carcinoma of the lung, head and neck cancer, olfactory neuroblastoma, and extrapulmonary small cell carcinomas), drugs (selective serotonin reuptake inhibitors, NSAIDs, certain anticonvulsants, certain chemotherapy agents), pulmonary disease (pneumonia, tuberculosis), and HIV infection.

In contrast, DI occurs either from lack of pituitary production of AVP (central DI) or renal unresponsiveness to AVP (nephrogenic DI). In either case, DI ultimately results in hypotonic polyuria (urine osmolality less than 250 mmol/kg) and hypernatremia. Central DI usually occurs due to traumatic, inflammatory, infectious, or cancer-related lesions that affect the neurohypophysis, whereas nephrogenic DI can either be inherited (e.g., mutations in the *AVP V2* receptor gene or mutations in the *AQP2* water channel gene) or acquired from hypokalemia, postobstructive polyuria, and medications such as lithium. DI results in polyuria with dilute urine and polydipsia.

Circulating concentrations of AVP under normal physiologic conditions range from less than 0.5 to 6 ng/L.[19] Although AVP is present in both the blood and urine, its quantification for diagnostic purposes can be difficult. Copeptin is a peptide derived from the C-terminus of the AVP prohormone that is more stable in plasma. Given that is it secreted in equimolar amounts as AVP from the posterior pituitary and can be measured more easily in plasma, copeptin has emerged as a promising surrogate marker for AVP in the diagnosis of AVP-dependent fluid disorders. Copeptin measurements allow accurate differentiation between various conditions within the polyuria–polydipsia syndrome. In the absence of prior fluid deprivation, baseline copeptin levels greater than 20 pmol/L reliably identifies patients with nephrogenic diabetes insipidus.[21]

General Treatment Considerations for Hyponatremia

Assessing the severity of hyponatremia based on a patient's symptoms, rather than the serum [Na^+] concentration alone, is critical prior to determining the initial therapy for hyponatremia.[14] Both the magnitude and rate of decrease in the serum [Na^+] concentration, as well as the chronicity of the hyponatremia, are correlated with the symptoms that a patient experiences. As discussed previously, symptoms related to acute hyponatremia are more severe than the symptoms of chronic hyponatremia. Altered mental status, seizures, focal neurologic deficits, coma, or other signs or symptoms of cerebral edema all meet criteria for hyponatremic encephalopathy (HNE). HNE is a medical emergency and should be treated urgently in order to prevent morbidity and mortality. Brain herniation from hyponatremia is seen almost exclusively in patients with acute hyponatremia or in patients with coexisting intracranial pathology. An increase in serum [Na^+] of 4 to 6 mEq/L is usually sufficient to reduce symptoms of acute hyponatremia.[22] Chronic hyponatremia, if not complicated by an acute episode, rarely presents as severely symptomatic HNE. This reflects the brain adaptation during chronic hyponatremia with a negligible brain volume increase.[23]

Acute hyponatremia with symptoms should be treated urgently with hypertonic (3%) saline, either via bolus or continuous infusion, in order to appropriately raise the serum [Na^+] and prevent catastrophic consequences such as cerebral edema, irreversible neurologic damage, respiratory arrest, brainstem herniation, and death.[24] Currently, vasopressin antagonists, such as vaptans, have no role in the treatment of severely symptomatic hyponatremia because of the uncertainty of increasing the serum [Na^+] sufficiently rapidly to alleviate the neurologic symptoms. Additionally, vasopressin antagonists should not be given in hyponatremia due to hypovolemic conditions, such as gastrointestinal or renal losses, as they can exacerbate hypotension and hypovolemia.[25]

Rapid correction of chronic severe hyponatremia may lead to osmotic demyelination syndrome (ODS; previously called central pontine myelinolysis) and even death.[26] The clinical course of ODS is biphasic, beginning with an initial phase of encephalopathy or seizures, which is caused by the hyponatremia. These symptoms improve with correction of the serum [Na^+]; however, a few days later, there is significant neurologic deterioration due to the osmotic myelinolysis. This second phase manifests as motor impairments leading to quadriparesis and pseudobulbar palsy in the most extreme form. It is usually only partially reversible, and leads to high morbidity and potential mortality, thus prevention is extremely important.[27] ODS can be confirmed with magnetic resonance imaging (MRI), as it can take the classic appearance of a hypointense pons on sagittal imaging but a hyperintense pons on coronal imaging. However, these changes may take 1 to 2 weeks to visualize by MRI.

In order to prevent the serious consequences of inadvertent overcorrection of serum [Na^+] in patients with acute hyponatremia, current guidelines recommend raising the serum [Na^+] concentration only by 6 to 8 mEq/L in the first 24-hour period. In symptomatic patients with acute hyponatremia or patients with severe symptoms, this goal should be achieved quickly (over 6 hours or less) with a constant serum [Na^+] level maintained for the remainder of the 24-hour period to avoid overly rapid correction.[25] Most cases of ODS have occurred in patients with severe hyponatremia whose serum [Na^+] concentration was raised by more than 10 to 12 mEq/L within 24 hours or more than 18 mEq/L within 48 hours. An important exception are patients with coexisting risk factors for ODS (serum [Na^+] less than 105 mEq/L, hypokalemia, alcoholism, malnutrition, or liver failure), who should be corrected no more than 8 mEq/L in any 24-hour period.[24,28] In cases of rapid serum [Na^+] overcorrection, hypotonic fluids such as 5% dextrose in water can be given to match the rate of urinary output in order to slow the rate of correction. In cases where the urine output is profound, this can be supplemented by administration of desmopressin.[25]

Hyponatremia in the Surgical and TBI Setting: Preoperative Hyponatremia

To date, most existing studies have focused primarily on hyponatremia in patients admitted to internal medicine services. The association between preoperative hyponatremia and perioperative outcomes in surgical patients remains less well known. However, one large-scale observational study evaluated the 30-day perioperative morbidity and mortality in patients who had documented preoperative hyponatremia. Out of 964,263 adult patients undergoing major surgery from more than 200 hospitals, 75,423 patients (7.8%) had preoperative hyponatremia (defined as a serum [Na^+] less than 135 mEq/L). The greatest prevalence of preoperative hyponatremia was seen in patients undergoing cardiac surgery (11.8%) and vascular surgery (11.2%), followed by general (7.5%), orthopedic (7.1%), and other (6.1%) surgical procedures. This study found that preoperative hyponatremia was associated with a higher risk of 30-day mortality, especially in patients undergoing nonemergency surgery. Furthermore, hyponatremia was associated with a greater risk of perioperative major coronary events, wound infections, and pneumonia. Lastly, perioperative hyponatremia prolonged median lengths of stay by approximately 1 day.[29] This illustrates the importance of careful evaluation of patients' electrolytes prior to surgery, and that even mild abnormalities in serum [Na^+] can have significant clinical consequences. Preoperative hyponatremia should be evaluated and treated prior to nonemergency surgical procedures if a reversible or treatable cause of the hyponatremia is found.

Hyponatremia in the Surgical and TBI Setting: Postoperative Hyponatremia

Postoperative patients represent another subset of patients who are vulnerable to the development of hyponatremia and its adverse consequences. Current knowledge of postoperative hyponatremia is based on small numbers of patients; therefore, more information is needed regarding the incidence, clinical setting, and outcome in larger surgical populations. Postoperative hyponatremia has previously been reported with prevalences of 1% to 5% in the United States and the European Union.[30] In another study, out of 1088 operative procedures performed (including cardiovascular, gastrointestinal-biliary tract, renal transplantation, and neurosurgical), there were 48 episodes (4.4% prevalence) of postoperative hyponatremia. Specifically, patients who underwent organ transplants, cardiovascular procedures, and surgery for trauma or gastroenterological conditions were at a high risk of developing hyponatremia.[31] Other studies have also shown a high frequency of postoperative hyponatremia in patients who have undergone spinal fusion surgery (20%), subtotal gastrectomy (67%), chronic biliary tube drainage (22%), mitral valve surgery (30%), and general surgery-trauma (40%).[32,33]

The development of hyponatremia after any type of surgical intervention is due to multiple factors. These factors include the stress response to the surgical procedure itself, the loss of blood and other bodily fluids, and the administration of intravenous fluids and blood products during preoperative, intraoperative, and postoperative periods. Potent nonosmotic stimuli to AVP secretion, such as positive pressure ventilation, stress, nausea and vomiting, hypoglycemia, fever, or decrease in intravascular volume, are common after surgery and can additionally increase the risk of hyponatremia.[34]

Numerous hormonal changes occur in response to surgery that influence salt and water metabolism during the postoperative time period. AVP release promotes water retention, and depending on the severity of the surgery and the development of complications, increased AVP secretion can continue for 3 to 5 days postoperatively. Additionally, renin is released from the juxtaglomerular cells of the kidney, partially due to increased sympathetic efferent activation. Renin stimulates the adrenal cortex to release aldosterone, which then leads to sodium reabsorption from the distal convoluted tubules in the kidney, with secondary water resorption.[35]

Aside from elevated plasma AVP levels, the most common precipitant of hyponatremia in patients after surgery is the iatrogenic infusion of hypotonic fluids (such as 0.45% sodium chloride [NaCl] or 5% dextrose in water). This is due to the dilutional effect on the serum [Na^+] levels that occurs with hypotonic fluid administration in the presence of nonosmotic AVP hormone release. Even administration of isotonic solutions (e.g., 0.9% NaCl) can result in a paradoxical fall in sodium concentration as the sodium contained in these solutions is excreted in the urine. This results in the net retention of electrolyte-free water and, subsequently, hyponatremia, a process that has been termed "desalination."[36]

Neurosurgical Patients

Hyponatremia is the most common electrolyte disorder encountered in neurosurgical patients.[37] It has been reported to occur in 50% of subarachnoid hemorrhage and 10% of transsphenoidal hypophysectomy cases.[38] The acute onset of most neurosurgical illnesses (e.g., subarachnoid hemorrhage and TBI) implies that the hyponatremia is acute, and therefore these patients are more likely to be symptomatic.[39] Patients' symptoms can be further exacerbated by other factors that produce cerebral irritation, including increased intracranial pressure or neurosurgical interventions. Hypovolemic volume status in neurosurgical patients can be clinically assessed by central venous pressure (CVP) or the presence of hypotension and/or tachycardia. Hypervolemic volume status usually shows elevated CVP with signs of fluid overload, such as peripheral and/or pulmonary edema and a positive fluid balance. However, most neurosurgical patients will be euvolemic with SIADH as the major etiology of their hyponatremia.[39]

Hyponatremia is also a frequently encountered complication after transsphenoidal pituitary surgery, commonly with a delayed fall of serum [Na^+] toward the end of postoperative week 1.[40] Given the potential delay in presentation of hyponatremia after surgery, this can present increased risk and complications for patients who are discharged early following surgery. Hyponatremia following transsphenoidal pituitary surgery has an incidence varying from 3% to 25%, depending on the study.[41,42] This hyponatremia is primarily due to SIADH; however, the presence of preoperative hypopituitarism makes postoperative hyponatremia more likely. The pathophysiology of SIADH in transsphenoidal pituitary surgery patients is due to the mechanical manipulation or irritation of the posterior pituitary or pituitary stalk. This pathology, responsible for fluctuating salt and water balance from the pituitary stalk injury, can be transient, triphasic, or permanent.[43]

Hyponatremia following pituitary surgery or TBI occurs as part of the triphasic response, which is characterized by acute DI, followed by SIADH, and then DI again (Fig. 18.1A). The initial phase of the triphasic response consists of central DI (which can last 5 to 7 days) due to "stunning" of the AVP neurons and the severing of downstream nerve terminals in the posterior pituitary.[44] Serum [Na^+] concentration increases at this time, and patients experience hypotonic polyuria and polydipsia if their thirst mechanism remains intact. Intravenous fluids are started during this phase in order to keep up with urinary losses and prevent or improve hypernatremia. The second phase (SIADH, which can last 2 to 14 days) results in hyponatremia due to the unregulated release of AVP either from the remaining degenerating neurons in the hypothalamus or from the remaining nerve terminals in the posterior pituitary.[45] This phase of SIADH should be treated by fluid restriction. Given the vastly different management between the first two phases of the triphasic response (intravenous fluid administration versus fluid restriction), judicious monitoring of the patient's urine output and serum [Na^+] concentration during all stages is pertinent in order to not paradoxically worsen the patients' hyponatremia. The third and final phase of the triphasic response results again in DI due to the release of the remaining AVP from the posterior pituitary gland and the inability of the hypothalamus to produce more AVP.[45] The major determinant of whether postoperative DI after transection of the pituitary stalk is transient or permanent depends to the level of the lesion: the closer the lesion is to the cell bodies of the AVP neurons in the hypothalamus, the more likely it is that the cell bodies will degenerate and permanent DI will ensue.[46]

Approximately 8% to 21% of patients with limited damage to the neurohypophysis experience an isolated second phase after pituitary surgery, resulting in hyponatremia secondary to SIADH without previous or subsequent DI.[47] These patients are thought to have significantly less posterior pituitary damage and undergo less stalk traction during the time of surgery compared with patients who develop the full triphasic response (Fig. 18.1B), and this is often seen following resection of pituitary microadenomas.[48]

A small population of patients who have TBI or a neurosurgical procedure may develop partial deficiency of AVP. Because they may experience less severe symptoms at first, the initial diagnosis may be missed. This can lead to a complicated clinical course and significant neurologic and cognitive disabilities.[49] Postneurosurgical patients and post-TBI patients should have careful monitoring of serum osmolality and urine output, even in the absence of initial symptoms, as rapid fluctuations in sodium and water homeostasis can be life-threatening. The triphasic response of

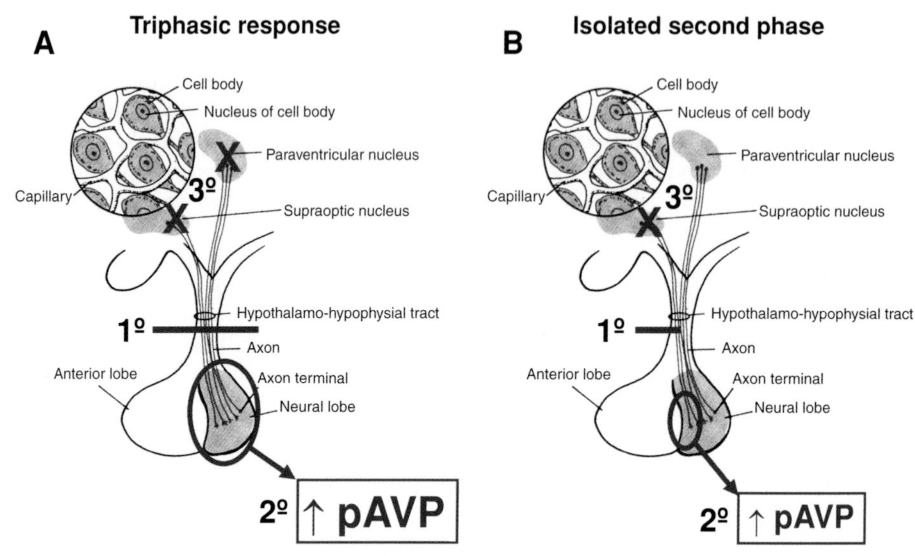

Fig. 18.1 Mechanisms underlying the pathophysiology of the triphasic pattern of diabetes insipidus (DI) and the isolated second phase. (A) In the triphasic response, the first phase of DI is initiated following a partial or complete pituitary stalk section, which severs the connections between the arginine vasopressin (AVP) neuronal cell bodies in the hypothalamus and the nerve terminals in the posterior pituitary gland, thus preventing stimulated AVP secretion *(1°)*. This is followed in several days by the second phase of syndrome of inappropriate antidiuretic hormone secretion (SIADH), which is caused by uncontrolled release of AVP into the bloodstream from the degenerating nerve terminals in the posterior pituitary *(2°)*. After all of the AVP stored in the posterior pituitary gland has been released, the third phase of DI returns if greater than 80% to 90% of the AVP neuronal cell bodies in the hypothalamus have undergone retrograde degeneration *(3°)*. (B) In the isolated second phase, the pituitary stalk is injured but not completely cut. Although maximum AVP secretory response will be diminished as a result of the stalk injury, DI will not result if the injury leaves intact at least 10% to 20% of the nerve fibers connecting the AVP neuronal cell bodies in the hypothalamus to the nerve terminals in the posterior pituitary gland *(1°)*. However, this is still followed in several days by the second phase of SIADH, which is caused by the uncontrolled release of AVP from the degenerating nerve terminals of the posterior pituitary gland that have been injured or severed *(2°)*. Because a smaller portion of the posterior pituitary is denervated, the magnitude of AVP released as the pituitary degenerates will be smaller and of shorter duration than with a complete triphasic response. After all of the AVP stored in the damaged part of the posterior pituitary gland has been released, the second phase ceases, but clinical DI will not occur if less than 80% to 90% of the AVP neuronal cell bodies in the hypothalamus undergo retrograde degeneration *(3°)*. (From Loh JA, Verbalis JG. Disorders of water and salt metabolism associated with pituitary disease. *Endocrinol Metab Clinics North Am.* 2008;37:213–234.)

pituitary stalk injury after neurosurgery or TBI emphasizes the importance of recognizing the signs and symptoms of each individual phase, and the need for close long-term patient monitoring for further signs and symptoms of sodium and water balance.

Lastly, cerebral salt wasting (CSW) is another potential cause of hyponatremia in those with underlying neurologic disease, particularly patients with subarachnoid hemorrhage (SAH), where either an impaired sympathetic output to the kidney and/or an unidentified natriuretic factor associated with the intracranial disorder causes renal sodium wasting.[18] CSW is characterized by hyponatremia and ECF depletion due to inappropriate sodium wasting in the urine (urinary [Na^+] greater than 40 mEq/L), high urine osmolality, and hypovolemia. In routine clinical practice, distinguishing CSW from SIADH can be difficult. The distinction is important, however, because in contrast to the use of fluid restriction to treat SIADH, CSW is treated by replacing the urine losses of water and sodium with isotonic, or in some cases hypertonic, saline. Although many studies have estimated widely different estimates on the prevalence of CSW, virtually all have been retrospective case reviews. The only study that prospectively evaluated the etiology of hyponatremia in patients with SAH was a study by Hannon et al.[50] Out of 100 consecutive SAH patients, 49% developed hyponatremia. Further analysis showed that the most common cause of hyponatremia was SIADH (71.4%), followed by adrenal insufficiency (8.2%). Interestingly, no cases of hyponatremia in these patients were determined to be due to CSW. This demonstrates that CSW is likely a very rare cause of hyponatremia following brain injury.

Traumatic Brain Injury Patients

An estimated 1.7 million people sustain a TBI annually. Of these 1.7 million people, 275,000 are hospitalized and 52,000 die. The greatest number of TBI-related emergency department visits and hospitalizations are due to falls.[51] Posttraumatic hypopituitarism (PTHP) can occur both with mild and severe TBI. The most common hormone abnormalities after TBI are gonadotropin and somatotropin deficiency, followed by corticotropin and thyrotropin deficiency.[52] However, these hormones are often difficult to interpret in the setting of acute stress, so their measurement is not clinically helpful in the first several weeks after the injury.[53] Patients who survive TBIs are prone to the development of hyponatremia due to a disruption in the CNS's ability to regulate sodium and water homeostasis, either due to direct damage to the neurohypophysis or secondary to blood loss (with resulting sodium and water retention to preserve intravascular volume and maintain organ perfusion). Additionally, the increased vascular permeability that occurs during TBI can cause third-space distribution of fluid, and treatment of brain edema may exacerbate sodium and water imbalances.[44,54] Disorders of sodium and water balance are especially common during the acute phase of TBI.[55] Previous literature has reported varying incidences of post-TBI hyponatremia, ranging from 9.6% to 51%.[38,56,57] Hyponatremia is also reported to occur in 50% of subarachnoid hemorrhage and 10% transsphenoidal hypophysectomy cases.[38] Usually, TBI-associated hyponatremia is transient and reversible if treated in an appropriate time frame.

Symptoms of hypothalamic-pituitary disruption after TBI can be subtle, ranging from headaches, nausea, and vomiting to more severe manifestations such as altered mental status and coma. Although the main cause of hyponatremia in post-TBI patients has primarily been thought to be SIADH, diagnosis of ACTH deficiency in post-TBI patients with resolution of hyponatremia after parental hydrocortisone has also been reported.[58] This is partially due to the fact that plasma cortisol levels are highly dynamic in the days following TBI, so a normal, single cortisol level may underestimate the presence of pituitary dysfunction immediately following TBI.[59] Other etiologies for post-TBI hyponatremia include CSW, hypovolemia, inappropriate administration of intravenous fluids, and inadequate dietary intake of salt.[60]

Post-TBI hyponatremia can have detrimental consequences ranging from physical disability to long-term cognitive and psychological defects. The resulting hypothalamic-pituitary dysfunction can further delay recovery from TBI. A study by Hannon et al. showed that in 100 patients with moderate to severe TBI (defined as a Glasgow Coma Scale score of less than 13), both free and total plasma cortisol levels were lower on days 1 to 3 after the initial brain injury; 51% of these patients developed central DI with resulting hypernatremia (mostly transient, with a median duration of 4 days), whereas only 15% developed hyponatremia. Of the patients who were hyponatremic, 13 out of 15 patients improved with administration of glucocorticoids and the other 2 patients had transient SIADH.[58] This study shows that patients with TBI often have low plasma cortisol concentrations, which may be inappropriate for their acute illness. Because the cosyntropin (synthetic ACTH) test cannot be used to diagnose secondary adrenal insufficiency in the setting of acute ACTH deficiency, some have suggested measuring serial plasma morning cortisol levels in patients with moderate to severe TBI and replacing hydrocortisone for levels less than 300 nmol/L,[61] while others recommend checking cortisol levels only in patients with clinical suspicion for adrenal insufficiency,[53,62] which most certainly should include any degree of hyponatremia.

Evaluation of Postoperative and Post-TBI Hyponatremia

The evaluation for postoperative and post-TBI hyponatremia is similar to the initial evaluation of generalized hyponatremia in nonsurgical patients, as described previously in this chapter. After a patient is found to be hyponatremic, first and foremost, the patient should be assessed for neurologic symptoms. Next, the chronicity of hyponatremia should be determined (either acute, less than 48 hours in duration, or chronic, greater than 48 hours in duration). Having a previous serum [Na^+] level is helpful in providing a baseline with which to compare subsequent [Na^+] levels. If no previous [Na^+] level is available, the patient's neurologic symptoms should be used as a surrogate for estimation of the duration of hyponatremia.[15] Clinically, the patient's ECF volume status should then be assessed (hypovolemic, euvolemic, or hypervolemic). The best discriminator of ECF volume is the urine [Na^+] concentration.[25] Urine [Na^+] less than 30 mmol/L is considered low and is usually indicative of hypovolemia, unless the patient has heart failure or cirrhosis (because low urine [Na^+] can be present in these conditions as well due to renal hypoperfusion despite ECF volume expansion from the underlying volume overloaded state). Hypovolemia should be suspected in surgical patients who have vomiting or diarrhea. Urine [Na^+] greater than 30 mmol/L with serum hypoosmolality (less than 275 mOsm/kg) is usually indicative of SIADH or renal sodium losses. It is important to mention that common postoperative symptoms, such as pain, gastrointestinal distention, or nausea, can lead to the nonosmotic secretion of AVP and the development of euvolemic hyponatremia. When further evaluating euvolemic hyponatremia, hypothyroidism and adrenal insufficiency should be assessed with thyroid function tests and cortisol levels and/or an ACTH stimulation test before confirming a diagnosis of SIADH.

Especially in the acute postoperative and post-TBI setting, patients should additionally have careful observation of their fluid balance. Using a staggered intravenous fluid regimen, which involves the administration of isotonic fluids during the immediate postoperative period (when there is a high degree of non–osmotically-stimulated AVP secretion), and hypotonic fluids only later if the patient develops hypernatremia, is one strategy to avoid hyponatremia.[63] Daily monitoring of renal function, serum [Na^+] levels, and other electrolytes in patients receiving intravenous fluids is essential. Coexistent renal dysfunction may result in the inability to excrete free water in the urine, making patients more susceptible to hyponatremia.

Treatment of Postoperative and Post-TBI Hyponatremia

Mild postoperative hyponatremia generally resolves without any specific intervention. However, treatment is indicated with moderate or severe hyponatremia when neurologic symptoms occur. In cases in which a patient is experiencing symptoms such as unexplained nausea, disorientation, seizures, obtundation, or coma, urgent treatment with hypertonic (3%) NaCl, either via bolus or continuous infusion, should be initiated. Boluses of 100 mL of hypertonic saline, repeated two to three times if there is no clinical improvement, has previously been recommended,[25] and a recent study has shown this to be safe and effective at improving the Glasgow Coma Score in neurologically damaged patients.[64] There is currently no consensus on the optimal infusion rate of hypertonic saline. Current guidelines recommend raising the serum [Na^+] concentration only by 4 to 8 mEq/L in a 24-hour period, with this goal achieved quickly in patients who are symptomatic in order to reverse cerebral edema, reduce intracranial pressure, and prevent seizures.[39] This recommendation is based on data that has shown that a 5-mmol/L increase in serum [Na^+] can reduce intracranial pressure and resolve the neurologic symptoms of herniation by nearly 50% within an hour.[65]

BOX 18.1 ■ General Recommendations for Employment of Fluid Restriction and Predictors of the Increased Likelihood of Failure of Fluid Restriction

General Recommendations

- Restrict *all* intake that is consumed by drinking, not just water.
- Aim for a fluid restriction that is 500 mL/day *below* the 24-hour urine volume.
- Do not restrict sodium or protein intake unless indicated.

Predictors of the Likely Failure of Fluid Restriction

- High urine osmolality (>500 mOsm/kg H_2O).
- Sum of the urine Na^+ and K^+ concentrations exceeds the serum Na^+ concentration.
- 24-hour urine volume <1,500 mL/day.
- Increase in serum Na^+ sodium concentration <2 mmol/L per day in 24 hours on a fluid restriction of ≤1 L/day.

H_2O, water; *K,* potassium; *kg,* kilogram; *L,* liter; *mL,* milliliter; *mmol,* millimole; *mOsm,* milliosmole; *Na,* sodium. (From Verbalis JG, Goldsmith SR, Greenberg A, et al. Diagnosis, evaluation, and treatment of hyponatremia: expert panel recommendations. *Am J Med*. 2103;126(10 Suppl 1):S1–S42.)

In iatrogenic hyponatremia due to the administration of hypotonic intravenous fluids, either isotonic or hypertonic fluids can be administered for treatment. If hypovolemic hyponatremia is suspected (urine [Na^+] less than 30 mEq/L and/or signs of hypovolemia on physical examination), volume repletion with isotonic saline (0.9% NaCl) should be given in order to replace the ECF volume and restore organ perfusion. Isotonic saline should also be given to patients with suspected CSW, although this entity is rare, as noted previously.

If the diagnosis of SIADH is clinically suspected and supported with the biochemical parameters of low plasma osmolality, inappropriate urine concentration, and elevated urine [Na^+], a daily fluid restriction of 500 to 1000 mL should be instituted. The fluid restriction includes all fluids ingested by the patients, not just water. There are certain predictors, if present, that can predict the likely failure of serum [Na^+] improvement after a fluid restriction is put in place (Box 18.1).[25] These patients are candidates for vasopressin receptor agonists ("vaptans") that act to improve hyponatremia by inhibiting AVP-mediated receptor activation. Treatment of hypervolemic hyponatremia should be directed at correcting the underlying disorder, along with sodium and fluid restriction and loop diuretics. Patients with hypervolemic hyponatremia may additionally be candidates for vaptan therapy. At high doses, vaptans have been associated with reversible liver injury, and consequently they are contracted in patients with underlying severe liver disease.

For patients who experience the triphasic response after pituitary stalk injury or TBI, the management can be divided into the following: expectant monitoring, antidiuretic hormone therapy, maintenance of fluid balance, monitoring for resolution of transient DI, and management of anterior pituitary insufficiency.[45] Strict surveillance of fluid intake and output with measurement of serum [Na^+], urine osmolality, and urine specific gravity every 6 hours is necessary. Desmopressin should be administered if a patient is suspected to have DI, as evidenced by polyuria (greater than 200 mL/hour for more than 2 hours) with urine specific gravity of less than 1.005 or urine osmolality less than 200 mOsm/kg H_2O, in addition to an elevated serum [Na^+]. During this time, the patient should also be allowed to drink to thirst and/or given hypotonic intravenous fluid such as 5% dextrose in water or 5% dextrose in 0.45% saline if unable to maintain normal serum [Na^+] during the DI phase. Fluid restriction, on the other hand, should be used to maintain eunatremia during the SIADH phase. Lastly, if there is concern for anterior pituitary hormone deficits with resulting secondary adrenal insufficiency, corticosteroids should be administered.[44] Timely diagnosis and administration of desmopressin (dDAVP) and/or hypertonic saline versus fluid restriction, depending on the clinical symptoms and phase of presentation, are critical for the maintenance of fluid homeostasis and symptom management. Long-term follow-up of all patients who experience a TBI is crucial in order to monitor for PTHP, regardless of clinical symptoms that reflect pituitary dysfunction.

For cases of hyponatremia following pituitary or suprasellar surgery, the isolated second phase of the triphasic response, prevention is the most efficacious strategy. A recent cohort-control study has suggested that use of a mandatory fluid restriction of 1000 mL/day during the first week following discharge can reduce the frequency of readmission for severe hyponatremia.[66] Whether this is done or not, all patients should be instructed to drink only when thirsty and have serum [Na^+] checked 1 week postoperatively. If severely symptomatic, patients with an isolated second phase should be treated with hypertonic saline as other cases of acute hyponatremia. However, if symptoms are mild to moderate, they should simply be observed because the SIADH generally dissipates spontaneously in 3 to 7 days as the posterior pituitary degeneration is completed.[47]

Summary

Hyponatremia is a common electrolyte disorder that affects multiple patient populations, including the elderly, those with multiple comorbidities, and, as described in this chapter, preoperative, postoperative, and TBI patients. Given its wide prevalence and its clinical implications, all medical providers, including surgeons, should be aware of the evaluation, diagnosis, and appropriate treatment of hyponatremia in order to prevent morbidity and mortality. The questions one must always ask during the initial recognition of hyponatremia are: (1) Is the patient symptomatic? (2) Is the hyponatremia acute or chronic in duration? (3) What is the patient's ECF volume status? These questions will facilitate the necessary further evaluation and appropriate treatment of the patient to avoid complications from the hyponatremia, as well as from adverse effects as a result of overly rapid correction of the hyponatremia.

References

1. Upadhyay A, Jaber BL, Madias NE. Epidemiology of hyponatremia. *Semin Nephrol.* 2009;29(3):227–238.
2. Wald R, Jaber BL, Price LL, Upadhyay A, Madias NE. Impact of hospital-associated hyponatremia on selected outcomes. *Arch Intern Med.* 2010;170(3):294–302.
3. Mohan S, Gu S, Parikh A, Radhakrishnan J. Prevalence of hyponatremia and association with mortality: results from NHANES. *Am J Med.* 2013;126(12):1127–1137.
4. Peri A. Morbidity and mortality of hyponatremia. *Front Horm Res.* 2019;52:36–48.
5. Boscoe A, Paramore C, Verbalis JG. Cost of illness of hyponatremia in the United States. *Cost Eff Resour Alloc.* 2006;4(1):10.
6. Gill G, Huda B, Boyd A, et al. Characteristics and mortality of severe hyponatraemia—a hospital-based study. *Clin Endocrinol (Oxf).* 2006;65(2):246–249.
7. Goel A, Farhat F, Zik C, Jeffery M. Triphasic response of pituitary stalk injury following TBI: a relevant yet uncommonly recognised endocrine phenomenon. *BMJ Case Rep.* 2018;2018.
8. Renneboog B, Musch W, Vandemergel X, Manto MU, Decaux G. Mild chronic hyponatremia is associated with falls, unsteadiness, and attention deficits. *Am J Med.* 2006;119(1):71.
9. Kinsella S, Moran S, Sullivan MO, Molloy MG, Eustace JA. Hyponatremia independent of osteoporosis is associated with fracture occurrence. *Clin J Am Soc Nephrol.* 2010;5(2):275–280.
10. Gunathilake R, Oldmeadow C, McEvoy M, et al. Mild hyponatremia is associated with impaired cognition and falls in community-dwelling older persons. *J Am Geriatr Soc.* 2013;61(10):1838–1839.
11. Verbalis JG, Barsony J, Sugimura Y, et al. Hyponatremia-induced osteoporosis. *J Bone Miner Res.* 2010; 25(3):554–563.
12. Usala RL, Fernandez SJ, Mete M, et al. Hyponatremia is associated with increased osteoporosis and bone fractures in a large us health system population. *J Clin Endocrinol Metab.* 2015;100(8):3021–3031.
13. Stelfox HT, Ahmed SB, Khandwala F, Zygun D, Shahpori R, Laupland K. The epidemiology of intensive care unit-acquired hyponatraemia and hypernatraemia in medical-surgical intensive care units. *Crit Care.* 2008;12(6):R162.
14. Verbalis JG. Emergency management of acute and chronic hyponatremia. In: Matfin G, ed. *Endocrine and Metabolic Emergencies.* Hoboken, NJ: John Wiley and Sons; 2019:679–699.

15. Verbalis JG. Euvolemic hyponatremia secondary to the syndrome of inappropriate antidiuresis. *Front Horm Res.* 2019;52:61–79.
16. Garrahy A, Thompson CJ. Hyponatremia and glucocorticoid deficiency. *Front Horm Res.* 2019;52:80–92.
17. Gaglio P, Marfo K, Chiodo III J. Hyponatremia in cirrhosis and end-stage liver disease: treatment with the vasopressin V(2)-receptor antagonist tolvaptan. *Dig Dis Sci.* 2012;57(11):2774–2785.
18. Rondon-Berrios H, Berl T. Physiology and pathophysiology of water homeostasis. *Front Horm Res.* 2019;52:8–23.
19. Thompson CJ, Verbalis JG. Posterior pituitary. In: Melmed S, Auchus RJ, Goldfine AB, Koenig RJ, Rosen C, eds. *Williams Textbook of Endocrinology*. Philadelphia: Elsevier; 2020:303–329.
20. Knepper MA. Molecular physiology of urinary concentrating mechanism: regulation of aquaporin water channels by vasopressin. *Am J Physiol.* 1997;272(1 Pt 2):F3–F12.
21. Christ-Crain M, Bichet DG, Fenske WK, et al. Diabetes insipidus. *Nat Rev Dis Primers.* 2019;5(1):54.
22. Sterns RH, Silver SM. Complications and management of hyponatremia. *Curr Opin Nephrol Hypertens.* 2016;25(2):114–119.
23. Verbalis JG. Brain volume regulation in response to changes in osmolality. *Neuroscience.* 2010;168(4): 862–870.
24. Sterns RH. Treatment of severe hyponatremia. *Clin J Am Soc Nephrol.* 2018;13(4):641–649.
25. Verbalis JG, Goldsmith SR, Greenberg A, et al. Diagnosis, evaluation, and treatment of hyponatremia: expert panel recommendations. *Am J Med.* 2013;126(10 Suppl 1):S1–S42.
26. Tandukar S, Rondon-Berrios H. Treatment of severe symptomatic hyponatremia. *Physiol Rep.* 2019; 7(21):e14265.
27. Sterns RH. Severe symptomatic hyponatremia: treatment and outcome. A study of 64 cases. *Ann Int Med.* 1987;107:656–664.
28. Sterns RH. Adverse consequences of overly-rapid correction of hyponatremia. *Front Horm Res.* 2019; 52:130–142.
29. Leung AA, McAlister FA, Rogers Jr SO, Pazo V, Wright A, Bates DW. Preoperative hyponatremia and perioperative complications. *Arch Intern Med.* 2012;172(19):1474–1481.
30. Ayus JC, Wheeler JM, Arieff AI. Postoperative hyponatremic encephalopathy in menstruant women. *Ann Int Med.* 1992;117:891–897.
31. Chung HM, Kluge R, Schrier RW, Anderson RJ. Postoperative hyponatremia. A prospective study. *Arch Int Med.* 1986;146:333–336.
32. Bruce RA, Merendino KA, Dunning MF, et al. Observations on hyponatremia following mitral valve surgery. *Surg Gynecol Obstet.* 1955;100(3):293–302.
33. Furey AT. Hyponatremia after choledochostomy and T tube drainage. *Am J Surg.* 1966;112(6):850–855.
34. Cuesta M, Thompson C. The relevance of hyponatraemia to perioperative care of surgical patients. *Surgeon.* 2015;13(3):163–169.
35. Desborough JP. The stress response to trauma and surgery. *Br J Anaesth.* 2000;85(1):109–117.
36. Steele A, Gowrishankar M, Abrahamson S, Mazer CD, Feldman RD, Halperin ML. Postoperative hyponatremia despite near-isotonic saline infusion: a phenomenon of desalination [see comments]. *Ann Intern Med.* 1997;126(1):20–25.
37. Upadhyay UM, Gormley WB. Etiology and management of hyponatremia in neurosurgical patients. *J Intensive Care Med.* 2012;27(3):139–144.
38. Sherlock M, O'Sullivan E, Agha A, et al. Incidence and pathophysiology of severe hyponatraemia in neurosurgical patients. *Postgrad Med J.* 2009;85(1002):171–175.
39. Hannon MJ, Thompson CJ. Hyponatremia in neurosurgical patients. *Front Horm Res.* 2019;52:143–160.
40. Lee JI, Cho WH, Choi BK, Cha SH, Song GS, Choi CH. Delayed hyponatremia following transsphenoidal surgery for pituitary adenoma. *Neurol Med Chir (Tokyo).* 2008;48(11):489–492.
41. Janneck M, Burkhardt T, Rotermund R, Sauer N, Flitsch J, Aberle J. Hyponatremia after trans-sphenoidal surgery. *Minerva Endocrinol.* 2014;39(1):27–31.
42. Jahangiri A, Wagner J, Tran MT, et al. Factors predicting postoperative hyponatremia and efficacy of hyponatremia management strategies after more than 1000 pituitary operations. *J Neurosurg.* 2013; 119(6):1478–1483.
43. Hollinshead WH. The interphase of diabetes insipidus. *Mayo Clin Proc.* 1964;39:92–100.
44. Goel A, Farhat F, Zik C, Jeffery M. Triphasic response of pituitary stalk injury following TBI: a relevant yet uncommonly recognised endocrine phenomenon. *BMJ Case Rep.* 2018;2018.

45. Loh JA, Verbalis JG. Diabetes insipidus as a complication after pituitary surgery. *Nat Clin Pract Endocrinol Metab*. 2007;3(6):489–494.
46. Lipsett MB, Maclean JP, West CD, Li MC, Pearson OH. An analysis of the polyuria induced by hypophysectomy in man. *J Clin Endocrinol Metab*. 1956;16(2):183–195.
47. Loh JA, Verbalis JG. Disorders of water and salt metabolism associated with pituitary disease. *Endocrinol Metab Clin North Am*. 2008;37(1):213–234.
48. Olson BR, Gumowski J, Rubino D, Oldfield EH. Pathophysiology of hyponatremia after transsphenoidal pituitary surgery. *J Neurosurg*. 1997;87(4):499–507.
49. Agha A, Thornton E, O'Kelly P, Tormey W, Phillips J, Thompson CJ. Posterior pituitary dysfunction after traumatic brain injury. *J Clin Endocrinol Metab*. 2004;89(12):5987–5992.
50. Hannon MJ, Behan LA, O'Brien MM, et al. Hyponatremia following mild/moderate subarachnoid hemorrhage is due to SIAD and glucocorticoid deficiency and not cerebral salt wasting. *J Clin Endocrinol Metab*. 2014;99(1):291–298.
51. Coronado VG, Xu L, Basavaraju SV, et al. Surveillance for traumatic brain injury-related deaths—United States, 1997-2007. *MMWR Surveill Summ*. 2011;60(5):1–32.
52. Bondanelli M, Ambrosio MR, Zatelli MC, De ML, degli Uberti EC. Hypopituitarism after traumatic brain injury. *Eur J Endocrinol*. 2005;152(5):679–691.
53. Tan CL, Alavi SA, Baldeweg SE, et al. The screening and management of pituitary dysfunction following traumatic brain injury in adults: British Neurotrauma Group guidance. *J Neurol Neurosurg Psychiatry*. 2017;88(11):971–981.
54. Rhoney DH, Parker Jr D. Considerations in fluids and electrolytes after traumatic brain injury. *Nutr Clin Pract*. 2006;21(5):462–478.
55. Kaufman HH, Timberlake G, Voelker J, Pait TG. Medical complications of head injury. *Med Clin North Am*. 1993;77(1):43–60.
56. Meng X, Shi B. Traumatic brain injury patients with a Glasgow Coma Scale score of </=8, cerebral edema, and/or a basal skull fracture are more susceptible to developing hyponatremia. *J Neurosurg Anesthesiol*. 2016;28(1):21–26.
57. Yumoto T, Sato K, Ugawa T, Ichiba S, Ujike Y. Prevalence, risk factors, and short-term consequences of traumatic brain injury-associated hyponatremia. *Acta Med Okayama*. 2015;69(4):213–218.
58. Hannon MJ, Crowley RK, Behan LA, et al. Acute glucocorticoid deficiency and diabetes insipidus are common after acute traumatic brain injury and predict mortality. *J Clin Endocrinol Metab*. 2013;98(8):3229–3237.
59. Della CF, Mancini A, Valle D, et al. Provocative hypothalamopituitary axis tests in severe head injury: correlations with severity and prognosis. *Crit Care Med*. 1998;26(8):1419–1426.
60. Rajagopal R, Swaminathan G, Nair S, Joseph M. Hyponatremia in traumatic brain injury: a practical management protocol. *World Neurosurg*. 2017;108:529–533.
61. Quinn M, Agha A. Post-traumatic hypopituitarism—who should be screened, when, and how. *Front Endocrinol (Lausanne)*. 2018;9:8.
62. Hamrahian AH, Fleseriu M. Evaluation and management of adrenal insufficiency in critically ill patients: disease state review. *Endocr Pract*. 2017;23(6):716–725.
63. Hilton AK, Pellegrino VA, Scheinkestel CD. Avoiding common problems associated with intravenous fluid therapy. *Med J Aust*. 2008;189(9):509–513.
64. Garrahy A, Dineen R, Hannon AM, et al. Continuous versus bolus infusion of hypertonic saline in the treatment of symptomatic hyponatremia caused by SIAD. *J Clin Endocrinol Metab*. 2019;104(9):3595–3602.
65. Koenig MA, Bryan M, Lewin III JL, Mirski MA, Geocadin RG, Stevens RD. Reversal of transtentorial herniation with hypertonic saline. *Neurology*. 2008;70(13):1023–1029.
66. Burke WT, Cote DJ, Iuliano SI, Zaidi HA, Laws ER. A practical method for prevention of readmission for symptomatic hyponatremia following transsphenoidal surgery. *Pituitary*. 2018;21(1):25–31.

CHAPTER 19

Diabetes Insipidus and Acute Hypernatremia

Chelsi Flippo ■ Christina Tatsi ■ Constantine A. Stratakis

Funding. The work was supported by the Intramural Research Program, *Eunice Kennedy Shriver* National Institute of Child Health & Human Development (NICHD), National Institutes of Health.

Disclosure Statement: Dr. Stratakis holds patents on technologies involving *PRKAR1A, PDE11A, GPR101* genes and/or their function; his laboratory has received research funding support by Pfizer Inc. for work unrelated to this project.

CHAPTER OUTLINE

Introduction

Serum sodium is tightly regulated by water homeostasis, which is primarily mediated by arginine vasopressin (AVP), thirst, and the kidneys. If water balance is disrupted, abnormalities in serum sodium concentration may occur. Hypernatremia, defined as a serum sodium above 145 mmol/L (145 mEq/L), is a common electrolyte disorder. As sodium is a functionally impermeable solute and is the major solute contributing to osmolality, hypernatremia results in cellular dehydration. Hypernatremia may result from excess loss of solute-free water, decreased solute-free water intake, or excess sodium administration. Although correction of transient hypernatremia is usually well tolerated, correction of chronic hypernatremia (with resultant chronic plasma hypertonicity) should be administered slowly and cautiously to avoid serious or even life-threatening consequences.[1,2]

Physiology of Water and Sodium Homeostasis

Serum osmolality, determined primarily by serum sodium, is tightly regulated by water homeostasis. This balance is maintained by thirst, AVP, and the kidneys. In normal humans, osmolality, or the concentration of osmotically active solutes in body fluids, is remarkably constant despite large variations in water and solute intake and excretion. Every kilogram of body water contains 285 to 290 mOsm of solute, consisting primarily of salts of sodium in extracellular fluid and of potassium in intracellular fluid. The identical osmolality of intracellular and extracellular fluids is produced by free movement of water across cellular and subcellular membranes, governed by the physical forces of osmosis and diffusion. A gain or loss of free water will be shared by all major body compartments (vascular, interstitial, and intracellular) in proportion to their relative sizes. The single exception to this free movement is the control of water permeability of the distal portion of the nephron by AVP (or antidiuretic hormone). This ability to excrete a hyperosmotic urine allows conservation of free water when the supply of available water is limited.[3]

The day-to-day fluctuations in total body water in a healthy individual are very small, amounting to approximately 0.2% of body weight per 24 hours. Although infants have a relative excess of body water and extracellular volume as related to total body weight, the surface area, oxygen consumption, cardiac output, insensible water loss, renal water excretion, and overall metabolism are all high in relation to total body water. Therefore, infants and young children are more vulnerable to water deficit and dehydration than adults.[4] Even with maximal renal conservation of water, the body is unable to prevent a continuous loss of insensible fluid through the skin, lungs, and gastrointestinal tract. For the replacement of this extrarenal loss, a person must rely on adequate water ingestion, with thirst playing an essential role in the regulation of tonicity and volume of body fluids.[3]

The major stimulus to thirst is increased osmolality of body fluids as perceived by osmoreceptors in the periventricular nucleus of the hypothalamus. Hypovolemia also has an important effect on thirst which is mediated by arterial baroreceptors and by the renin-angiotensin system. Although thirst is a conscious sensation, hypothalamic stimulating and inhibitory impulses are transmitted to the cerebral cortex and consciousness, which transforms the need, or lack of need, for water into appropriate behavior. Furthermore, impulses of cortical or voluntary origin can readily condition the sensation of thirst and create what might be called the thirst appetite, or voluntary habits of drinking. These vary greatly from individual to individual, with psychogenic polydipsia representing the extreme form of excessive ingestion. Conversely, in humans, injury to these centers, or failure of these hypothalamic-cortical impulses to stimulate thirst in a patient with altered mental status, may cause inadequate water ingestion despite need.[3]

Similar to thirst, change in body fluid osmolality is the most potent factor affecting AVP secretion. However, hypovolemia, the renin-angiotensin system, hypoxia, hypercapnia, hyperthermia, physical stress, and pain also have important effects, and many drugs have been shown to stimulate the release of AVP as well. AVP is a hormone produced by magnocellular neurons of the supraoptic and paraventricular nuclei of the hypothalamus. AVP is produced as a pre-prohormone, pre-proAVP. After cleavage of pre-proAVP, AVP is produced, along with neurophysin II and copeptin. Whereas neurophysin II functions as carrier protein for AVP, the function of copeptin has yet to be understood. AVP then travels in neurosecretory granules along the axons of the magnocellular neurons via the neurohypophyseal tract of the pituitary stalk and terminates at the posterior pituitary, where AVP is released into circulation. When serum osmolality rises above approximately 284 mOsm/kg H_2O, AVP is released into circulation from the posterior pituitary.[5] AVP then acts at the renal collecting ducts where it binds to its receptor, AVPR2 (or V2 receptor), which is expressed at the basolateral surface of the principal cells of the collecting ducts. Binding of AVP to its receptor results in translocation of aquaporin 2 to the apical membrane, allowing water to move from the lumen of the collecting ducts into the principal cell and then enter the interstitium through aquaporin 3 and 4 channels. The overall effect is resorption of solute-free water with concentrated urine and decreased urine output. Small changes in plasma AVP concentration of 0.5 to 4 μU/mL have major effects on urine osmolality and renal water handling.[3]

Whereas renal water handling is primarily determined by circulating AVP and renal perfusion, reabsorption of sodium throughout the nephron is facilitated by several luminal sodium transporters along the nephron, which take advantage of low concentrations of sodium within the cells maintained by sodium/potassium-ATPase (Na/K-ATPase) on the basolateral membrane. In the proximal tubule, the majority of the sodium is reabsorbed via the sodium/hydrogen exchanger NHE3, and angiotensin II increases sodium reabsorption by NHE3. The Na/K/Cl cotransporter in the thick ascending limb of Henle is the primary transporter. In the collecting duct, aldosterone activity promotes sodium reabsorption and, as mentioned previously, vasopressin activity promotes reabsorption of water.[6]

Etiologies of Hypernatremia

Hypernatremia may occur due to an excess loss of solute-free water, decreased solute-free water intake, or excess sodium administration (Fig. 19.1). Although solute loss may occur with excess solute-free water loss, decreased solute intake may occur with decreased solute-free water intake, and solute-free water intake may occur with excess sodium administration, the balance of solute and solute-free water changes will determine the serum osmolality. This balance is also important to recognize clinically, because the balance of solute and solute-free water changes will impact the assessment of volume status during physical examination (discussed in more detail in the "Clinical Presentation of Hypernatremia" section).

The most common cause of hypernatremia is lack of adequate free water intake. As serum sodium is tightly regulated, persistent hypernatremia should not occur in an individual with access to free water, who is alert, and has an intact thirst mechanism. Those at highest risk of hypernatremia are infants, elderly persons, those with altered mental status or neurologic impairment, or intubated patients. In these patients, although their thirst mechanism is intact, they cannot independently access fluids and are unable to communicate their need for fluids. Infants, especially those born preterm, are at particularly high risk for the development of hypernatremia because of their relatively small mass-to-surface area ratio and their dependency on a caretaker to administer fluids. Additionally, ineffective breastfeeding is a rare cause of hypernatremia in neonates, and it may be accompanied by significant vascular complications, such as venous thrombosis.[1,7–10] Close medical follow-up after birth with careful attention to weight loss and breastfeeding adequacy has been shown to prevent potentially devastating complications of hypernatremia in these young patients.[11] In elderly individuals, hypernatremia is often associated with infirmity or febrile illness. Thirst impairment also occurs in elderly patients, and nursing home residents and hospitalized patients are prone to hypernatremia because they depend on others for their water requirements.[1] Additionally, in a patient who is fluid restricted (e.g., nothing by mouth), hypernatremia may occur. Critically ill patients are also at higher risk of hypernatremia with approximately 2% to 6% hypernatremic on intensive care unit (ICU) admission and 4% to 26% becoming hypernatremic during the course of an ICU admission.[12] Patients with a lack of intact thirst mechanism (adipsia/hypodipsia) due to hypothalamic defects or with an altered set point for thirst and AVP release (termed "essential hypernatremia"), hypernatremia may occur due to lack of adequate free water intake.

Excess free water loss is another important cause of hypernatremia and includes both renal and insensible losses of water. Renal losses of excess water include central diabetes insipidus (DI), nephrogenic DI, primary polydipsia, osmotic diuresis, diuretic use, intrinsic renal disease, postobstructive diuresis, and the diuretic phase of acute tubular necrosis. Central DI occurs due to deficient AVP synthesis or secretion, and it results in the inability to maximally concentrate urine, resulting in water diuresis. Central DI may be hereditary, such as from autosomal dominant variants in *AVP* or autosomal recessive variants in the *AVP*, *WFS1*, or *PCSK1* genes. In general, however, central DI is most often acquired, resulting from hypothalamic, pituitary stalk, or posterior pituitary involvement of intracranial neoplasia, infiltrative lesions, inflammatory processes, or traumatic injury; central nervous system (CNS) infections; or drug or toxin exposure. Nephrogenic DI is due to renal resistance of AVP, and it presents clinically identical to central DI with water diuresis. Nephrogenic DI may be hereditary, such as from X-linked variants in the receptor gene *AVPR2* or autosomal recessive or autosomal dominant *AQP2* gene variants. Acquired causes of nephrogenic DI include drug exposure (e.g., lithium, cisplatin, demeclocycline), hypokalemia, hypercalcemia, infiltrative lesions, vascular disorders (e.g., sickle cell anemia), or mechanical

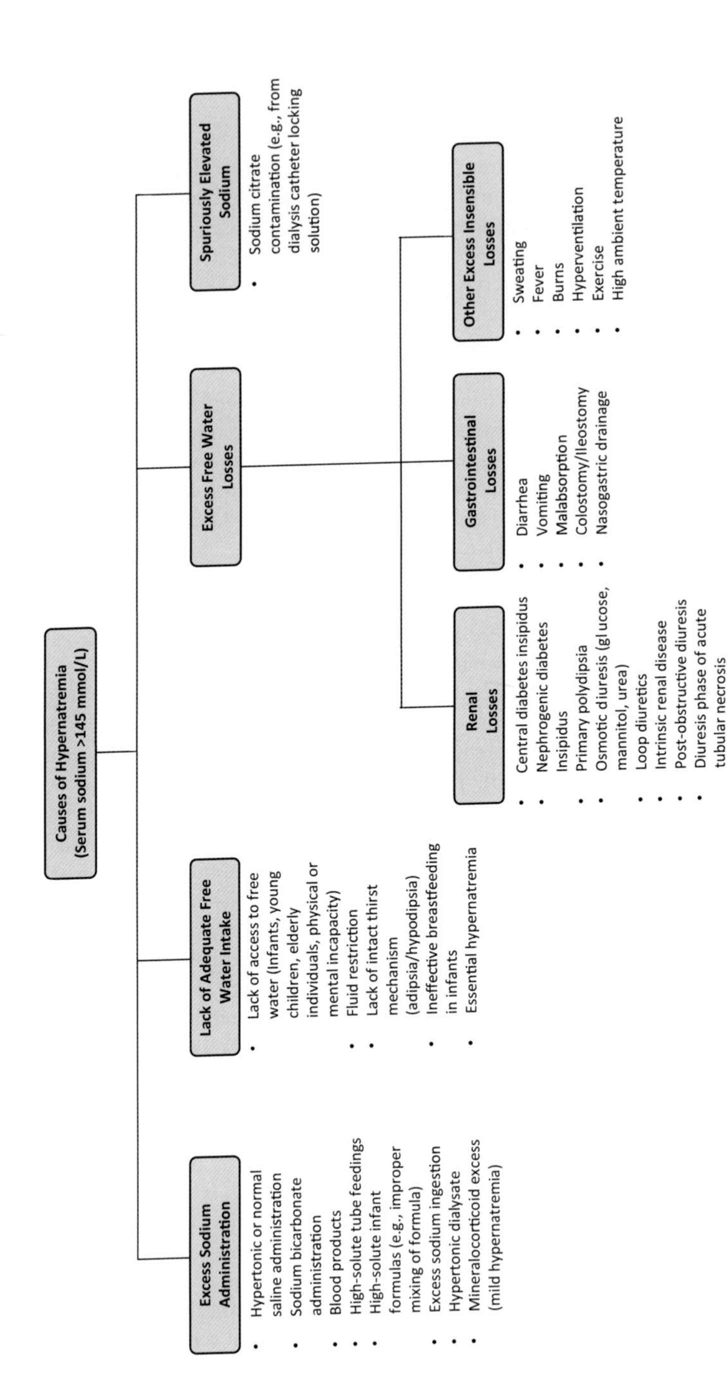

Fig. 19.1 . Causes of hypernatremia.

(e.g., polycystic kidney disease, urinary tract obstruction). Gestational DI may occur during pregnancy and is due to increased placental vasopressinase activity with increased breakdown of AVP. Primary polydipsia is a primary excess fluid intake, and it is associated in some with psychiatric conditions, though may also be seen in compulsive water drinking or due to an abnormally low thirst threshold (termed "dipsogenic DI"). Although hyponatremia may also occur in primary polydipsia, hypernatremia may occur due to tonicity of body fluids stabilizing at a new set point around the osmotic threshold for AVP secretion, due to depletion of renal medullary solute ("renal washout" effect), and due to downregulation of aquaporin 2 channels. Similar to all forms of DI, these mechanisms in primary polydipsia may prevent maximal concentration of urine with resultant water diuresis. Osmotic diuresis may also result in excess renal water losses and may be due to glucosuria (e.g., diabetes mellitus, sodium-glucose cotransporter 2 inhibitors), mannitol, or urea. Gastrointestinal losses of water are a common cause of excess water loss. Infants, young children, elderly patients, patients with DI, or other preexisting risk factors for hypernatremia are at the highest risk of severe hypernatremia from gastrointestinal losses, especially diarrhea. Other causes of excess insensible water losses include fever, hyperventilation, burns, exercise, excess sweating, and high ambient temperatures.

Hypernatremia may also occur due to excess sodium intake, such as from hypertonic or even normal saline infusions, sodium bicarbonate administration, blood products, high-solute tube feedings, or excess salt ingestion (e.g., salt tablets). High-solute infant formulas may also contribute to hypernatremia in infants, which may occur with improper mixing of formula. Mineralocorticoid excess may also result in hypernatremia, together with hypokalemia and hypertension, though hypernatremia is typically mild with serum sodium typically less than 150 mEq/L due to persistent volume expansion resulting in increasing the set point for AVP and thirst.[13]

Clinical Presentation of Hypernatremia

The signs and symptoms of acute hypernatremia largely reflect CNS involvement and are more prominent when the increase in the serum sodium concentration is large or occurs rapidly over a period of hours. Most outpatients with hypernatremia are either very young or very old, due to the previously mentioned risk factors for decreased free water intake. Common symptoms in infants include nonspecific manifestations such as tachypnea, weakness, muscle twitching, irritability, a characteristic high-pitched cry, vomiting, insomnia, and fever.[14] Unlike infants, adults and geriatric patients generally have fewer symptoms until serum sodium exceeds 160 mmol/L. Because the most common cause of hypernatremia is excessive solute-free water loss, patients may also have evidence of hypovolemia, including tachycardia, orthostatic blood pressure changes, or decreased blood pressure, dry mucous membranes, and delay in capillary refill.[1,7] However, volume depletion is variable, depending on the balance of water deficit and sodium excess. As water moves out of brain cells leading to contraction of cells of the brain, vascular rupture may occur in severe cases, with cerebral bleeding, subarachnoid hemorrhage, and progressive neurologic decline, including altered mental status, lethargy, coma, seizures, irreversible neurologic injury, and death.[1,7,15] As can be seen in rapid correction of hyponatremia, if serum sodium rises quickly, central pontine myelinolysis may also occur in hypernatremia.[16]

In chronic hypernatremia, defined as hypernatremia present more for than 1 day, patients may be asymptomatic due to cerebral adaption.[1] In early adaptation (within a few hours), there is accumulation of electrolytes into cells of the brain, pulling water into the cells. In chronic adaptation (occurs in hours to days), normalization of brain volume occurs as a result of accumulation of organic osmolytes. These solutes were historically termed "idiogenic osmoles" because they were unidentified and thought to be produced by the brain cells themselves.[1,17,18] Because of the adaptation that occurs, neurologic symptoms are less likely to be induced compared to acute hypernatremia. However, assessment of patients with chronic hypernatremia can be complicated by comorbid neurologic disease, as patients with an intact thirst mechanism (assuming access to free water) would have a compensatory increase in thirst preventing sustained hypernatremia, even for individuals with DI.

The concept of cerebral adaptation to hyperosmolality becomes clinically relevant regarding management of hypernatremia (discussed in detail later). Although normalization of brain volume occurs, this cerebral adaptation does not correct the hyperosmolality in the brain. Therefore, in patients with chronic hyperosmolality, aggressive treatment with hypotonic fluids may cause cerebral edema as water uptake by brain cells occurs more rapidly than osmolytes leave the brain cells, which can lead to coma, convulsions, and death.[1] This devastating consequence has been primarily described in children and highlights the importance of slower corrections of hyperosmolality.[2]

Diagnostic Evaluation

Hypernatremia is often multifactorial, and a thorough history is key to narrow down the differential, including a review of fluid intake to determine if the patient has an intact thirst mechanism, has restricted access to fluids, or is not being provided adequate free water in intravenous fluids. Patients should be evaluated for gastrointestinal losses, dermal losses from fever or burns, diet history (including enteral feedings, mixing of formula, breastfeeding adequacy), medication history (including diuretics), and sources of exogenous sodium. Strict intake and output should be followed to assess for polyuria (suggestive of DI, primary polydipsia, osmotic diuresis, or intrinsic renal disease) or oliguria (suggestive of hypovolemia or acute kidney injury). Serum sodium, glucose, blood urea nitrogen, creatinine, calcium, potassium, serum osmolality, urine osmolality, and urinalysis for glucose and specific gravity should be measured. Serum sodium should be measured to confirm the presence of hypernatremia and to calculate the free water deficit.[1] Urine osmolality and urine specific gravity should be determined to assess if the renal concentrating ability is appropriate, as urine should be maximally concentrated (urine osmolality greater than 800 mOsm/kg H_2O) in the setting of hypernatremia because hyperosmolality results in a maximal stimulus for AVP release.[1,7,19]

If the hypernatremic patient is determined to have polyuria, defined as urine output of greater than 2 L/m^2 per 24-hour (approximately 150 mL/kg per 24-hour at birth, 100 to 110 mL/kg per 24-hour until the age of 2 years, and 40 to 50 mL/kg per 24-hour in the older child and adult), then the patient should be assessed for causes of osmotic diuresis (e.g., glucosuria, uremia, mannitol use). Serum calcium and potassium should also be evaluated as hypercalcemia and hypokalemia can result in acquired nephrogenic DI. Serum and urine creatinine, as well as urine sodium, should be assessed to determine if there is renal failure or inappropriately low or normal urinary sodium.

Serum osmolality and urine osmolality should also be assessed if polyuria is present, with a high serum osmolality (greater than 300 mOsm/kg H_2O) with an inappropriately low urine osmolality (less than 300 mOsm/kg H_2O) being consistent with the diagnosis of DI, though it does not distinguish between nephrogenic and central DI. A low or normal serum osmolality (less than 270 mOsm/kg H_2O), which would not be expected in the setting of hypernatremia, with an appropriately high urine osmolality (greater than 800 mOsm/kg H_2O) may be consistent with primary polydipsia. A serum osmolality between 270 and 300 mOsm/kg H_2O with a urine osmolality less than 800 mOsm/kg H_2O is nondiagnostic, and an indirect water deprivation test may be indicated to differentiate between DI and primary polydipsia, though it has limited diagnostic accuracy, particularly for distinguishing primary polydipsia from partial central DI.[19] A random plasma copeptin may be considered, with a high diagnostic accuracy of a plasma copeptin level greater than 21.4 pmol/L in identifying nephrogenic DI from central DI and primary polydipsia.[20,21] Additionally, two new promising diagnostic tests, the hypertonic saline test and arginine-stimulated copeptin test, both of which utilize stimulated plasma copeptin measurements, have been proposed as alternative diagnostic tests for differentiating central DI and primary polydipsia.[19,22,23] However, these latter tests have not yet been validated in the pediatric population.

Management

The initial step in management of patients with hypernatremia is to determine the volume status. Although isotonic saline is not appropriate for correcting hypernatremia, the exception to this is in the initial management of hypovolemia and replacement with 0.9% saline to improve hemodynamic stability. However, after circulatory stabilization, fluids should then be switched to a hypotonic solution (e.g., oral free water or intravenous 0.45% saline) to continue correction of the free water deficit.[24] The free water deficit is determined as follows:

Free Water Deficit = Body weight in kg × 0.6 × (Measured Na/Ideal Na – 1)

As 60% of body mass is water (50% in female adults and 45% to 50% elderly individuals), multiplying 0.6 times the body weight allows for calculation of total body water.[1] Importantly, the free water deficit is an estimate of the free water deficit with its own limitations (e.g., lack of knowledge of premorbid body weight, estimation of approximately 60% of body mass being water), and serum sodium should be closely monitored during the correction to prevent too rapid a decrease in sodium.[25] Additionally, the free water deficit does not account for ongoing urinary and insensible losses, which should be added amount of fluids to be given.

Once the free water deficit is determined, the next step is to determine the rate to replace the free water deficit. The rate at which the deficit may be safely administered depends on how quickly hypernatremia developed. If the hypernatremia developed within only a few hours, then likely only early cerebral adaptation has occurred, and with correction of hypernatremia, the brain cells can rapidly lose potassium and sodium in response to decreasing serum osmolality. Therefore, correction of hypernatremia may safely be provided more quickly than in chronic hypernatremia. An appropriate correction of acute hypernatremia would be decreasing serum sodium by 1 mEq/L per hour.[1] However, with chronic hypernatremia, loss of accumulated organic osmolytes in brain cells occurs more slowly as hypernatremia is corrected. As fluids are given to correct the hypernatremia, more water is pulled into the brain cells still containing the organic osmolytes, which may result in cell swelling and cerebral edema, with potentially devastating neurologic consequences.[2,17] This development of cerebral edema has been primarily described in children in whom the hypernatremia was corrected at a rate exceeding 0.7 mEq/L per hour. In comparison, no neurologic sequelae were induced if the plasma sodium concentrations were lowered at 0.5 mEq/L per hour. Often it is unclear when the hypernatremia began to develop, in which case a slower correction should be given, as in chronic hypernatremia, for which serum sodium should be lowered by no more than 0.5 mEq/L per hour and no more than by 12 mEq/L per day.[26–28] Additionally, the free water deficit correction does not include urine output and insensible losses, so maintenance fluids should be given in addition to the free water deficit.

The rate of fluids also depends on the choice of fluids given. If the patient is able to tolerate enteral fluids, free water given by mouth or by tube is the preferred method to correct hypernatremia. However, if the hypernatremic patient is unable to tolerate enteral fluids, then the free water deficit correction may be given with hypotonic intravenous fluids (e.g., 0.2% saline or 0.45% saline). If free water by mouth is given, then a free water deficit may be calculated that aims for a goal sodium that is 12 mEq/L or less, then dividing that rate by 24 hours, which would give a rate that is estimated to decrease serum sodium by no more 12 mEq/L in a 24-hour period. If intravenous fluids are given, then a greater volume of fluids would be needed to correct the same free water deficit for increasing concentrations of saline. For example, 0.2% sodium chloride in water is approximately 75% free water, and 0.45% sodium chloride in water is approximately 50% water. Therefore, it would require more 0.45% sodium chloride in water to correct the same free water deficit as compared with 0.2% sodium chloride in water.[7] Importantly, serial serum sodium levels should be assessed to confirm that serum sodium is not decreasing more quickly than expected to allow titration of the free water deficit correction accordingly.

For treatment of central DI desmopressin is given, either as intranasal spray or tablets. Careful monitoring is needed to avoid the complications of water intoxication and hyponatremia, which may be prevented by allowing polyuria and thirst to "breakthrough" approximately once a day, or at least once a week at a minimum. However, in infants central DI is often managed with a low-solute infant formula and a thiazide, though polyuria will persist with this regimen, and desmopressin may become necessary. Management of nephrogenic DI includes removal of precipitating drugs (if possible) and sometimes initiation of thiazide diuretics, or nonsteroidal anti-inflammatory drugs.[2] For patients with a lack of intact thirst mechanism or for young infants, a water prescription may be needed in addition to the aforementioned management.

Prognosis

The morbidity and mortality associated with hypernatremia varies widely according to the severity of the condition, the rapidity of its onset, and the underlying condition resulting in hypernatremia.[1,7,29] Most deaths seem to be independent of the severity of hypernatremia and not directly related to CNS complications. Patients who develop hypernatremia following hospital admission and patients in whom treatment is delayed have the highest mortality.[7,29,30]

References

1. Adrogue HJ, Madias NE. Hypernatremia. *New Engl J Med.* 2000;342(20):1493–1499.
2. Kim SW. Hypernatremia: successful treatment. *Electrolyte and Blood Pressure.* 2006;4:66–71.
3. Weitzman RE, Kleeman CR. The clinical physiology of water metabolism. Part 1: the physiologic regulation of arginine vasopressin secretion and thirst. *West J Med.* 1979;131:373–400.
4. Institute of Medicine of the National Academies. *Water. Dietary Reference Intakes for Water, Sodium, Chloride, Potassium and Sulfate.* Washington, DC: National Academy Press; 2005:73–185.
5. Ball S. Vasopressin and disorders of water balance: the physiology and pathophysiology of vasopressin. *Ann Clin Biochem.* 2007;44:417–431.
6. Danziger J, Hoenig MP. The role of the kidney in disorders of volume: core curriculum 2016. *Am J Kidney Dis.* 2016;68(5):808–816.
7. Moritz ML, Ayus JC. Disorders of water metabolism in children: hyponatremia and hypernatremia. *Pediatrics in Review.* 2002;23(11).
8. Fitzgerald KC, Williams LS, Garg BP, Carvalho KS, Golomb MR. Cerebral sinovenous thrombosis in the neonate. *Arch Neurol.* 2006;63(3):405–409.
9. Gebara BM, Everett KO. Dural sinus thrombosis complicating hypernatremic dehydration in a breastfed neonate. *Clinical Pediatrics.* 2001;40:45–48.
10. Hbibi M, Abourazzak S, Babakhouya A, et al. Severe hypernatremic dehydration associated with cerebral venous and aortic thrombosis in the neonatal period. *BMJ Case Reports.* 2012;2012.
11. Iyer NP, Srinivasan R, Evans K, Ward L, Cheung W-Y, Matthes JWA. Impact of an early weighing policy on neonatal hypernatraemic dehydration and breast feeding. *Arch Dis Child.* 2008;93:297–299.
12. Lindner G, Funk G. Hypernatremia in critically ill patients. *J Critical Care.* 2013;28:216e11–216e20.
13. Gregoire JR. Adjustment of osmostat in primary aldosteronism. *Mayo Clin Proc.* 1994;69(11):1108–1110.
14. Morris-Jones PH, Houston IB. Prognosis of the neurological complications of acute hypernatremia. *Lancet.* 1967;2:1385–1389.
15. Finberg L, Kiley J, Luttrell CN. Mass accidental salt poisoning in infancy. *JAMA.* 1963;184(3):187–190.
16. Sterns RH. Disorders of plasma sodium—causes, consequences, and correction. *New Engl J Med.* 2015; 372:55–65.
17. Strange K. Regulation of solute and water balance and cell volume in the central nervous system. *J Am Soc Nephrol.* 1992;3(1):12–27.

18. McDowell ME, Wolf AV, Steer A. Osmotic volumes of distribution. *American Journal of Physiology-Legacy Content.* 1955;180(3):545–558.
19. Christ-Crain M, Bichet DG, Fenske WK, et al. Diabetes insipidus. *Nat Rev Dis Primers.* 2019;5(1):54.
20. Fenske W, Quinkler M, Lorenz D, et al. Copeptin in the differential diagnosis of the polydipsia-polyuria syndrome—revisiting the direct and indirect water deprivation tests. *J Clin Endocrinol Metab.* 2011;96(5):1506–1515.
21. Timper K, Fenske W, Kühn F, et al. Diagnostic accuracy of copeptin in the differential diagnosis of the polyuria-polydipsia syndrome: a prospective multicenter study. *J Clin Endocrinol Metab.* 2015;100(6):2268–2274.
22. Fenske W, Refardt J, Chifu I, et al. A copeptin-based approach in the diagnosis of diabetes insipidus. *New Engl J Med.* 2018;379:428–439.
23. Winzeler B, Cesana-Nigro N, Refardt J, et al. Arginine-stimulated copeptin measurements in the differential diagnosis of diabetes insipidus: a prospective diagnostic study. *Lancet.* 2019;394(10198):587–595.
24. Lin M, Liu SJ, Lim IT. Disorders of water imbalance. *Emerg Med Clin North Am.* 2005;23(3):749–770 ix.
25. Cheuvront SN, Kenefick RW, Sollanek KJ, Ely BR, Sawka MN. Water-deficit equation: systematic analysis and improvement. *Am J Clin Nutr.* 2013;97(1):79–85.
26. Blum D, Brasseur D, Kahn A, Brachet E. Safe oral rehydration of hypertonic dehydration. *J Pediatr Gastroenterol Nutr.* 1986;5(2):232–235.
27. Kahn A, Blum D, Casimir G, Brachet E. Controlled fall in natremia in hypertonic dehydration: possible avoidance of rehydration seizures. *Eur J Pediatr.* 1981;135(3):293–296.
28. Kahn A, Brachet E, Blum D. Controlled fall in natremia and risk of seizures in hypertonic dehydration. *Intensive Care Med.* 1979;5(1):27–31.
29. Bataille S, Baralla C, Torro D, et al. Undercorrection of hypernatremia is frequent and associated with mortality. *BMC Nephrology.* 2014;15(1):37.
30. Arampatzis S, Frauchiger B, Fiedler GM, et al. Characteristics, symptoms, and outcome of severe dysnatremias present on hospital admission. *Am J Med.* 2012;125(11):1125e1–1125e7.

CHAPTER 20

Hypopituitarism

Sara E. Lubitz

CHAPTER OUTLINE

Introduction

Hypothalamic stimulatory and inhibitory hormones traverse the hypophyseal-portal circulation to target specific cells of the pituitary gland. The pituitary cells synthesize and secrete trophic hormones, which target organs to secrete hormones, which then affect peripheral tissues (Figs. 20.1 and 20.2). Hypopituitarism, also known as pituitary insufficiency, refers to one or more pituitary deficiencies caused by pituitary or hypothalamic disease.

Hypopituitarism can be congenital or acquired and transient or permanent. The clinical manifestations may vary depending on the severity of the hormone deficit. In most scenarios, the secretion of gonadotropins and growth hormone (GH) is more likely to be affected than adrenocorticotropic hormone (ACTH) and thyroid-stimulating hormone (TSH), but isolated deficiencies of any hormone can occur. Posterior pituitary insufficiency, characterized by decreased

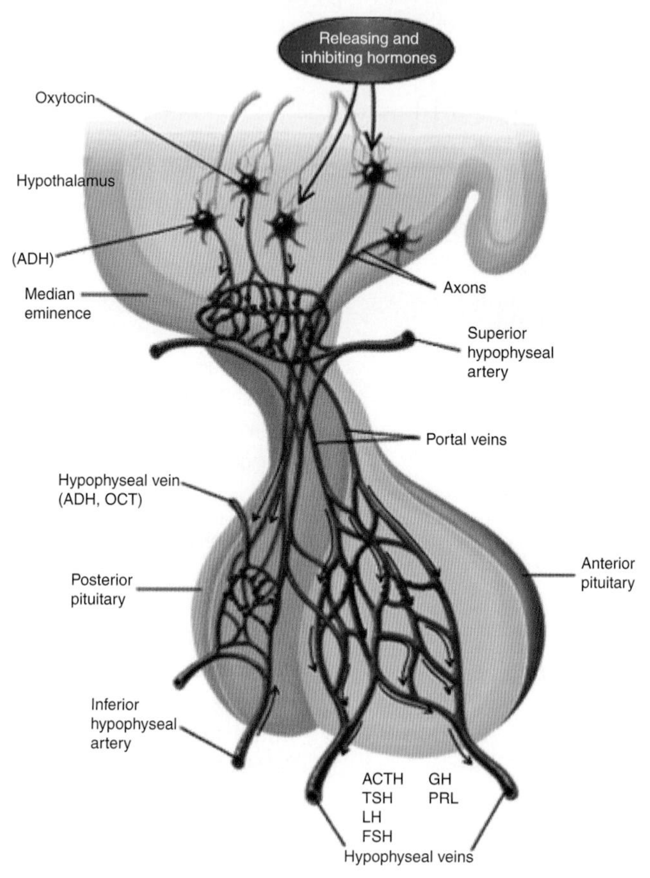

Fig. 20.1 Hypothalamic regulation of anterior pituitary function. (From Anat B-S, Melmed S. Hypothalamic regulation of anterior pituitary function. In: Melmed S, ed. *The Pituitary*, 4th ed. Academic Press, 2017. Adapted from Melmed S. Pituitary. In Dale DC, Federman DD, eds. *ACP Medicine*, vol. 1. 2006, 571–586.)

circulating antidiuretic hormone (ADH), leading to central diabetes insipidus (DI), will be discussed in Chapter 19.

EPIDEMIOLOGY

The prevalence of hypopituitarism is approximately 450 cases per million with an incidence of about 40 new cases per million per year.[1,2] There is high mortality associated with hypopituitarism.[3–5]

ETIOLOGIES

Hypopituitarism can be congenital or acquired and can arise from structural or functional disruption of the hypothalamus, portal system, or pituitary gland (Table 20.1). Patients with hypothalamic or pituitary masses, developmental craniofacial abnormalities, inflammatory disorders, neuro-granulomatous disease, head trauma, prior brain irradiation, or prior skull base surgery, and

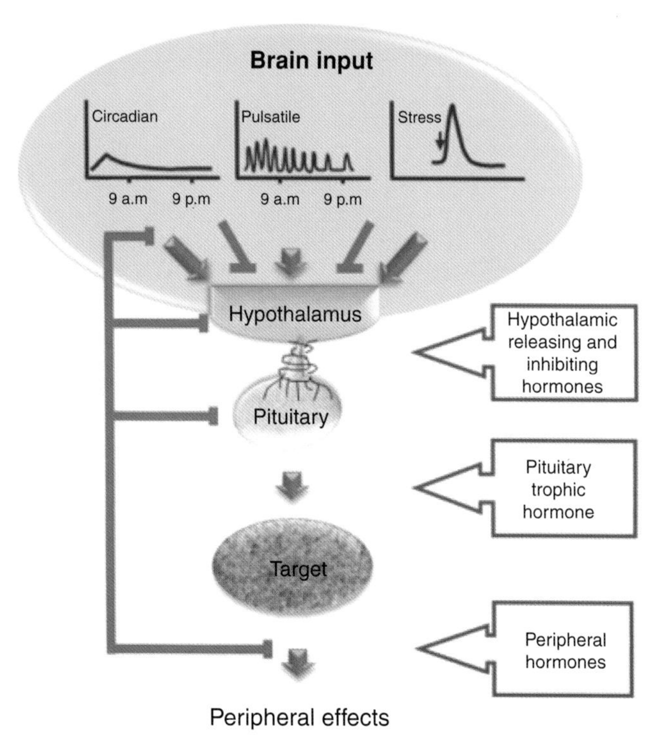

Fig. 20.2 The hypothalamic-pituitary axes. (From Anat B-S, Melmed S. Hypothalamic regulation of anterior pituitary function. In: Melmed S, ed. *The Pituitary*, ed 4. Academic Press, 2017.)

those who have previously experienced pregnancy-associated hemorrhage, should be screened for hypopituitarism.

DIAGNOSIS

The diagnosis of hypopituitarism relies on the measurement of basal and stimulated secretion of anterior pituitary hormones and the hormones secreted by the target glands. Magnetic resonance imaging (MRI) of the hypothalamus and pituitary with and without gadolinium contrast is the imaging test of choice. Genetic testing may be indicated in congenital or syndromic disease.[2]

Central Adrenal Insufficiency

INTRODUCTION

Hypothalamic corticotropin-releasing hormone (CRH) stimulates ACTH secretion by pituitary corticotroph cells. ACTH stimulates cortisol synthesis and secretion from the adrenal gland. ACTH is secreted in a pulsatile manner and follows a circadian rhythm, reaching peak levels in the early morning and nadirs around midnight. Cortisol exerts negative feedback inhibition on pituitary ACTH and hypothalamic CRH secretion (Fig. 20.3). Central adrenal insufficiency (AI) occurs when there is loss of hypothalamic CRH (tertiary adrenal insufficiency)

TABLE 20.1 ■ **Causes of Hypopituitarism**

Neoplastic
Pituitary adenoma or carcinoma
Metastatic disease
Craniopharyngioma
Lymphoma
Parasellar masses (meningioma, germinoma, glioma)
Traumatic
Surgery
Radiation
Traumatic brain injury
Vascular
Sheehan's syndrome
Apoplexy
Carotid aneurysm
Subarachnoid hemorrhage
Infiltrative/Inflammatory
Hypophysitis
Sarcoidosis
Wegner granulomatosis
Histiocytosis X
Hemochromatosis
Infectious
Bacterial infections
Fungal infections
Parasitic infections
Congenital
Mutations of *PROP1, HESX1, LHX3, LHX4, POU1F1, POMC, TPIT*
Drug-Induced
Glucocorticoids
Opiates
Bexarotine

or pituitary release of ACTH (secondary adrenal insufficiency). The most common cause of central AI is iatrogenic due to suppression of the hypothalamic-pituitary-adrenal (HPA) axis after glucocorticoid administration.

Acute adrenal insufficiency is a life-threatening emergency presenting with hypotension or hypovolemic shock. It can occur abruptly (e.g., pituitary apoplexy) or insidiously during times of physical stress in previously undiagnosed patients or those with known AI who fail to properly increase their replacement doses.

CLINICAL PRESENTATION

Central AI results in decreased secretion of cortisol and adrenal androgens. It can present with lethargy, weakness, nausea, vomiting, and hypotension. Signs of mineralocorticoid deficiency

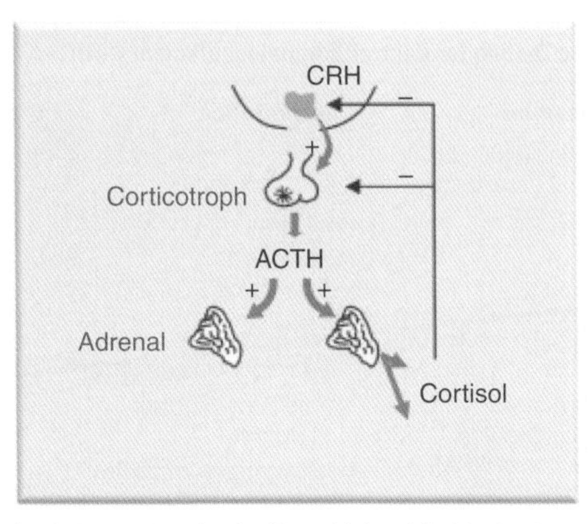

Fig. 20.3 The hypothalamic-pituitary-adrenal axis. (From Melmed S. Mechanisms for pituitary tumorigenesis: the plastic pituitary. *J Clin Invest*. 2003;112:1603–1618.)

(salt craving, hyperkalemia) are not present, as adrenal mineralocorticoid secretion is preserved. Hyponatremia can occur secondary to inappropriate secretion of ADH resulting from glucocorticoid deficiency (Box 20.1).

DIAGNOSTIC EVALUATION

We are unable to routinely measure CRH, and ACTH measurements are not very reliable because of the short plasma half-life, pulsatile secretion, and rigorous specimen handling requirements. Therefore we rely on cortisol testing for the diagnosis of adrenal insufficiency. However, due to the circadian changes in cortisol, a random cortisol level is not helpful. The first-line test for diagnosing central AI is measuring serum cortisol levels at 8:00 to 9:00 a.m. A cortisol level less than 3 g/dL is indicative of AI and a cortisol level greater than 15 g/dL likely excludes an AI diagnosis. For morning cortisol levels between 3 and 15 g/dL, stimulation testing is recommended.[1] Central AI can be diagnosed using insulin tolerance and the low-dose and standard-dose ACTH stimulation tests. The standard-dose test using 250 μg cosyntropin (synthetic ACTH 1-24) administered intravenously or intramuscularly is recommended. Peak cortisol levels less than 18.1 g/dL at 30 or 60 minutes indicate AI.[1] With the use of new cortisol assays using more specific monoclonal antibody immunoassays or liquid chromatography with tandem mass spectrometry (LC-MS/MS),

BOX 20.1 ■ Symptoms and Signs of Central Adrenal Insufficiency

Fatigue	Anorexia
Weight loss	Nausea
Vomiting	Muscle and joint pain
Dizziness	Hypotension
Fever	Abdominal pain
Hyponatremia	Blood count abnormalities (anemia, lymphocytosis, eosinophilia)
Hypoglycemia	Hypercalcemia

TABLE 20.2 ■ **Diagnostic Testing for Central Adrenal Insufficiency (AI)**

Test	Procedure	Interpretation	Comments
Serum cortisol	Morning (8:00–9:00 a.m.) basal testing	Normal: serum cortisol level >15 µg/dL Insufficient: <3 µg/dL Indeterminate: 3–15 µg/dL	Assumes normal CBG
Insulin tolerance test	Administer insulin (0.05–0.15 U/kg IV) Serum measurements of cortisol and glucose at 0, 30, 60 min	Blood glucose <40 mg/dL required for interpretation Normal: peak cortisol >18 µg/dL Insufficient: serum cortisol level <18 µg/dL	Symptomatic hypoglycemia contraindicated in elderly patients, those with seizure disorders, and cardiac disease Cortisol cut-off may be lower depending on assay
ACTH stimulation test (standard dose)	Administer synthetic ACTH 1-24 250 µg IV or IM Serum measurements of cortisol at 0, 30, 60 min	Normal: serum cortisol level <18 µg/dL Insufficient: serum cortisol level <18 µg/dL	Cortisol cut-off may be lower depending on assay False negative results in acute central AI

ACTH, Adrenocorticotropic hormone; *CBG,* cortisol-binding globulin; *IM,* intramuscular; *IV,* intravenous.

a lower cut-off for a normal response to ACTH testing of greater than 14.5 µg/dL has been proposed.[6] Furthermore, cortisol cut-offs for provocative testing are based on total cortisol levels and assume normal cortisol-binding globulin (CBG). Albumin is often used as a surrogate for CBG and lower cut-offs for normal cortisol response to ACTH testing or use of free cortisol levels may be considered in patients with low albumin.[7] Exogenous glucocorticoids should be withheld 18 to 24 hours prior to testing (Table 20.2).

MANAGEMENT

Central AI can lead to adrenal crisis, which is a life-threating emergency. Adrenal crisis occurs when the HPA axis cannot produce sufficient cortisol in response to an increased need (Box 20.2). Patients should be treated with aggressive hydration and stress-doses of glucocorticoids. For suspected adrenal crisis due to secondary AI, treat with an immediate parenteral injection of 50 to 100 mg hydrocortisone followed by 200 mg/day for the next

BOX 20.2 ■ Causes of Adrenal Crisis in Central Adrenal Insufficiency (AI)

- Acute stress in patient with known central AI
- Pituitary infarction/apoplexy
- After surgical cure of Cushing's syndrome
- Abrupt withdrawal of exogenous glucocorticoids

TABLE 20.3 ■ **Glucocorticoid Replacement Therapy**

Formulation	Dosing	Comments
Hydrocortisone	15–20 mg/day	Two or three times daily Potential for small dose adjustments
Prednisolone/Prednisone	2.5–7.5 mg/day	Long-acting physiologic effect Risk of overtreatment
Dexamethasone	0.25–0.75 mg/day	Long-acting physiologic effect Variable metabolism Risk of overtreatment

24 hours. The dose should be reduced to hydrocortisone 100 mg/day in divided doses the following day.[1] If the patient is improving, and without illness or planned-for invasive procedures, the goal should be to taper down to physiologic doses of glucocorticoids within 3 days.

For long-term treatment of central AI, hormonal replacement should try to mimic the physiologic cortisol pattern. Hydrocortisone 15 to 20 mg total daily dose should be given in divided doses two to three times a day. Patients should take the highest dose in the morning upon awakening, and the second in the afternoon (two-dose regimen) or the second and third at lunch and late afternoon, respectively (three-dose regimen).[1] Longer-acting glucocorticoids such as prednisone or prednisolone 2.5 to 7.5 mg/day or dexamethasone 0.25 to 0.75 mg/day may be used in selected patients for improved compliance or convenience (Table 20.3). Retrospective studies of patients taking higher doses and longer-acting glucocorticoids show a tendency toward adverse metabolic consequences including weight gain, dyslipidemia, and type 2 diabetes mellitus.[8] Slow-release preparations of hydrocortisone and hydrocortisone infusion pumps are in clinical development. Glucocorticoid dosing should be adjusted based on clinical symptoms, side effects, and comorbidities.

Because AI may mask the presence of partial DI, patients should be monitored for the development of DI after starting glucocorticoid replacement.

Once diagnosed with central AI, patient education is considered the key to preventing adrenal crisis. Patients should receive detailed information on their disease and learn how to self-adjust glucocorticoids during times of stress or illness (Table 20.4). Patients should carry an emergency card, bracelet, or necklace, and injectable glucocorticoids for emergency administration.[9]

Central Hypothyroidism

INTRODUCTION

Hypothalamic thyrotropin-releasing hormone (TRH) stimulates TSH secretion by pituitary thyrotroph cells. TSH binds to receptors on the thyroid gland and activates adenylyl cyclases, stimulates iodine uptake, and leads to the synthesis and secretion of thyroid hormones thyroxine (T4) and triiodothyroinine (T3). T4 and T3 exert negative feedback inhibition on pituitary TSH and hypothalamic TRH secretion (Fig. 20.4). Central hypothyroidism occurs when there is loss of hypothalamic TRH (tertiary hypothyroidism) or pituitary production and release of TSH (secondary hypothyroidism).

TABLE 20.4 ■ **Stress-Dosing Glucocorticoids**

Scenario	Change to Maintenance Dose
Febrile illness	Double or triple dose for 3 days
Minor trauma	Double or triple dose for 2–3 days
Minor surgical procedures	Double or triple dose for the day of surgery
Moderate surgical procedures	Doses equivalent to hydrocortisone 50–75 mg in divided doses for the day of surgery and the first postoperative day, with a return to the usual dose on the second postoperative day
Major surgical procedures	Doses equivalent to hydrocortisone 100–150 mg in divided doses for the day of surgery and the next 2–3 days, then return to the usual dose
Critical illness	Doses equivalent to hydrocortisone 200–300 mg/day in divided doses for 3–7 days, with tapered withdrawal guided by clinical response
Major trauma	Doses equivalent to hydrocortisone 100–150 mg in divided doses for the day of trauma and the next 2–3 days, then return to the usual dose

CLINICAL PRESENTATION

Central hypothyroidism can present with lethargy, constipation, cold intolerance, bradycardia, weight gain, and hyponatremia. The presentation is variable, with some patients being asymptomatic and others having profound symptoms of hypothyroidism (Box 20.3).

DIAGNOSTIC EVALUATION

Hypothalamic TRH testing is not readily available and TSH can be low, normal, or even elevated in central hypothyroidism. It is recommended to measure serum free T4 and TSH to evaluate

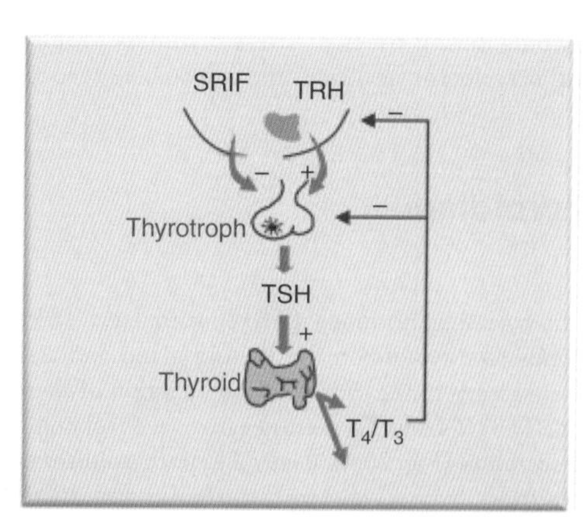

Fig. 20.4 The hypothalamic-pituitary-thyroid axis. (From Melmed S. Mechanisms for pituitary tumorigenesis: the plastic pituitary. *J Clin Invest*. 2003;112:1603–1618.)

BOX 20.3 ■ Symptoms and Signs of Central Hypothyroidism

Lethargy	Constipation
Cold intolerance	Bradycardia
Weight gain	Dry skin
Brittle hair	Delayed reflex relaxation time
Anemia	Hyponatremia
Thinning of the lateral eyebrows	Hyperlipidemia

central hypothyroidism. A free T4 level below the laboratory reference range in conjunction with a low, normal, or mildly elevated TSH in the setting of pituitary disease is consistent with a central hypothyroidism diagnosis.[1] Measurement of serum T3 is not helpful because it is often within the normal range even in patients with hypopituitarism.[2] One must use caution in diagnosing central hypothyroidism in a patient who is severely ill and could have nonthyroidal illness–induced changes in thyroid hormone levels.[1]

MANAGEMENT

Central hypothyroidism is treated with levothyroxine (L-T4). The dose can be calculated as 1.6 g/kg per day L-T4 and adjusted to achieve serum free T4 levels in the mid to upper half of the reference range.[1] TSH levels should not be used to adjust thyroid replacement dosing in patients with central hypothyroidism; almost all central hypothyroidism patients adequately treated with L-T4 will have undetectable TSH levels.[1,10,11]

Overtreatment with thyroid hormone can have adverse effects on the cardiovascular system and bone mineral density, which may already be compromised in patients with coexisting hypogonadism and GH deficiency.[2] Replacement of thyroid hormone should be done after assessment for adrenal insufficiency, as replacement of thyroid hormone without replacement of glucocorticoids can precipitate acute adrenal insufficiency.

Central Hypogonadism

INTRODUCTION

Hypothalamic gonadotropin-releasing hormone (GnRH) is secreted in a pulsatile manner and stimulates the pituitary gland to secrete follicle-stimulating hormone (FSH) and luteinizing hormone (LH) in a pulsatile manner. Feedback inhibition is regulated by the gonadal steroids estrogen and testosterone, and peptides inhibin and activin (Fig. 20.5). Gonadal steroids exert both positive and negative feedback on gonadotroph secretion. FSH stimulates Sertoli cell spermatogenesis in men and follicular development in women. In women, the ovulatory LH surge results in rupture of the follicle and then luteinization. LH stimulates the production of progesterone and estradiol by the luteinized follicle. In men, the primary role of LH is to stimulate testosterone synthesis by Leydig cells. Testosterone levels follow a circadian rhythm with peak serum values between 6:00 and 8:00 a.m. and trough levels in the evening.

Central hypogonadism, also called hypogonadotropic hypogonadism, occurs when there is loss of hypothalamic GnRH secretion or pulsatility or loss of pituitary LH and FSH pulsatile secretion. Elevated prolactin can also lead to central hypogonadism by interfering with GnRH pulse generation in the hypothalamus causing decreased gonadotropin secretion and a reduction in sex steroids.

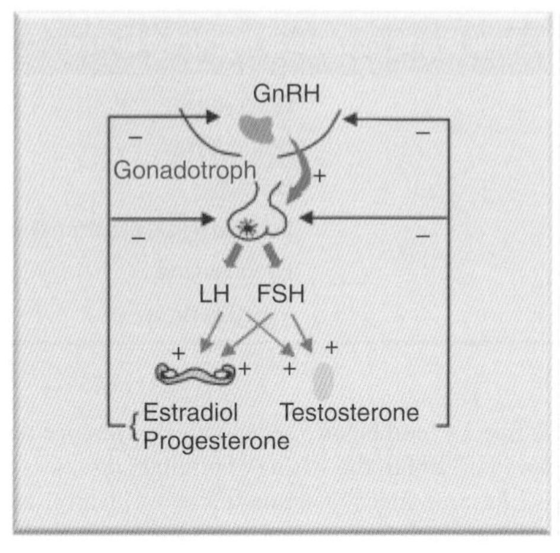

Fig. 20.5 The hypothalamic-pituitary-gonadal axis. (From Melmed S. Mechanisms for pituitary tumorigenesis: the plastic pituitary. *J Clin Invest*. 2003;112:1603–1618.)

CLINICAL PRESENTATION

Central hypogonadism in men presents with features of testosterone deficiency and/or impaired spermatogenesis (Box 20.4). Premenopausal women present with low estrogen and oligomenorrhea or amenorrhea (Box 20.5).

DIAGNOSTIC EVALUATION

LH and FSH levels vary with age and with the menstrual cycle in women. During the follicular phase of the menstrual cycle, LH levels rise steadily with a mid-cycle surge that stimulates ovulation. LH rises during the early follicular phase, falls in the late follicular phase, and peaks at mid-cycle. Both LH and FSH levels fall after ovulation (Fig. 20.6). Male FSH and LH levels are pulsatile but fluctuate less than those in women. Gonadotropin deficiency is best diagnosed by concurrent measurement of serum gonadotropins and gonadal steroids. Testing for central hypogonadism should be done in the absence of acute/subacute illness and combined with serum prolactin levels.[1]

Male central hypogonadism is diagnosed with low or normal FSH and LH in the setting of low, fasting, morning total testosterone levels. The diagnosis should be confirmed by repeating

BOX 20.4 ■ Symptoms and Signs of Hypogonadotropic Hypogonadism in Men

Testicular atrophy	Decreased libido
Erectile dysfunction	Osteoporosis
Gynecomastia	Loss of body hair
Small testes	Infertility
Anemia	Depressed mood
Fatigue	Decreased exercise capacity
Hypertension	Decreased lean body mass
Increased fat mass	

BOX 20.5 ■ Symptoms and Signs of Hypogonadotropic Hypogonadism in Women

Secondary amenorrhea	Osteoporosis
Decreased libido	Hot flashes
Night sweats	Vaginal atrophy

measurement of total testosterone. Measurement of free or bioavailable testosterone, using an accurate and reliable assay, is recommended for men in whom total testosterone concentrations are near the lower limit of normal range and in whom alterations of sex hormone–binding globulin (SHBG) are suspected.[12]

Females having regular menstrual cycles are unlikely to have central hypogonadism. Central hypogonadism in females can be diagnosed in the setting of low or normal FSH and LH levels

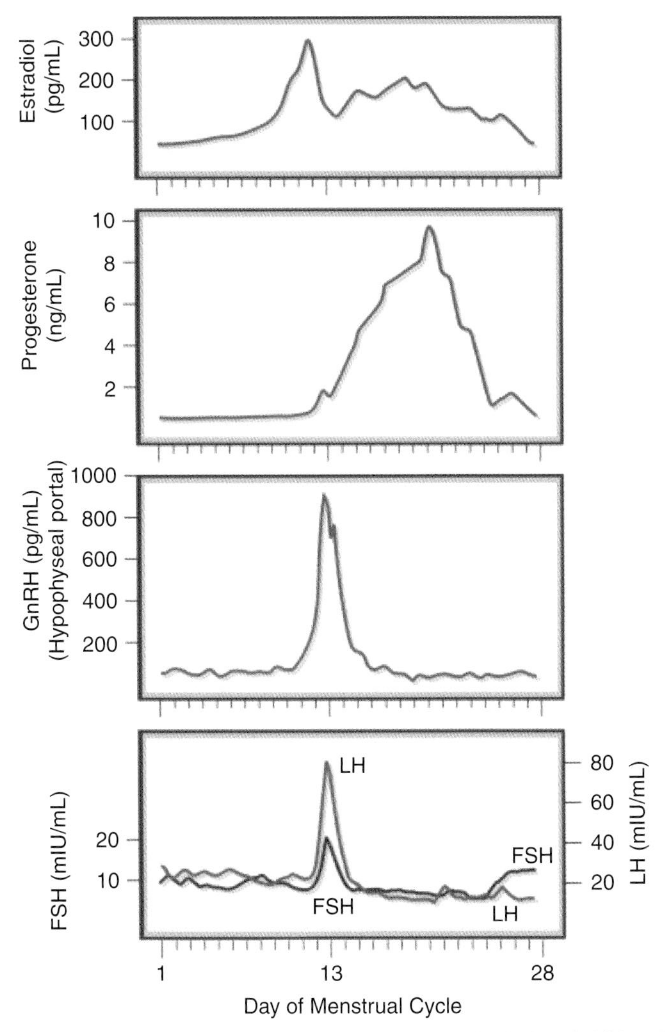

Fig. 20.6 Regulation of the ovarian cycle. (From Lechan RM. Neuroendocrinology. In Melmed S, Auchus RJ, Goldfine AB, Koenig RJ, Rosen CJ, eds. *Williams Textbook of Endocrinology*, 14th ed. Elsevier, Inc. 2020.)

TABLE 20.5 ■ **Testosterone Replacement Therapy**

Formulation	Dosing	Comments
Injection	75–100 mg of testosterone enanthate or cypionate administered SQ or IM weekly, or 150–200 mg administered IM every 2 weeks	Levels peak and nadir in between doses
Patch	2–4 mg testosterone patches applied daily over the skin of the back, abdomen, arms, or thighs	Delivers consistent levels Skin irritation and rash
Gel	20.25–100 mg of testosterone gel applied daily over the shoulders or arms	Delivers consistent levels Potential for transfer to another individual
Buccal	30 mg of a bioadhesive buccal testosterone tablet applied to buccal mucosa every 12 hours	Gum irritation
Nasal	11 mg of testosterone applied intranasally three times a day	Nasal and sinus symptoms
Pellets	150–450 mg testosterone implanted SQ at intervals of 3 to 6 months	Requires implantation by a health care provider Less flexible for dosage adjustment

IM, Intramuscular; *SQ,* subcutaneous.

in the presence of low estradiol. These findings are even more suggestive in a postmenopausal female who would be expected to have high FSH and LH levels in the presence of low estradiol.

MANAGEMENT

Untreated gonadotropin deficiency in both men and women is an independent risk factor affecting cardiovascular mortality; sex steroid replacement has been associated with significantly reduced standard mortality ratios.[5,13]

Testosterone replacement is recommended for adult males with central hypogonadism and no contraindications. The choice of testosterone replacement therapy depends on the risk of specific adverse effects, cost, patient convenience, and patient preferences (Table 20.5).[1] Doses are adjusted to keep serum testosterone levels in the normal range. Patients should be monitored with testosterone and hematocrit levels at 3 to 6 months, 12 months after starting testosterone therapy, and then annually thereafter. Prostate-specific antigen and digital rectal exam should be monitored in at-risk patients who agree to prostate cancer monitoring prior to starting testosterone therapy, and at 3 and 12 months after initiation of hormone replacement and then as per guidelines for prostate cancer screening. Exogenous testosterone therapy may suppress spermatogenesis, and should not be used in a man desiring fertility.[14] Fertility can be induced with use of gonadotropins; hCG is a long-acting LH analogue that stimulates the testes to produce testosterone and undergo spermatogenesis.

Gonadal hormone treatment is recommended in premenopausal women with central hypogonadism, provided there are no contraindications. Combined estrogen and progesterone hormone replacement is used for women with an intact uterus to prevent endometrial hyperplasia, and unopposed estrogens are used for women who have undergone hysterectomy. The choice of the estrogen and progestin preparation depends on the risk of adverse effects, cost, patient convenience, and

TABLE 20.6 ■ **Estrogen and Progestin Replacement Therapy**

Hormone	Formulation	Dosing	Comments
Estrogen and Progestin	Oral Synthetic Estrogen-Progestin Combination (oral contraceptive pill)	Ethinyl estradiol/progestin daily tablet	Pharmacologic rather than physiologic doses Hepatic first-pass effect
Estrogen and Progestin	Oral Estrogen-Progestin Combination	0.5 mg estradiol/0.1 mg norethindrone acetate or 1 mg estradiol/0.5 mg norethindrone acetate	Hepatic first-pass effect
Estrogen and Progestin	Combination Patch	0.05 mg estradiol/0.14–0.25 mg norethindrone per day patch applied twice a week 0.045 mg estradiol/0.015 mg levonorgestrel per day patch applied once a week	Skin irritation and rash
Estrogen	Oral 17-beta estradiol	0.5–2 mg daily estradiol tablet	Hepatic first-pass effect
Estrogen	Patch 17-beta estradiol	0.05–0.1 mg estradiol patch applied once or twice a week	Skin irritation and rash
Estrogen	Vaginal 17-beta estradiol	0.05–0.1 mg estradiol/day vaginal ring applied every 3 months	
Progestin	Oral Micronized Progesterone	200 mg for 12 days every month or 100 mg daily	Peanut allergy
Progestin	Oral Medroxyprogesterone	5–10 mg for 10–14 days every month	

patient preference (Table 20.6). Transdermal estrogen is preferred in patients with hypopituitarism because oral estrogen administration has first-pass effects increasing the hepatic production of binding globulins, triglycerides, high-density lipoprotein, and clotting factors, whereas their production is only minimally increased by transdermal estrogen administration.[15]

It is recommended that women continue hormone replacement therapy until they reach menopausal age (~50 years of age). There are no studies on premenopausal women with central hypogonadism; therefore, published results from women with primary hypogonadism in which treatment prevents decreased bone mineral density, fractures, and cardiovascular mortality are often extrapolated to this group of female patients.[1] Fertility can be achieved in females with hypogonadotropic hypogonadism using pulsatile GnRH administration or gonadotropin analogues to induce ovulation.

Growth Hormone Deficiency

INTRODUCTION

Hypothalamic growth hormone–releasing hormone (GHRH) is secreted in a pulsatile manner and stimulates the pituitary gland to secrete growth hormone. GH is produced and secreted in

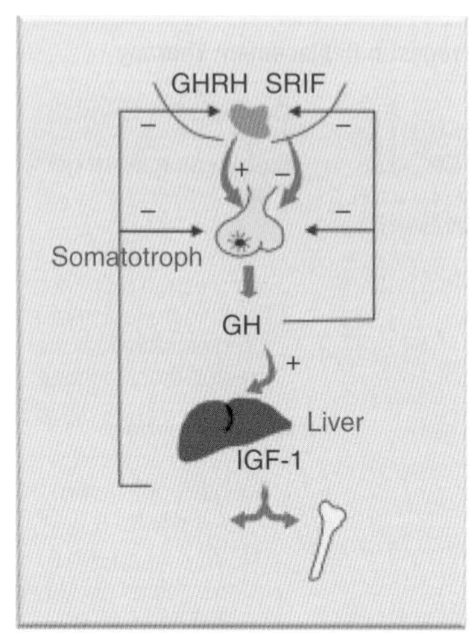

Fig. 20.7 The hypothalamic-pituitary-somatotropic axis. (From Melmed S. Mechanisms for pituitary tumorigenesis: the plastic pituitary. *J Clin Invest*. 2003;112:1603–1618.)

a pulsatile fashion under positive control of GHRH. Secretion is inhibited by somatostatin and negative feedback from GH and insulin-like growth factor 1 (IGF-1). GH stimulates IGF-1 production from the liver, controls release of fatty acids from adipose tissue, and directly works on cartilage cells in the growth plates of long bones (Fig. 20.7). IGF-1 is the major mediator of GH-stimulated somatic growth and has insulin-like effects. There is a physiologic decline in the GHRH-GH-IGF-1 axis with aging. Growth hormone deficiency occurs when there is loss of hypothalamic GHRH or pituitary release of GH.

CLINICAL PRESENTATION

Clinical features of adult GH deficiency are often subtle and may mimic metabolic syndrome or depression. GH deficiency is associated with adverse changes in body composition, muscle strength, quality of life, cardiovascular risk factors, and bone density[16] (Box 20.6).

DIAGNOSTIC EVALUATION

GH is secreted in a pulsatile manner and varies with nutritional status, exercise, sleep, weight, and age, and therefore random GH levels are not helpful for diagnosing GH deficiency. IGF-1 levels are more stable with a circulating half-life of 24 to 30 hours and age-adjusted values measured in

BOX 20.6 ■ Symptoms and Signs of Growth Hormone Deficiency

Fatigue	Decreased exercise capacity
Hypertension	Decreased lean body mass
Increased fat mass	Decreased bone mass
Hyperlipidemia	Insulin resistance
Impaired cardiac function	Depressed mood

TABLE 20.7 ■ **Diagnostic Testing for Growth Hormone (GH) Deficiency**

Test	Procedure	Interpretation	Comments
Serum insulin-like growth factor 1 (IGF-1)	Basal testing	Normal: serum IGF-1 within the age- and gender-adjusted normal range	Stimulation testing required for diagnosis of GH deficiency except persons with low IGF-1 and 3 or more additional pituitary deficits
Insulin tolerance test	Administer insulin 0.05–0.15 U/kg IV Serum measurements of GH and glucose at 0, 30, 60 min	Blood glucose <40 mg/dL required for interpretation Normal: peak GH response >5.1 µg/L Insufficiency: peak GH <5.1 µg/L	Symptomatic hypoglycemia contraindicated in elderly patients, those with seizure disorders, and cardiac disease
Glucagon stimulation test	Administer glucagon 1 mg IM; 1.5 mg IM if weight >90 kg Serum measurement of GH and glucose at 0, 30, 60, 90, 120, 150, 180, 210, and 240 min	Normal: peak GH >3 µg/L Insufficient: BMI <30: peak GH <3 µg/L BMI >30: peak GH <1 µg/L	Less accurate in patients with glucose intolerance
Macimorelin stimulation test	Administer Macimorelin 0.5 mg/kg orally after fasting Serum measurement of GH at 0, 30, 45, 60, 90 min.	Normal: peak GH >2.8 ng/mL	False-positive test results in patients using strong CYP3A4 inducers

BMI, Body mass index; *CYP3A4;* cytochrome P450 3A4; *IM,* intramuscular.

an accredited laboratory are a good screening test for GH deficiency. Growth hormone stimulation tests should be performed to confirm the diagnosis (Table 20.7).

Patients previously diagnosed with childhood GH deficiency should be retested as adults, as many of these patients prove to be GH sufficient on repeat testing.[1] Patients with low serum IGF-1 levels and clear-cut features of GH deficiency in the setting of known hypothalamic-pituitary disease and three other documented pituitary hormone deficiencies do not need to undergo stimulation testing for diagnosis.[1,17] Replacement of thyroid hormone and glucocorticoids should be done prior to testing for GH deficiency.

More recently, nontumoral causes of adult GH deficiency (e.g., traumatic brain injury [TBI], subarachnoid hemorrhage, ischemic stroke, and central nervous system infections) have been reported. However, the accuracy and reliability of GH stimulation tests have not been adequately studied in these populations.[17]

MANAGEMENT

GH replacement in patients with adult growth hormone deficiency improves lipoprotein metabolism, body composition, bone mineral density, and quality of life, but it remains unclear if there is a reduction in overall mortality.[1] GH replacement is available as a daily injection, and longer-acting preparations are in development. Dosing should be started at 0.2 to 0.4 mg/day for most patients and 0.1 to 0.2 mg/day for older patients and varied based on age-adjusted IGF-1 levels and symptoms. Initial low GH replacement doses are preferred because the side effect of fluid retention is dose dependent. Women on estrogen therapy and obese patients may require higher doses.[1]

Prolactin Deficiency

Prolactin deficiency is rare and seen in patients with hypothalamic-pituitary disease at presentation or after surgical and radiation treatment. It presents with the inability to lactate and may suggest global deficiency of pituitary hormones. However, many cases of hypopituitarism are associated with hyperprolactinemia that occurs due to pituitary stalk interruption.

Interactions Between Hormones

GLUCOCORTICOIDS AND THYROID HORMONE

Replacement of thyroid hormone without replacement of glucocorticoids can precipitate acute adrenal insufficiency. Patients with hypothyroidism should be evaluated for AI prior to initiating L-T4 therapy. If the diagnosis of AI cannot be excluded, patients should be started on empiric glucocorticoid therapy simultaneous with L-T4 therapy until a definitive diagnosis can be made.

GLUCOCORTICOIDS AND ESTROGEN

Oral estrogen therapy increases cortisol-binding globulin, leading to increased total cortisol levels.

GLUCOCORTICOIDS AND GROWTH HORMONE

GH suppresses the conversion of inactive cortisone to cortisol. Patients with partial or total ACTH deficiency who are receiving suboptimal glucocorticoid replacement may be at risk of developing AI when GH therapy is initiated.

GLUCOCORTICOIDS AND VASOPRESSIN

AI may mask the presence of partial diabetes insipidus. Patients should be monitored for DI after starting glucocorticoid replacement. Patients with unexplained improved DI should undergo testing for AI.[1]

THYROID HORMONE AND GROWTH HORMONE

Hypothyroidism alters GH and IGF-1 secretion. Hypothyroidism should be adequately treated prior to diagnosing GH deficiency. GH treatment can lower free T4. Patients should have thyroid function monitored 6 weeks after starting GH treatment, as new hypothyroidism may develop and patients on L-T4 hormone replacement may need dose adjustments.[1]

THYROID HORMONE AND ESTROGEN

Estrogen therapy increases thyroid binding globulin (TBG), leading to increased levothyroxine dose requirements.

GROWTH HORMONE AND ESTROGEN

Oral estrogen therapy leads to decreased circulating IGF-1 levels. Women on oral estrogen replacement require higher GH replacement doses compared with eugonadal females or males. This does not occur with transdermal administration of estrogen.[1]

Special Situations

PITUITARY SURGERY

All patients should be assessed for hypopituitarism prior to pituitary surgery. Thyroid hormone and glucocorticoids should be replaced prior to surgery with stress doses of glucocorticoids given perioperatively. Replacement of sex steroids and GH is typically deferred until the postoperative period.[18]

Pituitary surgery caries a reported risk of 3% to 14% for developing new-onset hypopituitarism.[19] The risk of developing postoperative pituitary failure depends on tumor size, surgical expertise, and the extent of surgery.[1] Immediately postoperative, it is most important to address glucocorticoid status and disturbances in sodium and fluid balance.

Disruption of the hypothalamus, the anterior pituitary, or the stalk, due to manipulation or damage at the time of surgery, may impair ACTH secretion.[20] There are two strategies for avoiding acute AI perioperatively: (1) glucocorticoids may be administered perioperatively to cover for potential iatrogenic AI and stopped once the HPA axis can be assessed; (2) a steroid-sparing protocol with assessment of the HPA axis both pre- and postoperative can be used to avoid unnecessary exposure to glucocorticoids. Perioperative steroids would be withheld entirely in a patient with normal preoperative adrenal function. In the next few days after surgery, early morning cortisol levels are measured and glucocorticoids initiated if the value is consistent with AI. The standard-dose ACTH stimulation test will not be able to diagnosis new-onset central AI in the immediate postoperative period. Glucocorticoids should be started empirically if there is clinical suspicion for AI. If glucocorticoids are initiated in the perioperative period, physiologic replacement doses (Table 20.3) should be maintained until further testing can be performed to assess the need for long-term replacement (Table 20.2).[18]

After pituitary surgery, either deficiency or excess of antidiuretic hormone can develop. DI occurs most commonly in the immediate period after pituitary or hypothalamic surgery and may be transient or permanent. Patients should be closely monitored with strict measurements of fluid intake, urine output, and electrolytes (see Chapters 18 and 19).

All pituitary axes should be reassessed starting at 6 weeks after pituitary surgery and then periodically to monitor for development or resolution of pituitary deficiencies.[1]

TRAUMATIC BRAIN INJURY

The high prevalence of hypopituitarism after head trauma has only recently been recognized. Hypopituitarism is thought to result from local trauma to the vasculature supplying the anterior pituitary gland. Hypopituitarism may manifest in the acute setting following head trauma, and after recovery, patients may have persistent deficiencies, or they may develop late-onset pituitary deficiencies after the head trauma. A systematic review of hypopituitarism following TBI reported a prevalence of 15% to 50% in patients with a history of head trauma. GH deficiency was the most common hormone abnormality, followed by gonadotropin, then ACTH, and then TSH deficiency.[21] The estimates of persistent hypopituitarism decrease to 12% if repeated testing is applied.[22]

In the acute situation, assessment should focus on the integrity of the HPA axis because of the essential role of glucocorticoids in the stress response. As pituitary impairment may recover, it is recommended to defer the assessment of the other anterior pituitary hormones to a time when the patient is recovered from the acute injury. Although common, GH deficiency may be transient in these patients; GH stimulation testing should be performed only after at least 12 months following the event.[17] Reevaluation of all anterior pituitary hormones and quality of life is recommended 6 to 12 months after TBI.[2] Further studies are needed to determine the optimal timing of pituitary hormone assessment and benefits of replacement in TBI patients.

RADIATION

Hypopituitarism is a well-described complication of radiation treatment of both pituitary tumors and other skull base lesions. Early radiation-induced hypopituitarism can present within months and is thought to be due to injury at the level of the hypothalamus, which results in secondary deficiencies of the anterior pituitary hormones. Late-onset hypopituitarism is likely caused by damage to the pituitary gland and can present more than 10 years after radiation. The risk of pituitary dysfunction after cranial radiation is dose and time dependent.

Prior long-term studies of conventional radiation therapy for pituitary adenomas have reported 40% to 100% prevalence of new pituitary deficits.[23–25] In a retrospective study of 748 survivors of childhood cancer who were treated with cranial radiation and followed for a mean of 27 years, the prevalence of anterior pituitary hormone deficiencies was 46.5%, 10.8%, 7.5%, and 4% for GH, LH/FSH, TSH, and ACTH, respectively.[26] In another study of 88 children with embryonal brain tumors treated with craniospinal irradiation and conformal primary site irradiation, the cumulative incidence of GH deficiency, ACTH deficiency, and central hypothyroidism at 4 years from diagnosis was 93%, 38%, and 23%, respectively.[27] Advances in stereotactic radiosurgery techniques may reduce radiation effects on normal surrounding tissue, but the robust long-term data is lacking. Patients who have had cranial radiation need lifelong screening for hormonal abnormalities.

APOPLEXY

Hemorrhage into the pituitary gland, or apoplexy, can cause hypopituitarism and will be discussed further in Chapter 21. Deficiencies of all pituitary hormones can occur, but the sudden onset of AI is the most serious because it can cause life-threatening hypotension.

IMMUNE CHECKPOINT INHIBITOR TOXICITY

Hypophysitis and resulting hypopituitarism can occur as a complication of anticytotoxic T lymphocyte–associated antigen 4 or anti-programmed cell death-1/ligand-1 antibodies and will be discussed in Chapter 24.

PREGNANCY

During pregnancy in a patient with hypopituitarism, we are most concerned about maintaining glucocorticoids, thyroid hormone, and ADH. There is no utility to measuring or replacing sex steroids, prolactin, or GH/IGF-1 during pregnancy.

Diagnosis of Hypopituitarism During Pregnancy

The diagnosis of lymphocytic hypophysitis should be strongly considered in patients who are pregnant or who have recently delivered and have symptoms of pituitary insufficiency. Hypophysitis typically presents with headache or visual disturbances and DI. It can be associated with partial or complete hypopituitarism. MRI may show a post-contrast homogenously enhancing pituitary mass or stalk thickening.

Sheehan's syndrome (postpartum pituitary necrosis) occurs in women who suffer large-volume hemorrhage during delivery. Hypopituitarism can be partial or complete and often presents with an inability to lactate or failure to resume menses postpartum.

The diagnosis of AI may be missed in the first trimester due to the overlapping symptoms of pregnancy. Furthermore, total cortisol levels may appear normal due to increased CBG. If unrecognized, AI can lead to maternal or fetal demise during gestation or in the puerperium.[28] A low morning cortisol of less than 3 μg/dL in the presence of clinical symptoms is diagnostic of AI.[1]

Central hypothyroidism may be very difficult to diagnose during pregnancy, as TSH measurements are unreliable and many free T4 assays do not perform well during pregnancy. Use of trimester-specific free T4 reference ranges are recommended.[29] Serum total T4 and T3 increase in parallel during early pregnancy due to increases in TBG and remain stable, ~1.5 times the nonpregnant reference range, by mid-second trimester. Therefore, a total T4 less than the upper limit of the nonpregnant reference range may be suggestive of central hypothyroidism. Estimation of free T4 concentrations can also be done by calculating a free thyroxine index.[29]

Treatment of Hypopituitarism During Pregnancy

Hydrocortisone is the preferred physiologic glucocorticoid replacement in pregnancy because it does not cross the placenta. Dose requirements may increase as the pregnancy progresses. Stress dose hydrocortisone is needed during the active phase of labor, similar to that used for surgery.[1] Following delivery, glucocorticoids should be rapidly tapered down to prepregnancy maintenance doses.

Thyroid hormone replacement is essential during pregnancy. The fetus is dependent on maternal free T4 in early pregnancy. The fetal thyroid begins concentrating iodine at 10 to 12 weeks and produces T3 and T4 at 15 to 18 weeks gestational age. The fetal pituitary begins producing TSH at 10 to 15 weeks, and the fetal hypothalamic-pituitary-thyroid axis is functional around 20 weeks, gestational age. Women may require a 20% to 30% increased dose of L-T4 during pregnancy, as the estrogen-induced increase in TBG requires an increased total body T4 pool to maintain a euthyroid state. Thyroid function should be monitored every 4 to 6 weeks for women with central hypothyroidism who become pregnant. Following delivery, maternal L-T4 dosing should be reduced to prepregnancy levels, and hypothalamic-pituitary-thyroid axis function assessed 6 weeks thereafter.[1,29]

References

1. Fleseriu M, Hashim IA, Karavitaki N, et al. Hormonal replacement in hypopituitarism in adults: an Endocrine Society clinical practice guideline. *J Clin Endocrinol Metab.* 2016;101(11):3888–3921.
2. Ascoli P, Cavagnini F. Hypopituitarism. *Pituitary.* 2006;9(4):335–342.
3. Bates AS, Van't Hoff W, Jones PJ, Clayton RN. The effect of hypopituitarism on life expectancy. *The Journal of Clinical Endocrinology & Metabolism.* 1996;81(3):1169–1172.
4. T. Rosén B-ÅB. Premature mortality due to cardiovascular disease in hypopituitarism. *The Lancet.* 336(8710):285-288.
5. Tomlinson JW, Holden N, Hills RK, et al. Association between premature mortality and hypopituitarism. *The Lancet.* 2001;357(9254):425–431.
6. Javorsky B, Carroll T, Algeciras-Schimnich A, Singh R, Colon-Franco J, Findling J. SAT-390 new cortisol threshold for diagnosis of adrenal insufficiency after cosyntropin stimulation testing using the elecsys cortisol II, access cortisol, and LC-MS/MS assays. *Journal of the Endocrine Society.* 2019;3(Supplement 1): SAT–390.
7. Hamrahian AH, Oseni TS, Arafah BM. Measurements of serum free cortisol in critically ill patients. *New England Journal of Medicine.* 2004;350(16):1629–1638.
8. Filipsson H, Monson JP, Koltowska-Haggstrom M, Mattsson A, Johannsson G. The impact of glucocorticoid replacement regimens on metabolic outcome and comorbidity in hypopituitary patients. *J Clin Endocrinol Metab.* 2006;91(10):3954–3961.
9. Bornstein SR, Allolio B, Arlt W, et al. Diagnosis and treatment of primary adrenal insufficiency: an Endocrine Society clinical practice guideline. *J Clin Endocrinol Metab.* 2016;101(2):364–389.
10. Shimon I, Cohen O, Lubetsky A, Olchovsky D. Thyrotropin suppression by thyroid hormone replacement is correlated with thyroxine level normalization in central hypothyroidism. *Thyroid.* 12(9):823–827.
11. Ferretti E, Persani L, Jaffrain-Rea M-L, Giambona S, Tamburrano G, Beck-Peccoz P. Evaluation of the adequacy of levothyroxine replacement therapy in patients with central hypothyroidism. *The Journal of Clinical Endocrinology & Metabolism.* 1999;84(3):924–929.
12. Bhasin S, Cunningham GR, Hayes FJ, et al. Testosterone therapy in men with androgen deficiency syndromes: an Endocrine Society clinical practice guideline. *The Journal of Clinical Endocrinology & Metabolism.* 2010;95(6):2536–2559.

13. Lindholm J, Nielsen EH, Bjerre P, et al. Hypopituitarism and mortality in pituitary adenoma. *Clin Endocrinol (Oxf)*. 2006;65(1):51–58.
14. Bhasin S, Brito JP, Cunningham GR, et al. Testosterone therapy in men with hypogonadism: an Endocrine Society clinical practice guideline. *The Journal of Clinical Endocrinology & Metabolism*. 2018;103(5): 1715–1744.
15. Chetkowski RJ, Meldrum DR, Steingold KA, et al. Biologic effects of transdermal estradiol. *New England Journal of Medicine*. 1986;314(25):1615–1620.
16. Capatina C, Wass JA. Hypopituitarism: growth hormone and corticotropin deficiency. *Endocrinol Metab Clin North Am*. 2015;44(1):127–141.
17. Yuen KCJ, Biller BMK, Radovick S, et al. American Association of Clinical Endocrinologists and American College of Endocrinology guidelines for management of growth hormone deficiency in adults and patients transitioning from pediatric to adult care. *Endocr Pract*. 2019;25(11):1191–1232.
18. Woodmansee WW, Carmichael J, Kelly D, Katznelson LAACE Neuroendocrine and Pituitary Scientific Committee. American Association of Clinical Endocrinologists and American College of Endocrinology disease state clinical review: postoperative management following pituitary surgery. *Endocr Pract*. 2015;21(7):832–838.
19. Dallapiazza RF, Jane JA, Jr. Outcomes of endoscopic transsphenoidal pituitary surgery. *Endocrinol Metab Clin North Am*. 2015;44(1):105–115.
20. Ausiello JC, Bruce JN, Freda PU. Postoperative assessment of the patient after transsphenoidal pituitary surgery. *Pituitary*. 2008;11(4):391–401.
21. Schneider HJ, Kreitschmann-Andermahr I, Ghigo E, Stalla GK, Agha A. Hypothalamopituitary dysfunction following traumatic brain injury and aneurysmal subarachnoid hemorrhage: a systematic review. *JAMA*. 2007;298(12):1429–1438.
22. Tanriverdi F, Schneider HJ, Aimaretti G, Masel BE, Casanueva FF, Kelestimur F. Pituitary dysfunction after traumatic brain injury: a clinical and pathophysiological approach. *Endocrine Reviews*. 2015;36(3):305–342.
23. Fernandez A, Brada M, Zabuliene L, Karavitaki N, Wass JAH. Radiation-induced hypopituitarism. 2009;16(3):733.
24. Snyder PJ, Fowble BF, Schatz NJ, Savino PJ, Gennarelli TA. Hypopituitarism following radiation therapy. *The American Journal of Medicine*. 1986;81(3):457–462.
25. McCord MW, Buatti JM, Fennell EM, et al. Radiotherapy for pituitary adenoma: long-term outcome and sequelae. *International Journal of Radiation Oncology • Biology • Physics*. 1997;39(2):437–444.
26. Chemaitilly W, Li Z, Huang S, et al. Anterior hypopituitarism in adult survivors of childhood cancers treated with cranial radiotherapy: a report from the St Jude Lifetime Cohort study. *J Clin Oncol*. 2015;33(5):492–500.
27. Laughton SJ, Merchant TE, Sklar CA, et al. Endocrine outcomes for children with embryonal brain tumors after risk-adapted craniospinal and conformal primary-site irradiation and high-dose chemotherapy with stem-cell rescue on the SJMB-96 trial. *Journal of Clinical Oncology*. 2008;26(7):1112–1118.
28. Lindsay JR, Nieman LK. The hypothalamic-pituitary-adrenal axis in pregnancy: challenges in disease detection and treatment. *Endocr Rev*. 2005;26(6):775–799.
29. Alexander EK, Pearce EN, Brent GA, et al. 2017 Guidelines of the American Thyroid Association for the diagnosis and management of thyroid disease during pregnancy and the postpartum. *Thyroid*. 2017;27(3):315–389.

CHAPTER 21

Pituitary Apoplexy

Alison P. Seitz ■ Makoto Ishii

CHAPTER OUTLINE

Introduction

Pituitary apoplexy is the potentially life-threatening hemorrhage or infarction of the pituitary gland leading to significant neurologic, neuro-ophthalmologic, and endocrine deficiencies. The classic triad of symptoms includes severe headache, vision loss or visual disturbances, and hypopituitarism with or without impaired consciousness that is acute and sudden in onset, but the symptoms can be mild and subacute in nature manifesting over days to even months.[1–3] Although pituitary apoplexy most commonly arises from an existing pituitary adenoma, it can rarely occur in a normal pituitary gland such as after significant postpartum hemorrhage and acute hypovolemic shock. Here, we review the epidemiology, pathophysiology, clinical presentation, diagnosis, and management of pituitary apoplexy.

Epidemiology

Pituitary apoplexy is rare, with a reported prevalence of 6.2 cases per 100,000 individuals and an incidence of 0.17 episodes per 100,000 per year.[3–5] Of patients with a known diagnosis of pituitary adenoma, the incidence of pituitary apoplexy ranged from 2% to 14.1% with a higher incidence in macrodaenomas than microadenomas.[3,6,7] Whereas pituitary adenomas such as prolactinomas are found more frequently in women than in men, pituitary apoplexy is seen in both sexes, with some studies finding a higher incidence in men.[3] Pituitary apoplexy is more frequent in the fifth or sixth decade but can be found at all ages.[3,8]

PRESENCE OF PITUITARY ADENOMA

Excluding incidental postmortem findings of pituitary apoplexy, 93% to 100% of reported pituitary apoplexy cases occur in patients with pituitary adenomas.[8–15] In rare cases, pituitary apoplexy arises from other pituitary and sellar lesions such as Rathke's cleft cyst (RCC),[12,14,16,17] craniopharyngioma,[16] sellar tuberculoma,[18] hypophysitis,[12,19,20] sellar abscess,[21] sellar metastasis,[22] or in normal pituitary gland postpartum, from acute hypovolemic shock (Sheehan's syndrome).[23–26] Apoplexy occurs in approximately 10% of existing, known pituitary adenomas, but estimates vary widely, as many pituitary tumors are undetected.[8,9,27,28] Apoplexy is the first presentation of pituitary disease in 73% to 97% of patients.[8,9,27] In incidentally detected pituitary adenomas, the risk of apoplexy is very low, with an incidence of only 0.2% of patients/year. The incidence increases to 0.83% to 1.1% in larger incidentally found pituitary tumors or macroincidentalomas; however, it may be higher in those with predisposing factors such as anticoagulation therapy or in faster-growing tumors.[28–30] Of note, subclinical (asymptomatic) pituitary apoplexy is frequent, affecting up to 25% of all pituitary tumors on imaging or at autopsy.[3]

Larger adenomas and nonfunctioning adenomas are most likely to apoplex. Of patients presenting with pituitary apoplexy related to an adenoma, 90% to 100% have adenomas measuring over 1 cm, and 6% to 38% over 2.5 cm.[1,8,9,11–13,15,16,31,32] In most studies, 10% to 24% of tumors are completely necrotic and cannot be typed on pathologic examination.[12,13,31,33] Of tumors that can be typed, 70% to 90% are nonfunctioning pituitary adenomas, most likely because they grow larger than secretory tumors while remaining asymptomatic.[1,8–11,13,15,31,32,34] Subtypes of nonfunctioning pituitary adenomas include silent gonadotropic hormone-expressing, null-cell (displaying no particular cell lineage differentiation), plurihormonal, silent adrenocorticotropic hormone (ACTH)-expressing, and growth hormone–expressing adenomas.[12,31,32] After nonfunctioning pituitary adenomas, prolactinomas result in 3% to 16%, growth hormone producing adenomas in 2% to 10%, and ACTH producing adenomas in 0% to 7% of pituitary apoplexy cases.[1,2,8–13,15,31,32,34] In children and adolescents, pituitary apoplexy is usually associated with prolactinomas rather than nonfunctioning adenomas.[35,36]

Pathophysiology

The pituitary gland is particularly prone to both bleeding and ischemic infarction, with a higher rate of spontaneous infarction than other central nervous system tumors.[37] Pituitary tumors require a significant amount of energy, are particularly sensitive to glucose deprivation, and contain few, fragile blood vessels compared with other tumors.[37] Pituitary tumors also tend to have high intratumoral pressure. Patients with small sellas may be more prone to pituitary apoplexy, likely because pressure on a pituitary tumor decreases blood flow and may precipitate apoplexy.[26,37] When a pituitary tumor infarcts or hemorrhages, it often leads to extensive coagulation necrosis of large parts of the normal pituitary gland.[38] The underlying molecular events leading to pituitary apoplexy are unclear and may include vascular endothelial growth factor, matrix metalloproteinases, hypoxia-inducing factor-1α, and inflammatory cytokines, among others; however, well-designed genomics, proteomic, and metabolomics studies using large sample sizes are lacking and are essential for the elucidation of the underlying molecular mechanisms of pituitary apoplexy.[39]

Precipitating Factors

Identifiable factors precipitate pituitary apoplexy in 15% to 40% of cases.[3,8,10,11] These potential precipitating factors can be broadly placed into two categories: (1) vascular causes such as blood pressure fluctuations and increased bleeding risk; and (2) increased pituitary demand such as during pregnancy, hormonal treatment, and pituitary testing. Additional precipitating factors may include radiation therapy and infiltrates like lymphocytic hypophysitis. However, for the majority of pituitary apoplexy cases, there is no clear underlying precipitant.

VASCULAR FACTORS: BLOOD PRESSURE FLUCTUATIONS AND BLEEDING RISK

Pituitary apoplexy often results from vascular factors such as (1) an acute decrease in perfusion of the pituitary leading to infarction, or (2) an increase in bleeding tendency or an acute increase in blood pressure leading to hemorrhage.

Any procedure that causes hemodilution, hypotension, or microemboli can potentially cause infarction of pituitary tissue, including surgical, angiographic, intravascular, and endoscopic procedures.[8,12,14,40,41] In a 2019 single-center retrospective study, 5% of patients had extracranial surgery within the past 24 hours before the pituitary apoplexy.[31] Cardiopulmonary bypass dynamics during cardiac surgery has been reported to cause infarction of the pituitary.[8,14,40] In one case report in a patient with atherosclerosis of the internal carotid arteries, lumbar fusion surgery in the prone position led to increased intraabdominal pressure and compression of the vena cava, lowering cardiac index, in addition to compressing the vertebral arteries, all leading to decreased perfusion to the pituitary, precipitating pituitary infarction.[42] Episodic hypotension from a variety of etiologies, including severe sepsis, hemodialysis, and phosphodiesterase type 5 (PDE5) inhibitors (e.g., vardenafil), may lead to pituitary apoplexy.[12,43,44] In one reported case, cardiac pharmacologic nuclear stress testing with regadenoson precipitated apoplexy, likely due to cerebral vasodilation and blood pressure fluctuation.[45]

Large, transient increases in blood pressure can precipitate pituitary hemorrhage. In one retrospective observational study of surgical cases, 2 out of 32 patients who presented with pituitary apoplexy were intoxicated with methamphetamine, possibly leading to acutely elevated blood pressure.[13] It is unclear if chronic hypertension also predisposes to pituitary apoplexy. A preceding diagnosis or acute presentation of hypertension (systolic BP greater than 140 mm Hg) is present in 5% to 48% of patients with pituitary apoplexy.[1,2,8,9,11,14,31,32,34]

Anticoagulation and thrombocytopenia are risk factors for hemorrhage, including in the pituitary gland. Between 5% and 25% of patients with pituitary apoplexy are on antiplatelet agents or anticoagulation. Use of aspirin, dabigatran, apixaban, rivaroxaban, warfarin, and heparin have all been implicated in pituitary apoplexy.[2,8,9,11,12,14,31,34,46–49] However, due to a lack of randomized studies, it is difficult to give evidence-based recommendations regarding the use of antiplatelet and anticoagulation agents in individuals with known pituitary adenomas. Head trauma, especially in patients on antiplatelet or anticoagulation therapy, can precipitate bleeding of pituitary tumors.[8,50,51] Cytotoxic chemotherapy resulting in thrombocytopenia may also predispose to pituitary apoplexy.[52,53]

INCREASED DEMAND: PREGNANCY, PITUITARY GLAND TESTING, AND HORMONAL THERAPY

Increases in pituitary demand, such as during pregnancy, pharmacologic stimulation, or pharmacologic treatment, can exceed available blood supply and lead to infarction of the pituitary.

Although this is most common in patients with pituitary adenomas, it can happen in a normal pituitary under special circumstances like pregnancy.

Pituitary demand increases in pregnancy, predisposing to infarction. Of women who present with pituitary apoplexy, 8% to 25% are pregnant or postpartum.[9,11,14] During pregnancy, placental estrogen stimulates lactotroph cells to secrete prolactin, resulting in lactotroph hyperplasia. This leads to increases in pituitary size, and therefore increases intracapsular pressure, compressing the blood supply to the pituitary, leaving it vulnerable to hypotension, while simultaneously increasing pituitary demand. The pituitaries of patients with small sellas are especially compressed. The increased metabolic demand combined with decreased blood supply can result in pituitary apoplexy.[26,54,55] In one study of women who presented with pituitary apoplexy in the third trimester, half had pre-eclampsia, indicating that hypertension or blood pressure fluctuations might also play a role.[9] In Sheehan's syndrome, severe postpartum hemorrhage leads to hypotension and infarction of the pituitary. Postpartum-disseminated intravascular coagulation can also lead to necrosis of the pituitary.[26]

Pharmacologic stimulation of the pituitary gland increases metabolic demand of the pituitary gland, and, especially in patients with existing pituitary tumors, can precipitate pituitary apoplexy. Inferior petrosal sinus sampling, in which ACTH is measured in petrosal and peripheral venous plasma from catheters inserted into both inferior petrosal veins before and within 10 minutes after administration of corticotropin-releasing hormone, can cause pituitary apoplexy in vulnerable patients.[56] Recent guidelines recommend against gonadotropin-releasing hormone (GnRH) or thyrotropin-releasing hormone stimulation tests given the rare but serious risk of apoplexy.[57]

Pituitary apoplexy has also been reported as a complication of hormonal treatments including use of the GnRH agonist leuprolide acetate for both prostate carcinoma and for fertility treatment,[58–61] and with use of the dopamine agonist cabergoline for prolactinoma in children and adults.[1,12,31,62] Unfortunately, there are no specific guidelines or biomarkers to help determine which patients with prolactinomas are at increased risk for developing pituitary apoplexy with dopamine agonist treatment. Additionally, at least two cases have been reported of children with prolactinomas who developed pituitary apoplexy 2 weeks after starting growth hormone.[35]

Clinical Presentation

As initially described by Brougham et al., the classic presentation of pituitary apoplexy is the sudden onset of impaired consciousness, headache and stiff neck, ocular palsies, and sometimes amblyopia or hemiparesis[63]; however, the actual neurologic signs and symptoms can vary widely (Table 21.1).[1,2,7–9,11–16,31–34,55] Additionally, a majority of patients with pituitary apoplexy will have significant endocrine dysfunction that could be life-threatening. Although the classic presentation of pituitary apoplexy is acute, symptoms may present in a subacute or chronic fashion with a range of hours to months from initial onset to progression of symptoms.[1,2]

HEADACHE AND IMPAIRED CONSCIOUSNESS

Headache due to meningeal irritation is the most prominent and common manifestation of pituitary apoplexy, reported to occur in 83% to 100% of cases.[1,2,7–9,11–15,31–34,55] The most classic presentation of the headache is severe and acute, often described as a "thunderclap" and easily confused with the headache of a subarachnoid hemorrhage, but the headache may have a more insidious, subacute onset.[1,3,9,12] There is no classic distribution for the headache: unilateral, frontal, temporal, occipital, and apical headaches have all been described.[1,9] Other signs and symptoms of meningeal irritation, including nuchal rigidity and photophobia, are often reported alongside the headache,[9,13,16] and 29% to 59% of patients report nausea and vomiting.[7–9,12–14,31,34]

TABLE 21.1 ■ **Clinical Manifestations of Pituitary Apoplexy**[a]

Symptom	Incidence (%)
Headaches	83–100
Visual acuity loss	23–55
Hypopituitarism	58–88
Visual field loss	22–63
Nausea	29–59
Ocular palsies	25–79
Altered level of consciousness/coma	3–19

[a]From references 1, 2, 7–9, 11–16, 31–34, and 55.

In the classic paper by Brougham et al., altered mental status was the most frequent neurologic abnormality found in pituitary apoplexy[63]; however, recent reports have found an overall lower incidence. Between 3% and 19% of patients present with altered level of consciousness ranging from lethargy to stupor and even coma.[8,12–16,31,33] In a review of patients with pituitary apoplexy during pregnancy and postpartum, 8% presented with altered mental status.[55] Altered mental status due to pituitary apoplexy can be subtle and masquerade as functional decline in older adults, especially in subacute presentations.[64]

VISUAL DISTURBANCES AND OTHER FOCAL NEUROLOGIC DEFICITS

Focal neurologic and neuro-ophthalmologic deficits occur in pituitary apoplexy from compression of cranial nerves and blood vessels. Visual disturbances, presenting acutely or progressively, are very common: 23% to 55% of patients have a visual acuity deficit and 22% to 63% have a visual field deficit.[9,11–14,27,31,34] Visual disturbances correlate with larger tumors.[12] Rarely, pituitary apoplexy presents with bilateral blindness, possibly accompanied by fixed dilated pupils and optic atrophy.[7,65]

Ocular palsies are present in 25% to 79% of patients, with involvement of oculomotor nerve palsy being most frequent resulting in limited adduction with exotropia and hypotropia, ptosis, and mydriasis.[8,9,11–13,15,27,34,66] Anisocoria or abnormal pupil responses occur in about 20% to 27% of cases.[9,34] Ocular palsies are correlated with larger tumors, panhypopituitarism, and tumor necrosis.[66]

Rarely, pituitary apoplexy can lead to compression of one or both internal carotid arteries, which can lead to infarction of large cerebral arterial territories or even bilateral cerebral hemispheres without early intervention.[1,50,67] Additionally, cerebral infarction secondary to arterial vasospasm has also been reported and should not be overlooked as a possible complication of pituitary apoplexy.[68,69]

ENDOCRINE DYSFUNCTION

On presentation with pituitary apoplexy, 58% to 88% of patients have some form of endocrine deficiency, often silent but sometimes leading to fatigue, menstrual disturbances, and reduced libido.[8,11,13,15,16,27,32,33] Cortisol deficiency is common, affecting 23% to 86% of all patients.[8,12–14,16,32,66,70] Cortisol deficiency leads to lack of suppression of ADH release, which results in hyponatremia (serum sodium less than 135 mmol/L) in 3% to 47% of patients.[9,11–13,16] In severe cases, patients can present with acute adrenal insufficiency, possibly leading to significant hyponatremia, hypotension, and loss of consciousness, requiring immediate empiric steroid replacement.[9,12,71,72] Other hormonal abnormalities are also common. From recent literature, 30% to 69% of patients present with hypogonadism,[8,9,12,14,16,32,66] 26% to 83% with hypothyroidism,[8,9,12,13,16,32,66] and 11% to 32% with growth hormone deficiency.[8,12,16,32,66] Occasionally, patients present with diabetes insipidus (1% to 3%)[2,8,13,16] or low serum prolactin.[9,32] Of note, the reported studies include only surgically managed patients, who tend to present with more severe deficits.[8]

Diagnosis

The diagnosis of pituitary apoplexy is made by clinical assessment and confirmed by radiologic detection of the pituitary apoplexy or pituitary tumor, even if no necrosis or hemorrhage is found.[3] Because pituitary apoplexy can present with headache and meningeal signs, the differential diagnosis often includes subarachnoid hemorrhage and bacterial meningitis. Less often, if the patient suffers from cerebral ischemia, then pituitary apoplexy may be mistaken for ischemic stroke or, if the patient presents with hypotension or other hemodynamic instability, for myocardial infarction. Diagnosis in pregnancy can be challenging. Lactotroph hyperplasia may lead to sudden-onset headache, visual changes, and hypopituitarism without apoplexy. In that case, magnetic resonance imaging (MRI) without contrast will show homogenous signal characteristics consistent with an enlarged pituitary, but will not show the ischemia or hemorrhage typical of pituitary apoplexy.[25,26]

CLINICAL ASSESSMENT

Lumbar puncture has limited utility in differentiating pituitary apoplexy from subarachnoid hemorrhage, as both will cause cerebrospinal fluid to have increased cerebrospinal fluid leukocytes, erythrocytes, and protein.[13] Lumbar puncture in pituitary apoplexy may also show aseptic meningitis.[38] However, lumbar puncture is essential if bacterial meningitis is suspected, in which case cerebrospinal fluid cultures should be obtained.[3,73]

Endocrine testing can also help differentiate pituitary apoplexy from other causes of headache and meningismus. Although a comprehensive hormone assessment will be important in guiding management of the endocrine dysfunction, it should not delay treatment, particularly with steroid therapy for presumed acute secondary adrenal insufficiency.

RADIOLOGIC IDENTIFICATION

In order to confirm the diagnosis, neuroimaging is used to detect pituitary apoplexy or the underlying pituitary tumor by computed tomography (CT) or MRI. Imaging of the pituitary gland can reveal a simple infarction, hemorrhagic infarction, mixed hemorrhagic infarction and clot, or pure clot with mixed features commonly seen.[3]

Computed Tomography

CT is fast and widely available but nonspecific. Acute hemorrhagic infarct of the pituitary gland may be seen on CT as a large heterogeneously hyperintense sellar mass, but aneurysms, meningiomas, RCC, germinomas, and lymphomas may also present similarly.[25,73] MRI is more sensitive for acute pituitary hemorrhage, and CT will fail to detect most nonhemorrhagic infarcts.[25,74] CT will, however, usually identify a pituitary or suprasellar mass.[74] In one study, 60% of patients were initially diagnosed on CT before a subsequent dedicated pituitary MRI.[9] In another, CT was very effective in showing a pituitary mass but could only identify hemorrhage in 40% of cases, whereas

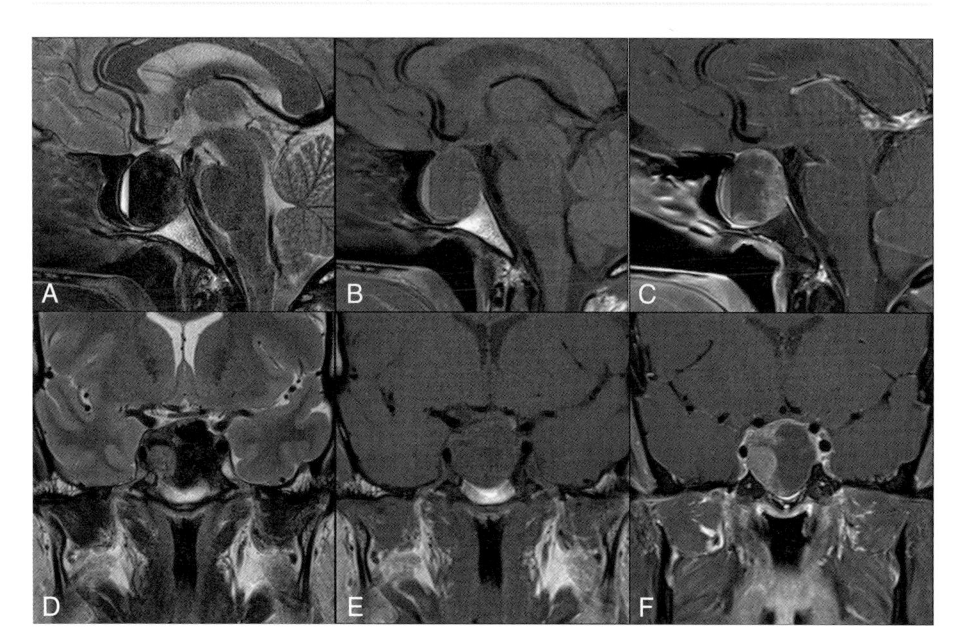

Fig. 21.1 MRI scans of pituitary apoplexy. Sagittal (A-C) and coronal (D-F) pituitary protocol MRI in a patient with acute pituitary hemorrhage (presented with clinical signs/symptoms of apoplexy). T2 (A, D), T1 (B, E), and postgadolineum T1 (C, F) images are displayed. Figure was adapted from Barkhoudarian, G., and Kelly, D.F., Neurosurgery Clinics of America, 2019.

MRI identified 89% of hemorrhages.[14] When a rapid diagnosis is needed, CT without contrast is most useful in the emergency setting to exclude a large bleed such as a subarachnoid hemorrhage or a large mass lesion before a dedicated pituitary MRI is obtained.[74]

Magnetic Resonance Imaging

The American College of Radiology (ACR) recommends MRI without contrast using a high-resolution pituitary protocol as the optimal first-line imaging test in pituitary apoplexy.[74] MRI without contrast is highly sensitive for both hemorrhage and infarction.[11] MRI can show tumor enlargement, sellar expansion, and intratumoral hemorrhage, which will appear as a T1 signal hyperintensity, a low T2 signal, or a hemorrhage fluid level (Fig. 21.1).[75] The radiologic differential diagnosis on MRI includes metastasis to the pituitary, pituitary abscess, craniopharyngioma, RCC, and sellar aneurysm, all of which may also present with headache and visual changes.[25,76] The ACR recommends including T1 fat saturation sequences in order to differentiate hemorrhage from fat in other soft-tissue masses such as craniopharyngiomas, RCC, dermoids, and teratomas.[74] During pregnancy, diagnosis of pituitary apoplexy on MRI can be especially difficult, because the pituitary gland enlarges and can appear similar to a pituitary adenoma, lymphocytic hypophysitis, and pituitary apoplexy.[26] MRI with IV contrast may be performed for use in operative guidance but is usually not necessary for diagnosis.[74]

Management

The management of pituitary apoplexy varies based on the acuity and severity of the neurologic or neuro-ophthalmologic deficits. For those with acute, severe, and worsening neurologic symptoms, surgical resection will be warranted, whereas those with minimal and stable symptoms may benefit from conservative medical management. However, whether surgical or medical management is indicated remains controversial, as a vast majority of patients fall between these two extremes. Guidelines for the management of pituitary apoplexy have been developed by various organizations, but the evidence supporting these guidelines has significant limitations, as there are no randomized controlled clinical trials comparing conservative medical management to surgical intervention in patients with pituitary apoplexy.

GRADING SYSTEM

There is no uniform grading system for pituitary apoplexy. The UK guidelines for management of pituitary apoplexy by the Pituitary Apoplexy Guidelines Development Group proposed the pituitary apoplexy score (PAS), as one possible scoring system that could serve as a uniform tool to monitor the conservatively managed patients in future clinical studies (Table 21.2).[70] However, this score has not been validated or used as a criterion for surgical or medication indication. In order to fill this gap, a comprehensive classification system has been proposed based on a retrospective series of 109 consecutive cases of pituitary apoplexy from a single institution.[16] Based on the clinical presentation, patients were classified into five grades with three modifiers ranging from grade 1 with no symptoms to grade 5 with acute visual deficits or impaired consciousness not allowing visual testing (Fig. 21.2). Higher-grade patients received urgent or timely surgical management, whereas lower-grade patients may have had elective surgical or conservative management.

TABLE 21.2 ■ **Pituitary Apoplexy Score (PAS)**[a]

Variable	Points
Level of consciousness	
Glasgow coma scale 15	0
Glasgow coma scale 8–14	2
Glasgow coma scale <8	4
Visual acuity	
Normal 10/10 (or no change from pre-pituitary apoplexy visual acuity)	0
Reduced, unilateral	1
Reduced, bilateral	2
Visual field deficits	
Normal	0
Unilateral defect	1
Bilateral defect	2
Ocular paresis	
Absent	0
Present unilateral	1
Present bilateral	2

[a]From reference 70.

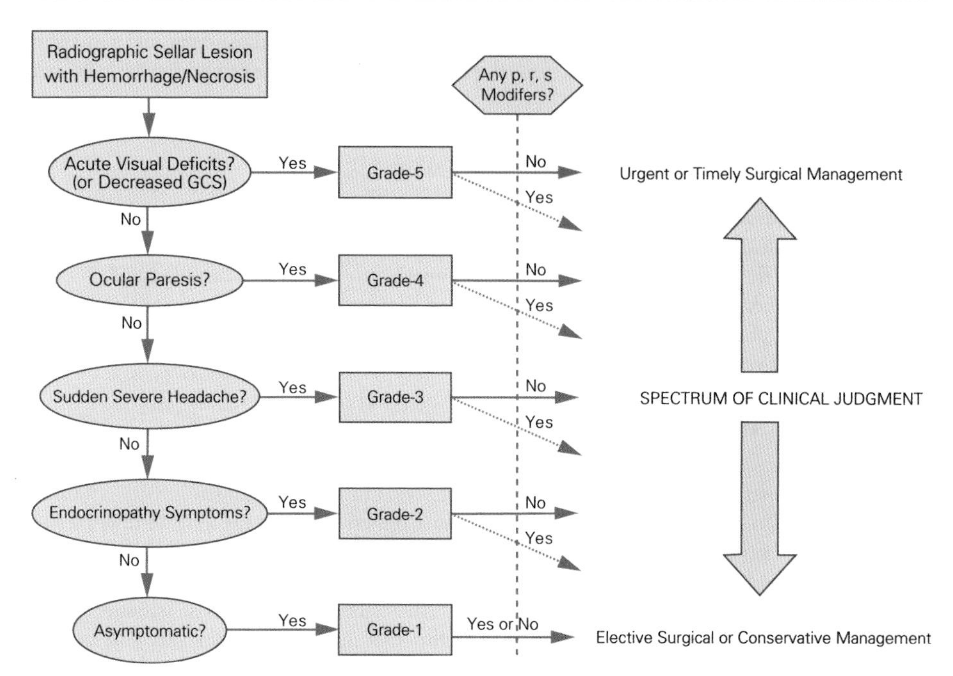

Fig. 21.2 Flow chart illustrating assessment using Pituitary Apoplexy Grading System. *GCS,* Glasgow Coma Scale; *p modifier,* prolactinoma; *r modifier,* hemorrhagic Rathke cleft cyst; *s modifier,* significant comorbidities. (Adapted from Jho DH, Biller BMK, Agarwalla PK, Swearingen B. Pituitary apoplexy: large surgical series with grading system. *World Neurosurg.* 2014;82(5):781–790.)

ACUTE MANAGEMENT

Regardless of whether a patient receives surgical or medical management, in the acute setting, particularly for those patients with hemodynamic instability, supportive care with fluid resuscitation, intravenous dextrose, and empiric hydrocortisone replacement should be started immediately after drawing blood to sample for hormonal assays.[57,70,73] Empiric steroid therapy (a bolus of intravenous hydrocortisone 100 to 200 mg followed by 50 to 100 mg every 6 hours or 2 to 4 mg/hour continuously) is mandatory in any patient with hemodynamic instability or signs of adrenal insufficiency, as corticotropic deficiency in patients with pituitary apoplexy can be life-threatening.[3]

SURGICAL MANAGEMENT

In pituitary apoplexy with severe neurologic or neuro-ophthalmologic deficits, surgical management is common and recommended based on guidelines from various endocrine and neurosurgical organizations.[70,77,78] A transsphenoidal resection performed by an experienced pituitary neurosurgeon is preferred, as it results in better neuro-ophthalmologic outcomes in most cases.[31,65] In surgically managed patients, overall reported rates of complications are low and include postoperative cerebrospinal fluid leaks (less than 5%), transient postoperative meningitis and confusion (less than 10%), transient epistaxis (less than 5%), impaired anterior pituitary function (less than 20% in one study), and diabetes insipidus (less than 5%).[2,9,14,15,34] In cases of postoperative hypopituitarism and diabetes insipidus, hormone deficiencies may be a consequence of apoplexy rather than of surgery. After resection, the Congress of Neurological Surgeons recommends those patients with residual or recurrent tumors have radiosurgery and radiation therapy, whereas those with no residual tumor or only a small intrasellar tumor may be followed with neuroimaging.[79]

CONSERVATIVE MEDICAL MANAGEMENT

Conservative medical management may be appropriate in pituitary apoplexy with absent or mild neuro-ophthalmic signs, as spontaneous recovery is seen in most patients with mild signs.[70,73,77] However, due to the fluctuating nature of pituitary apoplexy, patients who are managed conservatively need to be closely monitored for sequelae of hemorrhage, meningeal irritation, neuro-ophthalmologic deficits, and hormonal deficiencies, and surgical intervention considered if symptoms fail to improve or worsen.[70]

Outcomes

The majority of patients with pituitary apoplexy survive and live independently with minimal neurologic or neuro-ophthalmologic residual symptoms, though most require long-term hormone replacement.[14] Many of the recent retrospective studies have reported 0% mortality[8,9,11,13,34]; however, one 2015 study from Mayo Clinic reported 4 out of 87 patients died[14] and another from Essen, Germany reported 5 out of 60 patients died.[12] The cause of death in these patients varied. Based on these small numbers of reported cases, factors that may increase mortality risk include massive hemorrhage and medical comorbidities that preclude safe surgery or lead to postoperative cardiac or pulmonary complications.

NEURO-OPHTHALMOLOGIC AND NEUROLOGIC SYMPTOMS

Most patients with visual symptoms have at least partial resolution of visual field and visual acuity deficits, and many have complete resolution.[9] Ocular palsies tend to resolve at higher rates than visual deficits.[1,8,11,15,31,34,66]

Neurologic sequelae may appear much later than initial presentation. There is one case report of a young woman with a remote history of acute vision loss, partially resolved, who presented to an outpatient neurologist complaining of holocranial headaches. She was found to have herniation of the brain and optic chiasm into the empty sella left after she presumably suffered from pituitary apoplexy when she first had vision loss.[80] Most severe neurologic symptoms, such as altered mental status and nuchal rigidity, resolve after the acute period, but 20% to 37% of patients continue to have residual symptoms such as headaches.[12,13]

PITUITARY FUNCTION

Pituitary endocrine function rarely completely recovers in any patient with pituitary dysfunction on presentation.[9,11,15] After the acute period, most patients need long-term hormone replacement therapy. Rates of specific hormone replacement in recent studies vary widely: 46% to 78% need cortisol replacement, 5% to 74% need growth hormone replacement, 49% to 75% need thyroxine replacement, 5% to 12% need desmopressin, and 10% to 65% require gonadotropin, estrogen, or testosterone replacement.[8,9,11,12,14,34] Of surgically managed patients, about one-third of patients have global anterior pituitary deficiency.[12,34] Whereas one recent study found worse symptom progression (cranial nerve palsies, aseptic meningitis, and decreased consciousness levels) and higher rates of long-term hormonal deficiencies in patients with ischemic versus hemorrhagic pituitary apoplexy,[38] other studies found no differences.[13,32,81]

ASSESSING OUTCOMES BETWEEN SURGICAL AND MEDICAL MANAGEMENT

Several recent retrospective studies have analyzed outcomes between patients who underwent surgical versus medical management for pituitary apoplexy. In a recent large metaanalysis of 14 studies comprising of 259 surgically managed and 198 medically managed cases, there was no significant difference in the overall rates for any recovery (complete or partial) between surgical and medical management, with recovery rates in surgically versus conservatively managed patients of 35% versus 28% for endocrine function, 82% versus 85% for visual acuity, 82% versus 84% for visual field deficits, and 83% versus 95% for oculomotor dysfunction.[27] The rates for complete recovery in surgically versus conservatively managed patients were also similar: 39% versus 38% in endocrine function, 55% versus 61% in visual acuity, 49% versus 58% in visual field deficits, and 62% versus 60% for oculomotor dysfunction.[27] In contrast, an older metaanalysis comprising of 6 studies of surgically versus conservatively managed patients found a significantly higher rate of recovery of ocular palsy and visual fields among surgically managed patients, but no significant difference in the recovery of visual acuity and pituitary function.[82]

Other studies have examined early versus late surgery in pituitary apoplexy. In a study of patients undergoing surgery within 1 week versus after 1 week (range 8 to 210 days), rates of complete recovery in early versus late surgery were 100% versus 93% for ocular palsies, 56% versus 60% for visual acuity, 30% versus 44% for visual fields, and 59% versus 67% for full neurologic recovery, and none of the differences were statistically significant.[34] In another study of patients undergoing surgery within 72 hours versus later surgery, visual improvement was seen in 67% versus 84% of patients, complete resolution of preoperative decreased visual acuity or field cuts was seen in 33% versus 41%, cranial nerve palsies improved in 83% versus 80%, and no differences were significant.[13] A metaanalysis of 172 patients with pituitary apoplexy presenting with some visual deficit found 98% of patients who underwent surgery within 1 week experienced visual recovery versus 85% of patients who underwent surgery after 1 week, a difference that also did not reach statistical significance ($P = 0.07$).[83]

Most of the recent studies have shown no significant differences in outcomes between surgical and medical management of pituitary apoplexy, but none have been randomized controlled trials. Surgically managed patients tended to have more severe neuro-ophthalmologic deficits and larger tumors, which may have biased the results of these studies.[27,33] In one series, however, one-third of the patients treated conservatively presented with reduced level of consciousness and despite that severe presentation, four out of six had an excellent recovery.[14] The authors of that series concluded that conservative management is a good option for patients without severe neuro-ophthalmological deficits who respond quickly to early medical therapy.[14] Guidelines from most organizations recommend surgery within 1 week in patients with altered consciousness or worsening severe visual defect by an experienced pituitary surgeon.[57,70,77,84]

RECURRENCE AND FOLLOW-UP

Between 5% and 20% of patients have tumor recurrence or progression after apoplexy.[33,34] Most professional society guidelines recommend periodic surveillance imaging with MRI without contrast using a high-resolution pituitary protocol, with the first MRI 3 to 4 months after surgical intervention.[70,74,85] Whereas pituitary tumor progression is common, recurrent apoplexy is rarer and may depend on cavernous sinus involvement. In one study of surgically managed patients, recurrent pituitary apoplexy was seen in about 5% of patients, but almost a quarter of patients with adenoma remnants within the cavernous sinus after resection had multiple apoplexies.[31] In an older prospective study of a small number of medically managed pituitary apoplexy patients, one out of seven patients had a recurrence of apoplexy.[86] Patients with multiple apoplexies have significantly greater rates of ophthalmoplegia, likely because ophthalmoplegia is often due to cavernous sinus invasion.[31]

Conclusion

Pituitary apoplexy is a potentially life-threatening infarction or hemorrhage of pituitary tissue, usually of a pituitary tumor. Whereas the classic presentation is a sudden and severe headache with neuro-ophthalmologic deficits and hormone deficiencies, patients can also present with milder signs and symptoms over a subacute or chronic time period. When pituitary apoplexy is suspected, an MRI without contrast using a high-resolution pituitary protocol should be obtained to confirm the diagnosis as soon as possible. Hormonal assays should be drawn, and supportive care with intravenous fluids and dextrose and empiric steroid replacement should be started immediately. The decision to complete early transsphenoidal resection of the apoplectic tissue or conservatively manage remains controversial, and randomized controlled studies are clearly needed to help identify the optimal interventions for patients with pituitary apoplexy. Based on current guidelines, surgical intervention should be strongly considered in patients with severe neuro-ophthalmologic deficits or worsening clinical status. After the acute phase of the illness, most patients will at least partially recover from neurologic and neuro-ophthalmologic deficits, but most will need long-term hormone replacement in addition to periodic surveillance imaging with MRI scans.

References

1. Wang Z, Gao L, Wang W, et al. Coagulative necrotic pituitary adenoma apoplexy: a retrospective study of 21 cases from a large pituitary center in China. *Pituitary*. 2019;22(1):13–28.
2. Yang T, Bayad F, Schaberg MR, et al. Endoscopic endonasal transsphenoidal treatment of pituitary apoplexy: outcomes in a series of 20 patients. *Cureus*. 2015;7(10):e357.
3. Briet C, Salenave S, Bonneville J-F, Laws ER, Chanson P. Pituitary apoplexy. *Endocr Rev*. 2015;36(6):622–645.
4. Raappana A, Koivukangas J, Ebeling T, Pirilä T. Incidence of pituitary adenomas in Northern Finland in 1992–2007. *J Clin Endocrinol Metab*. 2010;95(9):4268–4275.
5. Fernandez A, Karavitaki N, Wass JAH. Prevalence of pituitary adenomas: a community-based, cross-sectional study in Banbury (Oxfordshire, UK). *Clinical Endocrinology*. 2010;72(3):377–382.
6. Ntali G, Wass JA. Epidemiology, clinical presentation and diagnosis of non-functioning pituitary adenomas. *Pituitary*. 2018;21(2):111–118.
7. Zhu X, Wang Y, Zhao X, et al. Incidence of pituitary apoplexy and its risk factors in Chinese people: a database study of patients with pituitary adenoma. *PLOS ONE*. 2015;10(9):e0139088.
8. Gondim JA, de Albuquerque LAF, Almeida JP, et al. Endoscopic endonasal surgery for treatment of pituitary apoplexy: 16 years of experience in a specialized pituitary center. *World Neurosurgery*. 2017;108:137–142.
9. Abbara A, Clarke S, Eng PC, et al. Clinical and biochemical characteristics of patients presenting with pituitary apoplexy. *Endocrine Connections*. 2018;7(10):1058–1066.
10. Bujawansa S, Thondam SK, Steele C, et al. Presentation, management and outcomes in acute pituitary apoplexy: a large single-centre experience from the United Kingdom. *Clinical Endocrinology*. 2014;80(3):419–424.
11. Giritharan S, Gnanalingham K, Kearney T. Pituitary apoplexy – bespoke patient management allows good clinical outcome. *Clinical Endocrinology*. 2016;85(3):415–422.
12. Grzywotz A, Kleist B, Möller LC, et al. Pituitary apoplexy – a single center retrospective study from the neurosurgical perspective and review of the literature. *Clinical Neurology and Neurosurgery*. 2017;163:39–45.
13. Rutkowski MJ, Kunwar S, Blevins L, Aghi MK. Surgical intervention for pituitary apoplexy: an analysis of functional outcomes. *Journal of Neurosurgery*. 2017;129(2):417–424.
14. Singh TD, Valizadeh N, Meyer FB, Atkinson JLD, Erickson D, Rabinstein AA. Management and outcomes of pituitary apoplexy. *Journal of Neurosurgery*. 2015;122(6):1450–1457.
15. Zoli M, Milanese L, Faustini-Fustini M, et al. Endoscopic endonasal surgery for pituitary apoplexy: evidence on a 75-case series from a tertiary care center. *World Neurosurgery*. 2017;106:331–338.

16. Jho DH, Biller BMK, Agarwalla PK, Swearingen B. Pituitary apoplexy: large surgical series with grading system. *World Neurosurgery*. 2014;82(5):781–790.
17. Kim E. A Rathke's cleft cyst presenting with apoplexy. *J Korean Neurosurg Soc*. 2012;52(4):404–406.
18. Verma R, Patil TB, Lalla R. Pituitary apoplexy syndrome as the manifestation of intracranial tuberculoma. *BMJ Case Rep*. 2014;2014.
19. Dan NG, Feiner RID, Houang MTW, Turner JJ. Pituitary apoplexy in association with lymphocytic hypophysitis. *Journal of Clinical Neuroscience*. 2002;9(5):577–580.
20. Husain Q, Zouzias A, Kanumuri VV, Eloy JA, Liu JK. Idiopathic granulomatous hypophysitis presenting as pituitary apoplexy. *Journal of Clinical Neuroscience*. 2014;21(3):510–512.
21. Kingdon C, Sidhu P, Cohen J. Pituitary apoplexy secondary to an underlying abscess. *Journal of Infection*. 1996;33(1):53–55.
22. Chhiber SS, Bhat AR, Khan SH, et al. Apoplexy in sellar metastasis: a case report and review of literature. *Turkish neurosurgery*. 2011;21(2):230–234.
23. Glezer A, Bronstein MD, Glezer A, Bronstein MD. Pituitary apoplexy: pathophysiology, diagnosis and management. *Archives of Endocrinology and Metabolism*. 2015;59(3):259–264.
24. González-González JG, Borjas-Almaguer OD, Salcido-Montenegro A, et al. Sheehan's syndrome revisited: underlying autoimmunity or hypoperfusion? *Int J Endocrinol*. 2018;2018.
25. Goyal P, Utz M, Gupta N, et al. Clinical and imaging features of pituitary apoplexy and role of imaging in differentiation of clinical mimics. *Quant Imaging Med Surg*. 2018;8(2):219–231.
26. Karaca Z, Tanriverdi F, Unluhizarci K, Kelestimur F. Pregnancy and pituitary disorders. *Eur J Endocrinol*. 2010;162(3):453–475.
27. Goshtasbi K, Abiri A, Sahyouni R, et al. Visual and endocrine recovery following conservative and surgical treatment of pituitary apoplexy: a meta-analysis. *World Neurosurgery*. 2019;132:33–40.
28. Kim JH, Dho Y-S, Kim YH, et al. Developing an optimal follow-up strategy based on the natural history of nonfunctioning pituitary adenomas. *Journal of Neurosurgery*. 2018;131(2):500–506.
29. Boguszewski CL, de Castro Musolino NR, Kasuki L. Management of pituitary incidentaloma. *Best Practice & Research Clinical Endocrinology & Metabolism*. 2019;33(2):101268.
30. Fernández-Balsells MM, Murad MH, Barwise A, et al. Natural history of nonfunctioning pituitary adenomas and incidentalomas: a systematic review and metaanalysis. *J Clin Endocrinol Metab*. 2011;96(4): 905–912.
31. Hosmann A, Micko A, Frischer JM, et al. Multiple pituitary apoplexy—cavernous sinus invasion as major risk factor for recurrent hemorrhage. *World Neurosurgery*. 2019;126:e723–e730.
32. Zaidi HA, Cote DJ, Burke WT, et al. Time course of symptomatic recovery after endoscopic transsphenoidal surgery for pituitary adenoma apoplexy in the modern era. *World Neurosurgery*. 2016;96:434–439.
33. Almeida JP, Sanchez MM, Karekezi C, et al. Pituitary apoplexy: results of surgical and conservative management clinical series and review of the literature. *World Neurosurgery*. 2019;130:e988–e999.
34. Kim Y-H, Cho YH, Hong SH, et al. Postoperative neurologic outcome in patients with pituitary apoplexy after transsphenoidal surgery. *World Neurosurgery*. 2018;111:e18–e23.
35. Culpin E, Crank M, Igra M, et al. Pituitary tumour apoplexy within prolactinomas in children: a more aggressive condition? *Pituitary*. 2018;21(5):474–479.
36. Jankowski PP, Crawford JR, Khanna P, Malicki DM, Ciacci JD, Levy ML. Pituitary tumor apoplexy in adolescents. *World Neurosurgery*. 2015;83(4):644–651.
37. Oldfield EH, Merrill MJ. Apoplexy of pituitary adenomas: the perfect storm. *Journal of Neurosurgery*. 2015;122(6):1444–1449.
38. Ogawa Y, Niizuma K, Mugikura S, Tominaga T. Ischemic pituitary adenoma apoplexy—clinical appearance and prognosis after surgical intervention. *Clinical Neurology and Neurosurgery*. 2016;148:142–146.
39. Gupta P, Dutta P. Landscape of molecular events in pituitary apoplexy. *Front Endocrinol*. 2018;9.
40. Aftab H, Zia B, Thim M, Malhotra N. Nonhemorrhagic pituitary apoplexy following CABG surgery. *J Endocr Soc*. 2019;3(Suppl 1):SUN–423.
41. Crisman C, Ward M, Majmundar N, et al. Pituitary apoplexy following endoscopic retrograde cholangiopancreatography. *World Neurosurgery*. 2019;121:201–204.
42. Joo C, Ha G, Jang Y. Pituitary apoplexy following lumbar fusion surgery in prone position. *Medicine (Baltimore)*. 2018;97(19).
43. Laluz V, Codorniz K. A case of pituitary apoplexy complicating the management of sepsis. *Loma Linda University Student Journal*. 2018;3(1).

44. Uneda A, Hirashita K, Yunoki M, Yoshino K, Date I. Pituitary adenoma apoplexy associated with vardenafil intake. *Acta Neurochir*. 2019;161(1):129–131.
45. Shetty S, Gnanaraj J, Jayamani Roshan S, El Accaoui R. Pituitary apoplexy after regadenoson myocardial perfusion scan. *J Nucl Cardiol*. 2020;27:336–339.
46. Abbott J, Kirkby GR. Acute visual loss and pituitary apoplexy after surgery. *BMJ*. 2004;329(7459):218–219.
47. Fanous N, Srihari A, Roper S, Woodmansee W. Pituitary apoplexy associated with apixaban. *J Endocr Soc*. 2019;3(Suppl 1):SUN–420.
48. Ly S, Naman A, Chaufour-Higel B, et al. Pituitary apoplexy and rivaroxaban. *Pituitary*. 2017;20(6):709–710.
49. Willamowicz AS, Houlden RL. Pituitary apoplexy after anticoagulation for unstable angina. *Endocrine Practice*. 1999;5(5):273–276.
50. Banerjee C, Snelling B, Hanft S, Komotar RJ. Bilateral cerebral infarction in the setting of pituitary apoplexy: a case presentation and literature review. *Pituitary*. 2015;18(3):352–358.
51. Billeci D, Marton E, Giordan E. Post-traumatic pituitary apoplexy: case presentation and review of literature. *Interdisciplinary Neurosurgery*. 2017;7:4–8.
52. Jang J-H, Ko YS, Hong EK, Gwak H-S. Extensive pituitary apoplexy after chemotherapy in a patient with metastatic breast cancer. *Brain Tumor Research and Treatment*. 2018;6(1):43–46.
53. Maki Y, Kurosaki Y, Uchino K, Ishibashi R, Chin M, Yamagata S. Pituitary apoplexy in long-term cabergoline user during thrombocytopenia due to chemotherapy for chronic myelocytic leukemia. *World Neurosurgery*. 2018;120:290–295.
54. Annamalai AK, Jeyachitra G, Jeyamithra A, Ganeshkumar M, Srinivasan KG, Gurnell M. Gestational pituitary apoplexy. *Indian J Endocrinol Metab*. 2017;21(3):484–485.
55. Grand'Maison S, Weber F, Bédard M-J, Mahone M, Godbout A. Pituitary apoplexy in pregnancy: a case series and literature review. *Obstet Med*. 2015;8(4):177–183.
56. Sangtian J, Ruanpeng D, Araki T. CRH induced pituitary apoplexy during IPSS in Cushing disease. *Endocrine Practice*. 2019;25:233–234.
57. Chanson P, Raverot G, Castinetti F, Cortet-Rudelli C, Galland F, Salenave S. Management of clinically non-functioning pituitary adenoma. *Annales d'Endocrinologie*. 2015;76(3):239–247.
58. Fabiano AJ, George S. Pituitary apoplexy after initial leuprolide injection. *World Neurosurgery*. 2016;95:616.
59. Jaggi S, Slone H, Strauss R, Zaeeter W, Palli V. Leuprolide injection induced pituitary apoplexy. *J Endocr Soc*. 2019;3(Suppl 1):SUN–421.
60. Keane F, Egan AM, Navin P, Brett F, Dennedy MC. Gonadotropin-releasing hormone agonist-induced pituitary apoplexy. *Endocrinol Diabetes Metab Case Rep*. 2016;2016:160021.
61. Sasagawa Y, Tachibana O, Nakagawa A, Koya D, Iizuka H. Pituitary apoplexy following gonadotropin-releasing hormone agonist administration with gonadotropin-secreting pituitary adenoma. *Journal of Clinical Neuroscience*. 2015;22(3):601–603.
62. Ghadirian H, Shirani M, Ghazi-Mirsaeed S, Mohebi S, Alimohamadi M. Pituitary apoplexy during treatment of prolactinoma with cabergoline. *Asian J Neurosurg*. 2018;13(1):93–95.
63. Brougham M, Heusner AP, Adams RD. Acute degenerative changes in adenomas of the pituitary body—with special reference to pituitary apoplexy. *Journal of Neurosurgery*. 1950;7(5):421–439.
64. Rais NC, Merchant RA, Seetharaman SK. Pituitary apoplexy masquerading as functional decline in an older person. *Age Ageing*. 2017;46(2):335–336.
65. Lubbe DE, Mankahla N, Carrara H, Semple P. Surgical intervention for binocular blindness in pituitary apoplexy. *Interdisciplinary Neurosurgery*. 2019;18:100490.
66. Hage R, Eshraghi SR, Oyesiku NM, et al. Third, fourth, and sixth cranial nerve palsies in pituitary apoplexy. *World Neurosurgery*. 2016;94:447–452.
67. Sussman ES, Ho AL, Pendharkar AV, Achrol AS, Harsh GR. Pituitary apoplexy associated with carotid compression and a large ischemic penumbra. *World Neurosurgery*. 2016;92:581.
68. Douleh DG, Morone PJ, Mobley B, Fusco MR, Chambless LB. Angioplasty is an effective treatment for vasospasm following pituitary apoplexy and tumor resection. *Cureus*. 2018;10(1).
69. Gambaracci G, Rondoni V, Guercini G, Floridi P. Pituitary apoplexy complicated by vasospasm and bilateral cerebral infarction. *BMJ Case Rep*. 2016;2016.
70. Rajasekaran S, Vanderpump M, Baldeweg S, et al. UK guidelines for the management of pituitary apoplexy. *Clinical Endocrinology*. 2011;74(1):9–20.

71. Watthanasuntorn K, Lertjitbanjong P, Hughes J. Pituitary apoplexy, an unexpected cause of syncope: case report. *J Endocr Soc.* 2019;3(Suppl 1):SUN–425.
72. Yoshino M, Sekine Y, Koh E, Hata A, Hashimoto N. Pituitary apoplexy after surgical treatment of lung cancer. *The Annals of Thoracic Surgery.* 2014;98(5):1830–1832.
73. Ishii M. Endocrine emergencies with neurologic manifestations. *Continuum (Minneap Minn).* 2017;23(3): 778–801.
74. Burns J, Policeni B, Bykowski J, et al. ACR appropriateness criteria® neuroendocrine imaging. *Journal of the American College of Radiology.* 2019;16(5, Supplement):S161–S173.
75. Barkhoudarian G, Kelly DF. Pituitary apoplexy. *Neurosurgery Clinics of North America.* 2019;30(4):457–463.
76. Ramos R, Machado MJ, Antunes C, Fernandes V, Marques O, Almeida R. Metastasis of a dorsal melanoma to a pituitary adenoma mimicking pituitary apoplexy. *Arq Bras Neurocir.* 2017;36(04):238–242.
77. Baldeweg SE, Vanderpump M, Drake W, et al. Society for Endocrinology Endocrine Emergency Guidance: emergency management of pituitary apoplexy in adult patients. *Endocr Connect.* 2016;5(5):G12–G15.
78. Lucas JW, Bodach ME, Tumialan LM, et al. Congress of Neurological Surgeons systematic review and evidence-based guideline on primary management of patients with nonfunctioning pituitary adenomas. *Neurosurgery.* 2016;79(4):E533–E535.
79. Sheehan J, Lee C-C, Bodach ME, et al. Congress of Neurological Surgeons systematic review and evidence-based guideline for the management of patients with residual or recurrent nonfunctioning pituitary adenomas. *Neurosurgery.* 2016;79(4):E539–E540.
80. Pineyro MM, Furtenbach P, Lima R, Wajskopf S, Sgarbi N, Pisabarro R. Brain and optic chiasm herniation into sella after pituitary tumor apoplexy. *Front Endocrinol.* 2017;8.
81. Patel DM, Miller JH, Omar NB, et al. Hemorrhagic and non-hemorrhagic pituitary apoplexy: clinical analysis. *Journal of Advances in Medicine and Medical Research.* 2016;12(7):1–9.
82. Tu M, Lu Q, Zhu P, Zheng W. Surgical versus non-surgical treatment for pituitary apoplexy: a systematic review and meta-analysis. *Journal of the Neurological Sciences.* 2016;370:258–262.
83. Sahyouni R, Goshtasbi K, Choi E, et al. Vision outcomes in early versus late surgical intervention of pituitary apoplexy: meta-analysis. *World Neurosurgery.* 2019;127:52–57.
84. Freda PU, Beckers AM, Katznelson L, et al. Pituitary incidentaloma: an Endocrine Society clinical practice guideline. *J Clin Endocrinol Metab.* 2011;96(4):894–904.
85. Ziu M, Dunn IF, Hess C, et al. Congress of Neurological Surgeons systematic review and evidence-based guideline on posttreatment follow-up evaluation of patients with nonfunctioning pituitary adenomas. *Neurosurgery.* 2016;79(4):E541–E543.
86. Maccagnan P, Macedo C, Kayath M, Nogueira R, Abucham J. Conservative management of pituitary apoplexy: a prospective study. *The Journal of clinical endocrinology and metabolism.* 1995;80:2190–2197.

PART 8

Endocrine Emergencies During Pregnancy

CHAPTER 22

Endocrine Emergencies in Obstetrics

Christopher G. Goodier ■ Aundrea Eason Loftley

CHAPTER OUTLINE

Thyroid Storm

Diabetic Ketoacidosis

Hyperparathyroidism

Thyroid Storm

Thyroid storm is a rare but life-threatening endocrine emergency occurring in 1% to 2% of pregnant women with hyperthyroidism. It typically has an acute onset and is associated with the following symptoms: fever, tachycardia, and central nervous system dysfunction (restlessness, altered mental status, and seizures). Untreated, it can lead to significant morbidity and mortality, including cardiac dysrhythmia, multiorgan failure, and even death. Case fatality rates range from 10% to 30% in the literature.[1] Given the severity of the disease process, a high clinical suspicion, rapid recognition, intervention, and supportive care are needed to maximize both maternal and fetal outcome.

Although the exact triggering mechanism is unknown, most cases are due to poorly controlled hyperthyroidism. Events such as pre-eclampsia, trauma, ketoacidosis, surgery, and infection have been associated with storm.[2,3] A careful search for underlying associated etiologies should be performed concurrent with treatment.

A high clinical suspicion is needed as the presenting signs and symptoms may be nonspecific enough to be confused with any number of other conditions.[4] Elevated blood pressure, headaches, abdominal pain, and even pulmonary edema or heart failure are features compatible with pre-eclampsia that may make the diagnosis of thyroid storm more difficult.[5]

The physiologic changes of pregnancy result in a compensated respiratory alkalosis, thus consultation with an obstetrician or Maternal Fetal Medicine specialist is suggested. Metabolic changes can lead to fetal heart rate tracing abnormalities, including tachycardia, loss of variability, and late decelerations, ultimately resulting in increased fetal morbidity and mortality.[6]

Laboratory analysis includes thyroid-stimulating hormone (TSH), free triiodothyronine (FT3) and free thyroxine (FT4), complete blood count (CBC), and complete metabolic panel (CMP). TSH is typically undetectable in thyroid storm, although cautious interpretation is required in the first trimester, as human chorionic gonadotropin (hCG) can bind to the TSH receptors present in thyroid tissue and act like a weak form of TSH. There are no generally accepted levels of thyroid hormone in maternal serum at which the diagnosis of thyroid storm is assured. FT4 and FT3 are often well above the upper limits of normal in pregnancy. Total hormone levels are also usually elevated, thus there may be significant laboratory overlap with simple hyperthyroidism. There is typically an associated leukocytosis as well as evidence of hyperglycemia, hypercalcemia, elevated liver enzymes, and electrolyte disturbances on metabolic panel screening.

Given a high incidence of case fatality rates and the need for early recognition, Burch and Wartofsky have outlined a commonly cited clinical scoring system for the probability of thyroid storm. Points are allocated for elevation in temperature, maternal pulse, and a number of organ system dysfunctions indicating a high, medium, or low probability of the diagnosis. A score of 45 or more is highly indicative of thyroid storm, a score of 25 or less makes the diagnosis unlikely and scores between 25 and 45 are suggestive and rely strongly on the use of clinical context.[7]

A diagnosis of thyroid storm requires prompt intervention for both mother and fetus, and treatment should not be delayed. A multidisciplinary approach to management is recommended, including Maternal Fetal Medicine, Endocrinology, Neonatology, and Critical Care specialists. In addition, preparation should be made for admission to an intensive care unit (ICU), with the availability of continuous fetal monitoring if the fetus has reached viability. Treating the underlying maternal metabolic derangement(s) is key to improving fetal status, thus it is important to exhaust all attempts to correct the underlying maternal abnormalities prior to intervening for the fetus.[8] The presence of a persistent fetal bradycardia or the development of category III fetal heart rate tracing that is unresponsive to resuscitative measures may require expedited delivery.

Intravenous access should be obtained, and cooling measures performed. Fluid balance and vital signs, including continuous pulse oximetry, need to be carefully monitored. An initial electrocardiogram (ECG) and continuous telemetry are recommended to identify arrhythmias. In addition, some patients can have thyrotoxic heart failure due to the myocardial effects of excess FT4, thus any cardiorespiratory complaints should be thoroughly evaluated, including echocardiography. Treatment is generally the same for thyroid storm and thyrotoxic heart failure, even in pregnancy.

The treatment of thyroid storm involves the use of several medications to decrease the level of thyroid hormone. Propylthiouracil (PTU) and methimazole (MMI) are thionamides and act within the thyroid gland to inhibit follicular growth and development, as well as the packaging of iodothyronines into T4 and T3.[9] PTU has the advantage of antithyroid effects within the thyroid gland as well as inhibiting the peripheral conversion at the tissue level, limiting the active form of thyroid hormone. However, there is a significant disadvantage of the use of PTU in that there have been rare cases of fulminate liver failure and death associated with its use, including instances in pregnancy. There is a Food and Drug Administration (FDA) "black box" warning for PTU concerning this link to hepatotoxicity. It is unclear how thyroid storm specifically affects this risk. MMI use in the first trimester of pregnancy has been linked to some teratogenic effects, specifically aplasia cutis and choanal atresia.[10] In addition, rarely a life-threatening agranulocytosis may develop after MMI and PTU use. Given these conflicting risks, there is no clear recommendation for which thionamide to initiate in thyroid storm in pregnancy; however, MMI is generally avoided in the first trimester.

Additionally, an iodide-containing medication to inhibit the further release of active thyroid hormone from the thyroid gland may be used. Oral potassium iodide, five drops every 8 hours, or intravenous sodium iodide 500 to 1000 mg every 8 to 12 hours may be used. It is important to be aware of the paradoxical release of thyroid hormone from the thyroid gland associated with iodide use; thus it is important to start iodine administration approximately 1 hour after the use of thionamides.[9] Corticosteroids are also an important treatment of thyroid storm, as they decrease systemic inflammation, as well as having the peripheral effects of decreasing T4 to T3 conversion. Beta-blockers such as propranolol or metoprolol will also reduce peripheral conversion of T4 to T3, and lessen the complications of tachycardia, such as high-output cardiac failure. Long-term use of beta-blockers has been associated with fetal growth restriction, but is generally considered safe in a risk/benefit consideration with the exception of atenolol. Other supportive medications include antipyretics such as acetaminophen (Table 22.1).

Conventional treatments may fail after trials of medical management in the most severe cases. There also may be adverse reactions to the thionamides, which may require discontinuation. Emergency thyroidectomy, with or without plasmapheresis, has been described successfully in thyroid storm, but must be considered high-risk and last-line treatment and can be performed in pregnancy.[11]

TABLE 22.1 ■ **Thyroid Storm Treatment**

	Treatment	Dose
MATERNAL	Supportive care	
	IV access	LR bolus then IVF at 150–250 mL/hour
		Continuous pulse oximetry, serial BP
	Consultation	ICU admission, Critical Care, Endocrine, Maternal Fetal Medicine
	Cooling measures	Acetaminophen 500 mg q6 hour
		Cooling blankets
	Testing	
	Laboratory	TSH, fT3/4, CBC diff, ABG, CMP
	Ancillary	ECG/telemetry, CXR, ECG
		Additional testing as needed (cultures, CT scan, etc.)
	Medications	
	First-line	Propylthiouracil (PTU) 300 mg PO or NG q6 hour
		Methimazole 20–25 mg PO q6–q8 hour (total daily dose 60–80 mg). Do not use methimazole during the first trimester
	Initial dose given 30–60 minutes after PTU	Potassium iodide (SSKI) 5 drops PO/NG q8 hour
	Block T4→T3 conversion	Dexamethasone 2 mg IV q6 hour × 4 doses
	Heart rate control (goal< 120 bpm)[a]	Propranolol 40–60 mg PO/NG q6 hour (IV alternative = propranolol prn or esmolol drip)
	Therapies not recommended	Radioiodine (contraindicated)
		Thionamide and levothyroxine combination therapy (insufficient evidence)
FETAL		
	Monitoring	Consult Maternal Fetal Medicine
		Initiate fetal monitoring if viability achieved
	Fetal optimization	Maternal left lateral decubitus
		Maternal O_2 supplementation
		Stabilize maternal condition PRIOR to delivery

[a]Ensure no evidence of heart failure or medical contraindication (e.g., asthma).
ABG, Arterial blood gas; *BP,* blood pressure; *bpm,* beats per minute; *CBC,* complete blood count; *CMP,* complete metabolic panel; *CT,* computed tomography; *CXR,* chest X-ray; *FT3/4,* free T3/T4; *ICU,* intensive care unit; *IVF,* intravenous fluid; *LR,* lactated Ringer's; *NG,* nasogastric; *PO,* by mouth; *prn,* as needed; *q,* every; *TSH,* thyroid-stimulating hormone.

In summary, thyroid storm is a rare, life-threatening condition that requires early recognition, multidisciplinary care, and aggressive therapy.

Diabetic Ketoacidosis

Like thyroid storm, diabetic ketoacidosis (DKA) is a medical emergency, which can result in both maternal and fetal morbidity and mortality. With early recognition and aggressive multidisciplinary management, the overall incidence has decreased from approximately 10% to 20% in the late 1970s to approximately 1% to 2% in most recent reports,[12–14] resulting in improved maternal and fetal mortality. Preterm birth, both from premature labor and from medical intervention, is a common occurrence after DKA.

The pathophysiology of DKA occurs due to the lack of insulin resulting in a perceived hypoglycemia at target cells. Glucagon is subsequently released, increasing serum glucose and leading to osmotic diuresis, which results in hypovolemia and electrolyte depletion.

Counterregulatory hormones release free fatty acids into the circulation, which are then oxidized to ketone bodies leading to a metabolic acidosis, which manifests as an anion gap. Ketoacids bind sodium and potassium, which are excreted in the urine, further worsening the electrolyte balance. If untreated, patients can experience cardiac dysfunction, decreased tissue perfusion, and worsened real function leading to shock, coma, and death.[12,15]

The normal physiologic changes of pregnancy increase the susceptibility to DKA. Insulin resistance, primarily due to human placental lactogen, cause insulin requirements to increase with advancing gestation. Respiratory adaptations during pregnancy result in a compensated maternal respiratory alkalosis. The associated decrease in serum bicarbonate reduces the body's normal buffering capacity, thus predisposing the patient to DKA.[12,13,15]

Although DKA more commonly affects those with type 1 diabetes, it can also be seen in patients with type 2 diabetes, ketosis prone diabetes, and latent autoimmune diabetes of adulthood (also known as LADA or "type 1.5"). Patients who are in DKA generally present with abdominal pain, malaise, persistent vomiting, increased thirst, hyperventilation, tachycardia, dehydration, and polyuria. Mental status changes can be seen as the level of acidosis worsens. The diagnosis is confirmed with documentation of hyperglycemia, acidosis, and ketonuria. Other laboratory findings include anion gap, ketonemia, renal dysfunction, and electrolyte abnormalities.[13,15] Typically, patients present with severely elevated serum glucose levels; however, DKA can occur with levels less than 200 mg/dL in pregnancy.[14] Euglycemic DKA (euDKA) and has been described in susceptible patient populations such as those with poor oral intake (prolonged period of fasting), pregnant patients, and nonpregnant patients who are treated with sodium-glucose cotransporter 2 (SGLT-2) inhibitors.[16]

Precipitating factors in pregnancy include emesis, infection, beta-sympathomimetic tocolytic agents, corticosteroids, poor compliance, and medical errors.[17,18] Although beta-sympathomimetics (e.g., terbutaline) are not routinely used for prolonged (greater than 48 hours) tocolysis due to the FDA safety communication in 2011, it is important to remember that they should be used very cautiously, if ever, for patients with diabetes.[12]

Although the mechanism is not clearly understood, DKA presents a significant risk to overall fetal well-being. The likely mechanism is related to maternal ketoacids that cross the placenta and lead to decreased fetal tissue perfusion and oxygenation.[15] The fetus has a limited ability to buffer significant acidemia, and therefore is quite sensitive to maternal acidosis. This often results in alterations of the fetal heart rate tracing, including decreased variability and/or late decelerations, which reflect fetal hypoxemia and acidosis. It is important to exhaust all attempts to correct the underlying maternal abnormalities prior to intervening for the fetus, as once maternal status stabilizes, the fetal status will generally follow.[14,15]

Like thyroid storm, DKA is considered a medical emergency and a multidisciplinary team, including Maternal Fetal Medicine, Endocrinology, Neonatology, and Critical Care, should be assembled. In addition, strong consideration should be made for admission to an ICU.

Treatment includes adequate intravenous access and placement of an indwelling urinary catheter. Significant fluid deficits should be anticipated and corrected. Insulin should be started and electrolyte abnormalities corrected. Fluid balance and vital signs need to be carefully monitored and documented.

A CMP with magnesium and phosphorous, CBC with differential, urinalysis, fingerstick blood glucose, arterial blood gas, and serum ketones should be collected. Additional testing (urine culture, blood culture, chest X-ray, etc.) should be performed based on clinical suspicion and any potential underlying processes. Initially, serum ketones, electrolytes, and maternal acid/base status

TABLE 22.2 ■ **Treatment of DKA**

	Treatment Modality	Plan
MATERNAL	Identify cause	H&P, rule out infection, place Foley catheter, serial vital signs, I/Os Consider ICU admission, Consult Critical Care, Endocrinology, Maternal Fetal Medicine
	Fluid replacement (estimated ~ 100 mL/kg)	Correct 75% total deficit in first 24 hours Begin with 0.9% normal saline Convert to D5 0.45% normal saline when FSBG < 250
	Insulin administration	Regular insulin via IV IV bolus 0.1 u/kg followed by 0.1 u/kg per hour continuous infusion
	Goal FSBG 150–200 in DKA	Goal reduction 20%–25% over 2 hours (if not increase IV infusion 1.5–2×) Continue IV insulin until acidosis and ketosis resolves Start SQ insulin therapy 1–2 hours PRIOR to stopping IV insulin
	Laboratory evaluation	CMP/Mg and Phos, pH, serum ketones every 2–4 hours initially Replete K+ once <5 mmol/L (goal 4–5) Replete HCO_3 if ph <6.9 with $NaHCO_3$ until pH >7.0
FETAL		
	Monitoring Fetal optimization	Consult Maternal Fetal Medicine Initiate fetal monitoring if viability achieved Maternal left lateral decubitus Maternal O_2 supplementation Stabilize maternal condition PRIOR to delivery

CMP, Complete metabolic panel; *DKA,* diabetic ketoacidosis; *FSBG,* finger stick blood glucose; *H&P,* history and physical; *HCO_3,* bicarbonate; *ICU,* intensive care unit; *I/Os,* input/output; *K+,* potassium; *Mg,* magnesium; *$NaHCO_3$,* sodium bicarbonate; *Phos.,* phosphorus; *SQ,* subcutaneous.

should be monitored every 2 hours until ketosis and acidosis resolved. Blood sugars should be collected hourly during this time to titrate insulin.[12,13,15–19]

Once viability is confirmed, fetal monitoring should be initiated. As noted, the fetal heart tracing will likely appear concerning during the initial phase of metabolic compromise. Maternal oxygen supplementation and left lateral decubitus positioning should be used to increase blood flow to fetus and improve oxygenation. Adequate hydration and correction of acid/base derangements must be started. Delivery is generally postponed until after the maternal metabolic condition is stabilized, as this will usually correct the fetal heart tracing abnormality. There are exceptions, including severely prolonged bradycardia or a persistent category III tracing.

Table 22.2 illustrates a general algorithm for the treatment of diabetic ketoacidosis in pregnancy, including rehydration, reduction of hyperglycemia, and correction of acid-base and electrolyte imbalance, while searching for and treating the underlying etiology.[12,13,15–19]

The hypovolemia associated with DKA is estimated at 100 mL/kg of total body weight and is typically 4 to 10 L.[20] Aggressive intravenous replacement with isotonic normal saline should be started with the goal to replace approximately 75% of the overall deficit within the first 24 hours. Hypotonic fluids (e.g., lactated ringers and 0.45% saline) should be avoided initially as they can cause a rapid decline in plasma osmolarity leading to maternal cerebral edema. Blood glucose values should be monitored hourly and once the serum glucose reaches less than 250 mg/dL, intravenous fluids should be switched to D5 – 0.45% normal saline.

Intravenous insulin administration should be undertaken immediately to aid in lowering blood glucose levels to an initial goal of 150 to 200 mg/dL in order to avoid rapid correction and resulting complications. Blood glucose levels should be monitored hourly while the patient is receiving intravenous insulin. Subcutaneous and intramuscular insulin are typically avoided due to the slower onset of action, which is worsened in DKA.[12] It is important to remember that insulin requirements can be significant, and most protocols suggest an initial bolus dose of 10 to 20 units of regular insulin, followed by an infusion rate of 5 to 10 units/hour. This amount should be increased if the blood glucose values do not fall by 20% to 25% over 2 hours. The amount of insulin required to achieve target blood sugar levels is largely affected by factors such as diabetes subtype and degree of hypovolemia present.

It is important to continue the insulin infusion until the anion gap is closed and acidosis is resolved. This can take significantly longer than correcting the hyperglycemia and typically takes 12 to 24 hours. Once it is deemed safe to transition to subcutaneous insulin, the first dose of a long- or intermediate-acting analog should be given 2 hours prior to the discontinuation of the intravenous infusion to decrease the risk of recurrent ketoacidosis.

Potassium is the most common electrolyte abnormality in DKA, although levels are often normal initially. The actual deficit is estimated at 5 to 10 mEq/kg. Once the serum potassium level falls below 5 mmol/L, intravenous replacement should begin with the goal to maintain potassium levels between 4 and 5 mmol/L. Adequate renal function should be documented prior to replacing potassium. Serum potassium levels should be checked every 2 to 4 hours as significant hypokalemia can precipitate a cardiac arrhythmia.

Replacement of low serum bicarbonate levels remain a source of controversy and replacement is generally agreed upon if the patient's pH is less than 7.0. Some studies have shown that routine replacement of low serum levels of bicarbonate have not proven beneficial in DKA and may cause unnecessary maternal and fetal complications. Replacement can delay the correction of ketoacidosis in the maternal bloodstream and, if corrected too rapidly, elevate fetal partial pressure of carbon dioxide (PCO_2) impairing fetal ability to maintain adequate O_2 transfer.[12,19]

The management approach that we have described for DKA is also applicable to the treatment of hyperosmolar hyperglycemic state (HHS). DKA and HHS differ based on the severity of hyperglycemia (more severe in HHS) and the presence of ketoacidosis (seen in DKA).

Effective management of hyperglycemic crises during pregnancy requires an interdisciplinary team approach. With the appropriate management strategies in place, the team can help reduce the likelihood of prenatal morbidity and mortality.

Hyperparathyroidism

Primary hyperparathyroidism (pHPT) is the third most common endocrine disorder (prevalence 0.1% to 0.4% in the general population) and is rare in pregnancy. In a review by Ruda et al., solid parathyroid disorders account for 80% of cases in the general population, with the remaining cases a result of diffuse hyperplasia and adenomas.[21]

Although the incidence of pHPT during pregnancy is rare, the maternal and fetal complications of moderate to severe disease can be significant in the absence of an appropriate management strategy. Maternal and fetal complications are rare when the degree of hypercalcemia is mild.

The diagnosis requires an elevated total calcium level adjusted for serum albumin (serum calcium + 0.8 × [4 – serum albumin]) or elevated serum ionized calcium level with an elevated parathyroid hormone level. Patients with hyperparathyroidism caused by a parathyroid adenoma or hyperplasia typically have inappropriately high PTH secretion in relation to the serum calcium concentration. It is important to mention that 10% of patients with pHPT have a normal-range PTH level in the setting of hypercalcemia.[22,23] This can lead to diagnostic uncertainly, as there is a smaller population of patients who will also have this laboratory pattern but have familial hypocalciuric hypercalcemia (FHH). FHH is a genetic disorder resulting in a mutation in the calcium sensing receptor and is characterized by mild hypercalcemia, a normal or slightly elevated PTH level, and hypocalciuria. It is important to distinguish pHPT from FHH because parathyroidectomy is not indicated in patients with FHH. The calcium/creatine clearance ratio can be calculated and is used to distinguish pHPT from FHH.[22,23]

In pregnancy, most patients with pHPT are asymptomatic and undiagnosed, as routine calcium levels are not checked. In addition, nausea and vomiting are common in pregnancy and more commonly associated with pregnancy associated physiologic changes.[24] Pregnancy tends to offer protection from maternal hypercalcemia, due to transplacental transport to meet fetal needs, especially during the third trimester. This protection is eliminated after delivery, and thus there is an increased risk of maternal hypercalcemia in the puerperal period. Pregnancy may also confer a physiologic benefit in women with underlying pHPT due to the reduction in serum calcium levels that occurs as a result of increased volume expansion, which is most significant during the third trimester. For this reason, nonpregnant reference ranges for serum calcium should not be used; however, the ionized calcium level is unaffected by the physiologic changes that occur during pregnancy, and nonpregnant reference ranges remain appropriate.[25]

Among women who are symptomatic and have mild to moderate disease, maternal symptoms typically include nausea, vomiting, anorexia, constipation, depression, and mental confusion. Kidney stones, pancreatitis, and abdominal pain as well as ECG changes including short QT interval and arrhythmia can be seen.

In pregnancy the most common presenting symptom is renal colic secondary to nephrolithiasis.[26] pHPT is more often associated with pancreatitis in the pregnant population (7% to 13%) than in the nonpregnant state. This is thought to be secondary to elevated serum calcium levels resulting in damaged pancreatic ducts.[27] Other clinical findings that can be seen in pregnancy include hypertension and preeclampsia. pHPT does not seem to be associated with increased risk of miscarriage; however, without treatment, fetal complications can be seen in up to 80% of pregnancies, specifically neonatal hypocalcemia, preterm birth, intrauterine growth restriction, and stillbirth. Elevated maternal PTH levels can result in suppression of fetal PTH production with subsequent neonatal hypocalcemia and tetany in pregnancies complicated with moderate to severe hypercalcemia.[28,29] These complications can be significantly reduced with maternal treatment and neonatal evaluation.[30,31]

Once the diagnosis of hyperparathyroidism is ascertained, a careful search for the underlying etiology should begin. In pregnant women who are appropriate candidates for parathyroidectomy, preoperative localization should be done with ultrasound. Sestamibi and computed tomography scans should be avoided due to radiation exposure. Surgical removal of the parathyroid glands is generally reserved for symptomatic hypercalcemia and preferred in the second trimester due to decreased maternal and fetal risks. It is the only definitive treatment.[32,33]

In asymptomatic patients with mild hypercalcemia, treatment of pHPT includes conservative therapy such as increased fluids and decreased calcium intake with vitamin D supplementation. Calcitonin does not cross the placenta and thus is likely safe; however, it is not generally effective. Bisphosphonates should be avoided unless absolutely necessary due to the effect on fetal bones.

In summary, the appropriate management of pHPT during pregnancy can help mitigate potential adverse maternal and fetal outcomes.

References

1. Tietgens ST, Leinung MC. Thyroid storm. *Med Clin North Am.* 1995;79:169–184.
2. Goldberg PA. Critical issues in endocrinology. *Clin Chest Med.* 2003;24:583–606.

3. Parker JA, Conway DL. Diabetic ketoacidosis in pregnancy. *Obstet Gynecol Clin N Am*. 2007;34:533–543.
4. Nayak B, Burman K. Thyrotoxicosis and thyroid storm. *Endocrinol Metab Clin N Am*. 2006;35:663–686.
5. Sugiyama Y, Tanaka R, Yoshiyama Y, et al. A case of sudden onset thyroid storm just before cesarean section manifesting congestive heart failure and pulmonary edema. *JA Clinical Reports*. 2017;3:20.
6. Delport EF. A thyroid-related endocrine emergency in pregnancy. *JEMDSA*. 2009;14(2):199–201.
7. Burch HB, Wartofsky L. Thyroid storm. *Endocrinol Metab Clin North Am*. 1993;22:266–277.
8. Rashid M, Rashid MH. Obstetric management of thyroid disease. *Obstet Gynecol Surv*. 2007;62(10): 680–688.
9. Bahn RS, Burch H, Copper D, et al. Hyperthyroidism and other causes of thyrotoxicosis: management guidelines of the ATA and the AACE. *Endocr Pract*. 2011;17(3):456–520.
10. Gianantonio E, Schaefer C, Mastroiacovo P. Adverse fetal effects of prenatal methimazole exposure. *Teratology*. 2001;64(5):262–266.
11. Vyas AA, Vyas P, Fillipon NP, et al. Successful treatment of thyroid storm with plasmapheresis in a patient with MMI-induced agranulocytosis. *Endocr Pract*. 2010;16(4):673–676.
12. Parker JA, Conway DL. Diabetic ketoacidosis in pregnancy. *Obstet Gynecol Clin N Am*. 2007;34:533–543.
13. Abdu TAM, Barton DM, Baskar V, Kamalakannan D. Diabetic ketoacidosis in pregnancy. *Postgrad Med J*. 2003;79(934):454.
14. Whiteman VE, Homko CJ, Reece EA. Management of hypoglycemia and diabetic ketoacidosis in pregnancy. *Obstet GynecolClinics*. 1996;23(1):88–107.
15. Carroll M, Yeomans ER. Diabetic ketoacidosis in pregnancy. *Crit Care Med*. 2005;33:S347–S353.
16. Peters AL, Buschur EO, Buse JB, et al. Euglycemic diabetic ketoacidosis: a potential complication of treatment with sodium-glucose cotransporter 2 inhibition. *Diabetes Care*. 2015;38:1687.
17. Rogers BD, Rogers DE. Clinical variable associated with diabetic ketoacidosis during pregnancy. *J Reprod Med*. 1991;36:797–800.
18. Montoro MN, Myers VP, Mestman JH, et al. Outcome of pregnancy in diabetic ketoacidosis. *Am J Peritanol*. 1993;10:17–20.
19. Foley MR, Strong TH, Garite TJ. *Obstetric Intensive Care Manual*. 2nd ed. New York: McGraw Hill Publishers; 2004.
20. Chauhan SP, Perry KG, McLaughlin BN, Roberts WE, Sullivan CA, Morrison JC. Diabetic ketoacidosis complicating pregnancy. *J Perinatol*. 1996;16(1):173–175.
21. Ruda JM, Hollenbeak CS, Stack BC. A systematic review of the diagnosis and treatment of primary hyperparathyroidism from 1995-2003. *Otolaryngol Head Neck Surg*. 2005;132(2):359–372.
22. Szalat A, Shpitzen S, Tsur A, et al. Stepwise CaSR, AP2S1, and GNA11 sequencing in patients with suspected familial hypocalciuric hypercalcemia. *Endocrine*. 2017;55:741.
23. Lee JY, Shoback DM. Familial hypocalciuric hypercalcemia and related disorders. *Best Pract Res Clin Endocrinol Metab*. 2018;32:609.
24. Schnatz PF, Curry SL. Primary hyperparathyroidism in pregnancy: evidence-based management. *Obstet Gynecol Surv*. 2002;57:365–376.
25. Dahlman T, Sjöberg HE, Bucht E. Calcium homeostasis in normal pregnancy and puerperium. A longitudinal study. *Acta Obstet Gynecol Scand*. 1994;73(5):393–398. doi:10.3109/00016349409006250.
26. Parks J, Coe F, Favus M. Hyperparathyroidism in nephrolithiasis. *Arch Intern Med*. 1980;140(11):1479–1481.
27. Jinhkate SN, Valand AG, Ansari S, Bharambe BM. Hyperparathyroidism complicating pregnancy: a diagnostic challenge? *J Postgrad Med*. 2014;63(3):329–331.
28. Truong MT, Lalakea ML, Robbins P, Friduss M. Primary hyperparathyroidism in pregnancy: a case series and review. *Laryngoscope*. 2008;118:1966.
29. McMullen TP, Learoyd DL, Williams DC, et al. Hyperparathyroidism in pregnancy: options for localization and surgical therapy. *World J Surg*. 2010;34:1811.
30. Delmonico FL, Neer RM, Cosimi AB, Barnes SB, Russell PS. Hyperparathyroidism during pregnancy. *Am J Surg*. 1976;131(3):328–337.
31. Kelly TR. Primary hyperparathyroidism during pregnancy. *Surgery*. 1991;110(6):1028–1033.
32. Dochez V, Ducarne G. Primary hyperparathyroidism during pregnancy. *Arch Gynecol Obstet*. 2015;291: 259–263.
33. Ramin K. Diabetic ketoacidosis in pregnancy. *Obstetrics and Gynecology Clinics*. 1999;26(3):481–488.

CHAPTER 23

Graves' Hyperthyroidism in Pregnancy

Caroline T. Nguyen ■ Jorge H. Mestman

CHAPTER OUTLINE

Background

Graves' hyperthyroidism (GH) in pregnancy affects less than 0.5% of pregnant women.[1] Prior to the advent of antithyroid drugs (ATDs) in the 1940s, GH perinatal mortality was as high as 45%.[2] Perinatal mortality has improved significantly and in 2011 was reported at 1.7%.[3] By making an early diagnosis of GH and maintaining euthyroidism during pregnancy, the physician can reduce the risk of complications to the mother, fetus, and newborn.

Pathophysiology and Natural History of Graves' Hyperthyroidism During Pregnancy

GH is an autoimmune condition in which thyroid-stimulating immunoglobulins (TSI) stimulate the thyroid-stimulating hormone receptor (TSHR), leading to increased thyroid hormone production and thyrotoxicosis.[4] In pregnancy, TSI cross the placenta and act on the fetus's thyroid. High titers of TSI may lead to fetal thyrotoxicosis. GH may worsen in early pregnancy, possibly secondary to human-chorionic gonadotropin (hCG) stimulation of the thyroid gland and/or elevation in TSI during the first trimester.[5–7] As pregnancy progresses, changes in the immunologic response lead to a decrease in TSI and improvement in GH.

Clinical Presentation of Graves' Hyperthyroidism in Pregnancy

Symptoms of hyperthyroidism may include palpitations, tremors, heat intolerance, weight loss, night sweats, moist skin, and loose bowel movements.[4] Signs of GH include ophthalmopathy, diffuse goiter, and pretibial myxedema. In the absence of signs of GH, a diagnosis of hyperthyroidism from clinical symptoms alone may be difficult as many symptoms are present in normal pregnancy.

Etiology of Hyperthyroidism in Pregnancy

The etiology of hyperthyroidism in pregnancy is broad (Box 23.1). GH is typically characterized by the signs and symptoms discussed above, often preceding pregnancy, a suppressed TSH, an elevated thyroxine (T4) outside of the pregnancy reference range, and presence of TSI. Laboratory tests will be discussed further later.

The most common etiology of hyperthyroidism in pregnancy is gestational transient thyrotoxicosis (GTT), which affects 1% to 5% of all pregnant women.[8] TSH is suppressed and T4 is elevated, but unlike GH, TSI is undetectable. GTT is most often associated with hyperemesis gravidarum, which typically occurs between 4 and 8 weeks of gestation and consists of persistent nausea, vomiting, greater than 5% weight loss, dehydration, ketonuria, and electrolyte disturbances that may require hospitalization.[9] Distinguishing between GTT and GH is important because GTT does not require treatment with ATDs and has not been associated with adverse pregnancy outcomes (Table 23.1).[10–13] The clinical course of GTT parallels the level of hCG, resolving by the end of the first or middle of the second trimester.[14,15] Women with a prior history of GTT are at increased risk for a repeat episode.[8]

BOX 23.1 ■ Etiologies of Hyperthyroidism in Pregnancy

- Graves' hyperthyroidism
- Painless thyroiditis
- Subacute thyroiditis
- Toxic adenoma
- Toxic multinodular goiter
- Gestational transient thyrotoxicosis (GTT)
  - Hyperemesis gravidarum
  - Multiple gestations
- Trophoblastic disease
- Hyperplacentosis
- Hyperreactio luteinalis
- Thyroid-stimulating hormone (TSH)-receptor mutation
- TSH-producing pituitary tumor
- Excessive levothyroxine (LT4) intake
- Drugs
  - Amiodarone
  - Lithium
  - Cysteine proteases (CP) inhibitors
  - Interferons
  - Iodine

Adapted with permission from reference 86.

TABLE 23.1 ■ **Differentiating GTT From GH**

	GTT	GH
Hyperthyroid symptoms prior to pregnancy	–	+
Hyperthyroid symptoms during pregnancy	+/–	+
Nausea/vomiting	++	–/+
Goiter/ophthalmopathy	–	+
Thyroid-stimulating immunoglobulins	–	+

GH, Graves' hyperthyroidism; *GTT*, gestational transient thyrotoxicosis
Adapted with permission from reference 87.

Laboratory Measurements and Considerations in Pregnancy

THYROID-STIMULATING HORMONE

Physiologic changes occur in normal pregnancy that lead to a decrease in TSH. hCG is secreted from the placenta and, due to a shared alpha subunit with TSH, acts on the TSHR. This leads to increased thyroxine hormone production, which feeds back to the pituitary and leads to a decrease in TSH. Consequently, the TSH reference range in pregnancy is shifted down by approximately 0.4 mIU/mL compared to the nonpregnancy reference range.[16] TSH is typically suppressed in GH.

Biotin, a water-soluble B vitamin (B7), is used in several hair and nail supplements. Biotin may interfere with biotin streptavidin immunoassays used in commercial assays to measure TSH and thyroid hormones.[17] Depending on the type of assay, biotin may cause a falsely depressed hormone level (TSH) or elevated free T4 (FT4) level, mimicking hyperthyroid laboratory tests. Withholding biotin for 8 hours may be sufficient to prevent interference with thyroid function laboratory testing. However, biotin is generally withheld for approximately 3 days prior to thyroid function tests (TFTs).[18]

THYROXINE

An increase demand in thyroid hormone requirement in pregnancy is met by an estrogen-mediated increase in hepatic thyroid-binding globulin (TBG) synthesis. Elevation in TBG, along with decreased albumin concentration in the latter half of pregnancy, may contribute to falsely low FT4 immunoassay levels. When using automated immunoassays by nonequilibrium methods, trimester-specific reference ranges should be applied. Alternatively, the FT4 index (FT4I) or total T4 have been shown to be reliable estimations of thyroxine concentration in the latter half of pregnancy.[19] The nonpregnant T4 reference range is adjusted by 1.5 to give the pregnancy reference range (i.e., 4 to 10 μg/dL becomes 6 to 15 μg/dL in pregnancy).

TRIODOTHYRONINE (T3)

T3 is rarely indicated in the assessment of patients with GH. An exception is if the TSH is suppressed in the setting of a normal T4 level, which can be seen in the case of exogenous T3 or autonomous functioning nodule.

THYROID-STIMULATING IMMUNOGLOBLULINS (TSI) AND THYROID-STIMULATING HORMONE RECEPTOR ANTIBODIES (TRAb)

There are two methods to measure antibodies of the TSH receptor: a bioassay, which measures TSI; and a competitive receptor immunoassay, which measures TSHR antibodies (TRAb). The difference between the two assays is that TSI measures only stimulating antibodies, whereas the TRAb assay measures all antibodies to the TSHR including stimulating, neutral, and blocking antibodies.[20] Although TSI is the pathogenetic hallmark of GH, TRAb may also be used in the diagnosis of GH because in a clinically hyperthyroid patient, the majority of the TRAb will be stimulating antibodies.[21]

The TSI bioassay is a functional assay that measures cyclic adenosine monophosphate (cAMP), a downstream product of TSI binding to the TSHR, by radioimmunoassay or chemiluminescent assay. The TRAb assay is a competitive immunoassay that detects antibodies by their capacity to compete for binding of radiolabeled TSH to the TSH receptor. Both assays have sensitivities and specificities greater than 98%.[20,22] The TSI bioassays have the advantage of detecting a functional property of the antibodies. The TRAb competitive receptor assay may be more readily available and less expensive (Table 23.2). Going forward in this chapter, the term *TSI* is interchangeable with *TRAb*.

TSI should be measured at presentation in pregnant women with active GH with or without ATD treatment, a history of GH previously treated with radioactive iodine ablation (RAIA) or surgery, or a past pregnancy with a fetus/neonate with thyroid dysfunction, because TSI greater than three times the upper limit of normal (ULN) is associated with increased risk of fetal and neonatal hyperthyroidism.[23–25] Women who are currently euthyroid or hypothyroid who were treated with surgery or RAIA may continue to have elevated TSI because TSI may remain elevated for years, especially after RAIA.[26–29] Women who are euthyroid secondary to treatment with ATDs at the time of diagnosis of pregnancy are unlikely to have elevated TSI levels.

Management and Treatment Options

The mainstay of treatment of GH in pregnancy is ATDs. The concern with ATDs in the setting of pregnancy is the association of both ATDs, propylthiouracil (PTU) and methimazole (MMZ), with congenital malformations (Table 23.3).[32,90–92] The maximum sensitivity to teratogenic effects

TABLE 23.2 ■ **Antibodies to the TSH Receptor: TRAb Versus TSI Assay**

	TRAb	TSI
Antibodies detected	Stimulating, neutral, blocking	Stimulating
Type of assay	• Competitive receptor immunoassay • Patient's sera TRAb competes with human monoclonal thyroid stimulating antibody (m22) to bind porcine TSH R-coated enzyme linked immune sorbent assay (ELISA)	• Bioassay • TSI interacts with TSHR leading to increased cyclic adenosine monophosphate (cAMP), corresponding luciferase activity and emission of light
Sensitivity and specificity	>98%[20,22]	>98%[20,22]
Considerations	• More readily available • Less expensive	• Functional assay • Measures only stimulating antibodies

TRAb, TSH receptor antibodies; *TSH,* thyroid-stimulating hormone; *TSI,* thyroid-stimulating immunoglobulins.
From references 1–3, 22, and 87–89.

TABLE 23.3 ■ **Complications Associated With Antithyroid Drugs**

Propylthiouracil (PTU)	Methimazole (MMZ)
Congenital malformations	

• Preauricular sinus, fistula, and cysts[32]
• Urinary tract abnormalities in males (e.g., kidney cysts, hydronephrosis)
	• Methimazole embryopathy[90,91]
	  • Aplasia cutis
	  • Choanal atresia[92]
	  • Esophageal atresia
	  • Omphalocele
	  • Dysmorphic facial features
	• Eye defects
	• Urinary tract malformations
	• Athelia
	• Ventral septal defects
	• Developmental delay

Maternal complications	
Skin rash, pruritus, migratory polyarthritis, lupus-like syndrome, cholestatic jaundice, agranulocytosis[46,93]	
• Fulminant liver failure[31,41,94]	

of ATDs is during organogenesis, gestational weeks 6 to 10.[30] If possible, ATDs should be avoided during this time. The physician may consider withholding ATDs at the time of diagnosis of pregnancy in certain patients. Women who have been treated for greater than 6 months, have a prepregnancy TSH within the reference range, and TSI levels less than three times ULN may be able to maintain euthyroidism without ATDs.[16] If ATD is withheld, TFTs should be monitored each week until week 12 then every 2 to 4 weeks as clinically indicated. If hyperthyroidism recurs in the first trimester, PTU should be started.

If ATDs may not be stopped, PTU is the drug of choice in the first trimester and is dosed at 50 to 150 mg orally every 8 hours, with TSH and T4 checked every 2 to 4 weeks as clinically indicated. Although both PTU and MMZ have similar effectiveness, rates of crossing the placenta, and incidence of congenital malformations (~2% to 4%),[31–35] the congenital malformations associated with PTU (e.g., preauricular cysts and urinary tract abnormalities), are considered less severe and surgically correctable compared with those of MMZ (e.g., aplasia cutis, choanal and esophageal atresia, omphalocele, dysmorphic facies, athelia, and ventral septal defects) (Table 23.2).[31–33,36–39,90–92] Both PTU and MMZ are associated with agranulocytosis, and patients should be educated to monitor for symptoms such as fever and sore throat.[93]

In the second trimester, PTU is often switched to MMZ (1 mg MMZ:20 mg PTU) given the ease of once-per-day dosing of MMZ and concern for the rare but serious complication of fulminant liver failure with PTU.[16,40,41,94] Monitoring hepatic enzymes has not been found to be effective for patients on ATDs. Propranolol 10 to 20 mg orally every 6 to 8 hours may be used to alleviate hyperadrenergic symptoms initially and should be titrated down as tolerated, with care to maintain a heart rate between 80 and 100 beats per minutes (bpm). Long-term use of beta-blockers has been associated with intrauterine growth restriction (IUGR), neonatal bradycardia, and hypoglycemia.[42]

The lowest dose of ATD necessary to maintain thyroxine levels in the ULN for the pregnancy reference range should be used. ATDs are not dosed based on maternal T3 levels, as this may lead to overtreatment and hypothyroidism in the fetus.[43] Furthermore, TSH may remain suppressed during treatment and throughout pregnancy. Indications that the ATD dose should be lowered include if TSH becomes detectable, the TSI levels are less than three times the ULN, FT4 or

BOX 23.2 ■ Potential Complications of Uncontrolled Hyperthyroidism in the Pregnant Patient

- Maternal congestive heart failure
- Thyroid storm
- Miscarriage
- Gestational hypertension
- Preeclampsia
- Premature delivery
- Placental abruption
- Premature rupture of membranes
- Intrauterine growth restriction
- Central hypothyroidism in the neonate
- Still birth
- Postpartum bleeding

FT4I is consistently below the ULN, or any sign of fetal hypothyroidism on fetal ultrasound (US) (discussed in further detail later).

As pregnancy progresses, TSI levels decrease and are generally below three times the ULN for the majority of women by gestational week 20.[23,24,44,45] Accordingly, ATD requirements decrease, and up to 40% of women will be able to titrate off ATDs in the third trimester.[46] If the dosage of ATD is low (e.g., MMZ 2.5 to 5 mg daily or PTU 50 to 100 mg daily) and TSI is less than three times ULN, it may be discontinued and TFTs monitored closely for recurrence. The risk of fetal and neonatal hyperthyroidism is low when TSI is less than three times ULN.[23]

Due to the associated congenital malformations and maternal complications associated with ATDs, alternative options have been considered. In Japan, potassium iodide has been used in lieu of ATDs to treat GH during pregnancy with decreased rates of congenital malformations compared to MMZ.[47] These studies have not been reproduced, and it is currently not recommended in the United States. Rarely, thyroidectomy is necessary in the setting of a large goiter causing compressive symptoms or patients who are intolerant to ATDs.[48] If surgery is indicated during pregnancy, the second trimester is considered the safest for the mother and fetus. In a woman undergoing surgery, TSI should be measured at the time of surgery because if greater than three times the ULN, TSI and fetal US to assess for fetal hyperthyroidism will need to be followed after surgery. ^{131}I RAIA is contraindicated in pregnancy.[16]

Complications of Graves' Hyperthyroidism in Pregnancy

Uncontrolled hyperthyroidism is associated with potential complications that may affect the mother, fetus, and neonate. In women with long-standing uncontrolled hyperthyroidism, complications include congestive heart failure and thyroid storm. In the pregnant woman with uncontrolled hyperthyroidism, possible complications include miscarriage, gestational hypertension, preeclampsia, premature delivery, placental abruption, premature rupture of membranes, and postpartum bleeding. Fetal complications may include IUGR, and developmental dysplasia of the hip associated with first-trimester maternal hyperthyroidism.[49,50] The neonate is at possible risk for prematurity, stillbirth, low birth weight, and central hypothyroidism in mothers who had uncontrolled hyperthyroidism throughout pregnancy (Table 23.3).[50–57]

Women with controlled hyperthyroidism have significantly reduced risk of complications compared to those who remain uncontrolled. Pregnancy-induced hypertension, low birth weight, and preterm delivery were 5 times, 9 times, and 16 times greater, respectively, in women with uncontrolled hyperthyroidism compared with women with controlled hyperthyroidism.[55] However, women who are subsequently controlled in pregnancy still have an increased risk of complications compared with those controlled prior to pregnancy.[55,56]

THYROID STORM

TS in pregnancy is very rare. TS occurs in patients with long-standing uncontrolled hyperthyroidism who encounter a precipitating event (e.g., infection, pregnancy, surgery, drugs, etc.) that leads to decompensation. TS is characterized by altered mental status and hyperthermia. The patient in TS requires intensive care unit–level care, treatment with intravenous fluids, ATDs, beta-blockers, preferably nonselective propranolol, SSKI (potassium iodide or Lugol's solution), steroids, and empiric pregnancy-appropriate antibiotics. The care of the pregnant patient in TS is similar to that of the nonpregnant patient (see Chapter 1 on Thyroid Storm for more details).

FETAL THYROTOXICOSIS

Fetal thyrotoxicosis (FT) is caused by TSI crossing the placenta and acting on the TSHR of the fetal thyroid gland. FT typically occurs between gestational weeks 18 and 26 when the fetal TSH receptors appear to become significantly responsive to TSI.[58–60] Women who have TSI greater than three times ULN or a prior fetus or neonate with a thyroid disorder are at risk for FT.[23–25]

As was stated previously, TSI should be checked at the time of diagnosis of pregnancy in women at risk for FT. TSI should be repeated at 18 weeks' gestation. If TSI is greater than three times the ULN at that point, the fetus should have a fetal US to assess for evidence of fetal hyperthyroidism. Fetal US should be performed every 4 weeks to assess the gestational age, fetal viability, amniotic fluid volume, and fetal anatomy.[61,62] TSI should be repeated at 30 to 34 weeks, and if TSI remains greater than three times the ULN, close fetal and neonatal monitoring is warranted with frequent US as indicated.[16] In addition to an elevated TSI greater than three times ULN, other indications for a fetal US include a prior fetus or neonate with thyroid disorder, fetal tachycardia by doppler (heart rate greater than 160 bpm), history of poorly controlled hyperthyroidism, and concern for excessive treatment with ATDs.

Treatment of FT consists of adjusting maternal ATDs and following fetal signs of hyperthyroidism. If the mother is hypothyroid due to prior treatment of her GH with RAIA or surgery, the ATD is added to levothyroxine and doses are adjusted based on fetal tachycardia and goiter size.[26,63,64] The lowest dose of ATD to maintain normal fetal heart rate (110 to 160 bpm) should be used, with fetal assessment every 1 to 2 weeks.

FETAL HYPOTHYROIDISM

Fetal hypothyroidism may occur due to overtreatment with ATDs. Fetal goiter may present and lead to fetal, obstetric, and neonatal complications. The fetus may develop polyhydramnios from an inability to swallow. Labor dystocia may occur due to hyperextension of the fetal neck from the fetal goiter and C-section may be preferred.[65,66] Rarely, US-guided cordocentesis may be used to assess fetal thyroid status. Risk of complications is low (0.5% to 1%) when done at centers with experience.[58,65,67] If fetal hypothyroidism develops, the ATD is reduced or stopped with subsequent normalization of thyroid function and decreased fetal goiter size. In exceptional cases, intraamniotic levothyroxine may be necessary.[68] The goal is to maintain maternal T4 levels in the upper limit of pregnancy reference range.

NEONATAL HYPERTHYROIDISM

Neonatal hyperthyroidism occurs in 1% to 5% of offspring of pregnant women with GH.[59,69–71] Those with fetal hyperthyroidism should have thyroid tests checked at birth and every few days as clinically indicated. Neonatal hyperthyroidism may present with tachycardia, hyperactivity, small for gestational age, accelerated bone maturation, and rarely, premature craniosynostosis, microcephaly, and psychomotor disabilities may occur.[46,62,72,73]

Newborns without evidence of hyperthyroidism born to mothers with GH on ATD should be screened for thyroid dysfunction at 2 to 5 days of age as the transfer of ATD via the placenta may result in normal thyroid function laboratory tests at birth. A TSH level less than 0.9 mIU/L between days 3 and 7 of life predicts neonatal hyperthyroidism with a positive predictive value of 90%.[71] TSI may stay present for several months in the newborn's circulation.[72,74]

NEONATAL HYPOTHYROIDISM

Neonatal hypothyroidism may result from overtreatment with maternal ATD or central hypothyroidism from suppression of fetal TSH in uncontrolled GH.[75] Prompt treatment improves neurodevelopmental outcomes.[76]

Postpartum Considerations

Women who remain hyperthyroid in the postpartum period should be treated as per standard practices. This typically entails ATDs. RAIA is contraindicated in women who are breastfeeding and requires separation of the mother and newborn. Women who are euthyroid remain at risk for recurrence of GH in the first year postpartum.[6,77] Hyperthyroidism from recurrence of Graves' disease should be differentiated from postpartum thyroiditis (PPT), which occurs in 5% of pregnancies, often in women with thyroid peroxidase (TPO)-Ab positivity, and does not require treatment with ATDs.[78] Onset of hyperthyroid symptoms more than 4 months postpartum and elevated TSI titers would be suggestive of GH.

Women may continue to breastfeed while taking ATDs. Although PTU and MMZ have been found in breast milk at very small concentrations, they have not been shown to detrimentally affect the newborn.[79–84] The lowest effective dose should be used with maximum doses of MMZ being 20 mg daily and PTU 450 mg daily.[16]

Prevention—Preconception Counseling

Challenging clinical dilemmas in the pregnant patient with uncontrolled GH may be avoided with greater emphasis on preconception counseling. All women of reproductive age with GH or past history of GH should be advised to plan pregnancies and use contraception if sexually active. Women should be advised to contact their doctor immediately once pregnant.

Prepregnancy treatment options including ATDs, RAIA, and surgery should be discussed with women with GH of child bearing age. The potential risks and benefits of each option should be discussed in relation to the patient's desired timeline for pregnancy. Ideally, women should avoid pregnancy until hyperthyroidism has been controlled for several months. Women requiring high doses of ATD who want to become pregnant should consider definitive therapy prior to conception. If TSI is greater than three times the ULN and the patient would like to become pregnant soon, surgery may be the best option. TSI levels will decline immediately after surgery, whereas

TSI increases after RAIA and may stay elevated for years.[27] The rate of neonatal hyperthyroidism increases with the proximity of conception to RAIA. In Japan, 5.5% of pregnancies conceived within 2 years of RAIA were complicated by neonatal hyperthyroidism.[28]

As discussed previously, PTU is the preferred ATD in the first trimester due to the congenital malformations associated with MMZ. The physician has the option to switch the patient to PTU prior to or at time of diagnosis of pregnancy. However, frequently pregnancy may not be discovered or the patient may not present to the clinic until after the period of organogenesis (weeks 6 to 10). The rate of congenital malformations is higher in newborns born to women exposed to both PTU and MMZ in early pregnancy.[32,85] Therefore, although there is concern for PTU-associated hepatotoxicity, MMZ should be switched to PTU once contraception is stopped.

Summary

The successful treatment of a pregnant woman with GH depends on a timely and accurate diagnosis, maintenance of euthyroidism for the duration of pregnancy using the lowest dose of ATD necessary, education of the patient, and a collaborative effort of the endocrinologist, obstetrician-gynecologist, maternal fetal medicine, neonatologist, and pediatrician. Preconception counseling for women of child bearing age with GH should be a part of routine treatment plans. An understanding of the unique aspects of caring for a pregnant patient with GH will help achieve the goal of delivery of a healthy, euthyroid newborn.

References

1. Cooper DS, Laurberg P. Hyperthyroidism in pregnancy. *Lancet Diabetes Endocrinol.* 2013;1(3):238–249.
2. Davis LE, Lucas MJ, Hankins GD, Roark ML, Cunningham FG. Thyrotoxicosis complicating pregnancy. *Am J Obstet Gynecol.* 1989;160(1):63–70.
3. Luewan S, Chakkabut P, Tongsong T. Outcomes of pregnancy complicated with hyperthyroidism: a cohort study. *Arch Gynecol Obstet.* 2011;283(2):243–247.
4. Smith TJ, Hegedus L. Graves' disease. *N Engl J Med.* 2016;375(16):1552–1565.
5. Andersen SL, Olsen J, Carle A, Laurberg P. Hyperthyroidism incidence fluctuates widely in and around pregnancy and is at variance with some other autoimmune diseases: a Danish population-based study. *J Clin Endocrinol Metab.* 2015;100(3):1164–1171.
6. Amino N, Tanizawa O, Mori H, et al. Aggravation of thyrotoxicosis in early pregnancy and after delivery in Graves' disease. *J Clin Endocrinol Metab.* 1982;55(1):108–112.
7. Weetman AP. Immunity, thyroid function and pregnancy: molecular mechanisms. *Nat Rev Endocrinol.* 2010;6(6):311–318.
8. Goldman AM, Mestman JH. Transient non-autoimmune hyperthyroidism of early pregnancy. *J Thyroid Res.* 2011;2011:142413.
9. Goodwin TM, Montoro M, Mestman JH. Transient hyperthyroidism and hyperemesis gravidarum: clinical aspects. *Am J Obstet Gynecol.* 1992;167(3):648–652.
10. Casey BM, Dashe JS, Wells CE, McIntire DD, Leveno KJ, Cunningham FG. Subclinical hyperthyroidism and pregnancy outcomes. *Obstet Gynecol.* 2006;107(2 Pt 1):337–341.
11. Tong Z, Xiaowen Z, Baomin C, et al. The effect of subclinical maternal thyroid dysfunction and autoimmunity on intrauterine growth restriction: a systematic review and meta-analysis. *Medicine (Baltimore).* 2016;95(19):e3677.
12. Haddow JE, Craig WY, Neveux LM, et al. Implications of high free thyroxine (FT4) concentrations in euthyroid pregnancies: the FaSTER trial. *J Clin Endocrinol Metab.* 2014;99(6):2038–2044.
13. Kinomoto-Kondo S, Umehara N, Sato S, et al. The effects of gestational transient thyrotoxicosis on the perinatal outcomes: a case-control study. *Arch Gynecol Obstet.* 2017;295(1):87–93.
14. Glinoer D, de Nayer P, Bourdoux P, et al. Regulation of maternal thyroid during pregnancy. *J Clin Endocrinol Metab.* 1990;71(2):276–287.
15. Goodwin TM, Montoro M, Mestman JH, Pekary AE, Hershman JM. The role of chorionic gonadotropin in transient hyperthyroidism of hyperemesis gravidarum. *J Clin Endocrinol Metab.* 1992;75(5):1333–1337.

16. Alexander EK, Pearce EN, Brent GA, et al. 2017 Guidelines of the American Thyroid Association for the diagnosis and management of thyroid disease during pregnancy and the postpartum. *Thyroid*. 2017;27(3):315–389.
17. Elston MS, Sehgal S, Du Toit S, Yarndley T, Conaglen JV. Factitious Graves' disease due to biotin immunoassay interference—a case and review of the literature. *J Clin Endocrinol Metab*. 2016;101(9):3251–3255.
18. Holmes EW, Samarasinghe S, Emanuele MA, Meah F. Biotin interference in clinical immunoassays: a cause for concern. *Arch Pathol Lab Med*. 2017;141(11):1459–1460.
19. Lee RH, Spencer CA, Mestman JH, et al. Free T4 immunoassays are flawed during pregnancy. *Am J Obstet Gynecol*. 2009;200(3):260 e1-6.
20. Bucci I, Giuliani C, Napolitano G. Thyroid-stimulating hormone receptor antibodies in pregnancy: clinical relevance. *Front Endocrinol (Lausanne)*. 2017;8:137.
21. Diana T, Krause J, Olivo PD, et al. Prevalence and clinical relevance of thyroid stimulating hormone receptor-blocking antibodies in autoimmune thyroid disease. *Clin Exp Immunol*. 2017;189(3):304–309.
22. Tozzoli R, Bagnasco M, Giavarina D, Bizzaro N. TSH receptor autoantibody immunoassay in patients with Graves' disease: improvement of diagnostic accuracy over different generations of methods. Systematic review and meta-analysis. *Autoimmun Rev*. 2012;12(2):107–113.
23. Abeillon-du Payrat J, Chikh K, Bossard N, et al. Predictive value of maternal second-generation thyroid-binding inhibitory immunoglobulin assay for neonatal autoimmune hyperthyroidism. *Eur J Endocrinol*. 2014;171(4):451–460.
24. Banige M EC, Biran V, Desfrere L, et al. Study of the factors leading to fetal and neonatal dysthyroidism in children of patients with Graves disease. *J Endocr Soc*. 2017;1(6):751–761.
25. van Dijk MM, Smits IH, Fliers E, Bisschop PH. Maternal thyrotropin receptor antibody concentration and the risk of fetal and neonatal thyrotoxicosis: a systematic review. *Thyroid*. 2018;28(2):257–264.
26. Akangire G, Cuna A, Lachica C, Fischer R, Raman S, Sampath V. Neonatal Graves' disease with maternal hypothyroidism. *AJP Rep*. 2017;7(3):e181–e1e4.
27. Laurberg P, Wallin G, Tallstedt L, Abraham-Nordling M, Lundell G, Torring O. TSH-receptor autoimmunity in Graves' disease after therapy with anti-thyroid drugs, surgery, or radioiodine: a 5-year prospective randomized study. *Eur J Endocrinol*. 2008;158(1):69–75.
28. Yoshihara A, Iwaku K, Noh JY, et al. Incidence of neonatal hyperthyroidism among newborns of Graves' disease patients treated with radioiodine therapy. *Thyroid*. 2019;29(1):128–134.
29. Kautbally S, Alexopoulou O, Daumerie C, Jamar F, Mourad M, Maiter D. Greater efficacy of total thyroidectomy versus radioiodine therapy on hyperthyroidism and thyroid-stimulating immunoglobulin levels in patients with Graves' disease previously treated with antithyroid drugs. *Eur Thyroid J*. 2012;1(2):122–128.
30. Laurberg P, Andersen SL. Therapy of endocrine disease: antithyroid drug use in early pregnancy and birth defects: time windows of relative safety and high risk? *Eur J Endocrinol*. 2014;171(1):R13–R20.
31. Cooper DS, Rivkees SA. Putting propylthiouracil in perspective. *J Clin Endocrinol Metab*. 2009;94(6): 1881–1882.
32. Andersen SL, Olsen J, Wu CS, Laurberg P. Birth defects after early pregnancy use of antithyroid drugs: a Danish nationwide study. *J Clin Endocrinol Metab*. 2013;98(11):4373–4381.
33. Yoshihara A, Noh J, Yamaguchi T, et al. Treatment of Graves' disease with antithyroid drugs in the first trimester of pregnancy and the prevalence of congenital malformation. *J Clin Endocrinol Metab*. 2012;97(7):2396–2403.
34. Wing DA, Millar LK, Koonings PP, Montoro MN, Mestman JH. A comparison of propylthiouracil versus methimazole in the treatment of hyperthyroidism in pregnancy. *Am J Obstet Gynecol*. 1994; 170(1 Pt 1):90–95.
35. Momotani N, Noh JY, Ishikawa N, Ito K. Effects of propylthiouracil and methimazole on fetal thyroid status in mothers with Graves' hyperthyroidism. *J Clin Endocrinol Metab*. 1997;82(11):3633–3636.
36. Andersen SL, Olsen J, Wu CS, Laurberg P. Severity of birth defects after propylthiouracil exposure in early pregnancy. *Thyroid*. 2014;24(10):1533–1540.
37. Song R, Lin H, Chen Y, Zhang X, Feng W. Effects of methimazole and propylthiouracil exposure during pregnancy on the risk of neonatal congenital malformations: A meta-analysis. *PLoS One*. 2017; 12(7):e0180108.
38. Gianetti E, Russo L, Orlandi F, et al. Pregnancy outcome in women treated with methimazole or propylthiouracil during pregnancy. *J Endocrinol Invest*. 2015;38(9):977–985.

39. Barbero P, Valdez R, Rodriguez H, et al. Choanal atresia associated with maternal hyperthyroidism treated with methimazole: a case-control study. *Am J Med Genet A*. 2008;146A(18):2390–2395.
40. Andersen SL, Olsen J, Laurberg P. Antithyroid drug side effects in the population and in pregnancy. *J Clin Endocrinol Metab*. 2016;101(4):1606–1614.
41. Russo MW, Galanko JA, Shrestha R, Fried MW, Watkins P. Liver transplantation for acute liver failure from drug induced liver injury in the United States. *Liver Transpl*. 2004;10(8):1018–1023.
42. Rubin PC. Current concepts: beta-blockers in pregnancy. *N Engl J Med*. 1981;305(22):1323–1326.
43. Momotani N, Noh J, Oyanagi H, Ishikawa N, Ito K. Antithyroid drug therapy for Graves' disease during pregnancy. Optimal regimen for fetal thyroid status. *N Engl J Med*. 1986;315(1):24–28.
44. Gonzalez-Jimenez A, Fernandez-Soto ML, Escobar-Jimenez F, Glinoer D, Navarrete L. Thyroid function parameters and TSH-receptor antibodies in healthy subjects and Graves' disease patients: a sequential study before, during and after pregnancy. *Thyroidology*. 1993;5(1):13–20.
45. Kamijo K. TSH-receptor antibodies determined by the first, second and third generation assays and thyroid-stimulating antibody in pregnant patients with Graves' disease. *Endocr J*. 2007;54(4):619–624.
46. Patil-Sisodia K, Mestman JH. Graves hyperthyroidism and pregnancy: a clinical update. *Endocr Pract*. 2010;16(1):118–129.
47. Yoshihara A, Noh JY, Watanabe N, et al. Substituting potassium iodide for methimazole as the treatment for Graves' disease during the first trimester may reduce the incidence of congenital anomalies: a retrospective study at a single medical institution in Japan. *Thyroid*. 2015;25(10):1155–1161.
48. Bruner JP, Landon MB, Gabbe SG. Diabetes mellitus and Graves' disease in pregnancy complicated by maternal allergies to antithyroid medication. *Obstet Gynecol*. 1988;72(3 Pt 2):443–445.
49. Momotani N, Ito K, Hamada N, Ban Y, Nishikawa Y, Mimura T. Maternal hyperthyroidism and congenital malformation in the offspring. *Clin Endocrinol (Oxf)*. 1984;20(6):695–700.
50. Ishikawa N. The relationship between neonatal developmental dysplasia of the hip and maternal hyperthyroidism. *J Pediatr Orthop*. 2008;28(4):432–434.
51. Mannisto T, Mendola P, Grewal J, Xie Y, Chen Z, Laughon SK. Thyroid diseases and adverse pregnancy outcomes in a contemporary US cohort. *J Clin Endocrinol Metab*. 2013;98(7):2725–2733.
52. Andersen SL, Olsen J, Wu CS, Laurberg P. Low birth weight in children born to mothers with hyperthyroidism and high birth weight in hypothyroidism, whereas preterm birth is common in both conditions: A Danish national hospital register study. *Eur Thyroid J*. 2013;2(2):135–144.
53. Wang Y, Sun XL, Wang CL, Zhang HY. Influence of screening and intervention of hyperthyroidism on pregnancy outcome. *Eur Rev Med Pharmacol Sci*. 2017;21(8):1932–1937.
54. Zhang Y, Li Y, Shan Z, et al. Association of overt and subclinical hyperthyroidism during weeks 4-8 with adverse pregnancy outcomes. *J Womens Health (Larchmt)*. 2019;28(6):842–848.
55. Millar LK, Wing DA, Leung AS, Koonings PP, Montoro MN, Mestman JH. Low birth weight and preeclampsia in pregnancies complicated by hyperthyroidism. *Obstet Gynecol*. 1994;84(6):946–949.
56. Aggarawal N, Suri V, Singla R, et al. Pregnancy outcome in hyperthyroidism: a case control study. *Gynecol Obstet Invest*. 2014;77(2):94–99.
57. Kempers MJ, van Trotsenburg AS, van Rijn RR, et al. Loss of integrity of thyroid morphology and function in children born to mothers with inadequately treated Graves' disease. *J Clin Endocrinol Metab*. 2007;92(8):2984–2991.
58. Fisher DA. Fetal thyroid function: diagnosis and management of fetal thyroid disorders. *Clin Obstet Gynecol*. 1997;40(1):16–31.
59. Polak M, Le Gac I, Vuillard E, et al. Fetal and neonatal thyroid function in relation to maternal Graves' disease. *Best Pract Res Clin Endocrinol Metab*. 2004;18(2):289–302.
60. Donnelly MA, Wood C, Casey B, Hobbins J, Barbour LA. Early severe fetal Graves disease in a mother after thyroid ablation and thyroidectomy. *Obstet Gynecol*. 2015;125(5):1059–1062.
61. Luton D, Le Gac I, Vuillard E, et al. Management of Graves' disease during pregnancy: the key role of fetal thyroid gland monitoring. *J Clin Endocrinol Metab*. 2005;90(11):6093–6098.
62. King JR, Lachica R, Lee RH, Montoro M, Mestman J. Diagnosis and management of hyperthyroidism in pregnancy: a review. *Obstet Gynecol Surv*. 2016;71(11):675–685.
63. Joshi K, Zacharin M. Hyperthyroidism in an infant of a mother with autoimmune hypothyroidism with positive TSH receptor antibodies. *J Pediatr Endocrinol Metab*. 2018;31(5):577–580.

64. Kiefer FW, Klebermass-Schrehof K, Steiner M, et al. Fetal/neonatal thyrotoxicosis in a newborn from a hypothyroid woman with Hashimoto thyroiditis. *J Clin Endocrinol Metab*. 2017;102(1):6–9.
65. Nachum Z, Rakover Y, Weiner E, Shalev E. Graves' disease in pregnancy: prospective evaluation of a selective invasive treatment protocol. *Am J Obstet Gynecol*. 2003;189(1):159–165.
66. Aubry G, Pontvianne M, Chesnais M, Weingertner AS, Guerra F, Favre R. Prenatal diagnosis of fetal goitrous hypothyroidism in a euthyroid mother: a management challenge. *J Ultrasound Med*. 2017;36(11): 2387–2392.
67. Delay F, Dochez V, Biquard F, et al. Management of fetal goiters: 6-year retrospective observational study in three prenatal diagnosis and treatment centers of the Pays de Loire perinatal network. *J Matern Fetal Neonatal Med*. 2018:1–191.
68. Bliddal S, Rasmussen AK, Sundberg K, Brocks V, Feldt-Rasmussen U. Antithyroid drug-induced fetal goitrous hypothyroidism. *Nat Rev Endocrinol*. 2011;7(7):396–406.
69. Mitsuda N, Tamaki H, Amino N, Hosono T, Miyai K, Tanizawa O. Risk factors for developmental disorders in infants born to women with Graves disease. *Obstet Gynecol*. 1992;80(3 Pt 1):359–364.
70. Zakarija M, McKenzie JM, Hoffman WH. Prediction and therapy of intrauterine and late-onset neonatal hyperthyroidism. *J Clin Endocrinol Metab*. 1986;62(2):368–371.
71. Banige M, Polak M, Luton D. Research Group for Perinatal Dysthyroidism Study G. Prediction of neonatal hyperthyroidism. *J Pediatr*. 2018;197:249–254 e1.
72. McKenzie JM, Zakarija M. Fetal and neonatal hyperthyroidism and hypothyroidism due to maternal TSH receptor antibodies. *Thyroid*. 1992;2(2):155–159.
73. Leger J. Management of fetal and neonatal Graves' disease. *Horm Res Paediatr*. 2017;87(1):1–6.
74. van der Kaay DC, Wasserman JD, Palmert MR. Management of neonates born to mothers with Graves' disease. *Pediatrics*. 2016;137(4).
75. Kempers MJ, van Tijn DA, van Trotsenburg AS, de Vijlder JJ, Wiedijk BM, Vulsma T. Central congenital hypothyroidism due to gestational hyperthyroidism: detection where prevention failed. *J Clin Endocrinol Metab*. 2003;88(12):5851–5857.
76. Simpser T, Rapaport R. Update on some aspects of neonatal thyroid disease. *J Clin Res Pediatr Endocrinol*. 2010;2(3):95–99.
77. Rotondi M, Cappelli C, Pirali B, et al. The effect of pregnancy on subsequent relapse from Graves' disease after a successful course of antithyroid drug therapy. *J Clin Endocrinol Metab*. 2008;93(10):3985–3988.
78. Nguyen CT, Mestman JH. Postpartum thyroiditis. *Clin Obstet Gynecol*. 2019;62(2):359–364.
79. Cooper DS. Antithyroid drugs. *N Engl J Med*. 2005;352(9):905–917.
80. Eisenstein Z, Weiss M, Katz Y, Bank H. Intellectual capacity of subjects exposed to methimazole or propylthiouracil in utero. *Eur J Pediatr*. 1992;151(8):558–559.
81. Azizi F, Khoshniat M, Bahrainian M, Hedayati M. Thyroid function and intellectual development of infants nursed by mothers taking methimazole. *J Clin Endocrinol Metab*. 2000;85(9):3233–3238.
82. Kampmann JP, Johansen K, Hansen JM, Helweg J. Propylthiouracil in human milk. Revision of a dogma. *Lancet*. 1980;1(8171):736–737.
83. Johansen K, Andersen AN, Kampmann JP, Molholm Hansen JM, Mortensen HB. Excretion of methimazole in human milk. *Eur J Clin Pharmacol*. 1982;23(4):339–341.
84. Cooper DS, Bode HH, Nath B, Saxe V, Maloof F, Ridgway EC. Methimazole pharmacology in man: studies using a newly developed radioimmunoassay for methimazole. *J Clin Endocrinol Metab*. 1984;58(3):473–479.
85. Seo GH, Kim TH, Chung JH. Antithyroid drugs and congenital malformations: a nationwide Korean cohort study. *Ann Intern Med*. 2018;168(6):405–413.
86. Mestman JH. Hyperthyroidism in pregnancy. *Curr Opin Endocrinol Diabetes Obes*. 2012;19(5):394–401.
87. Nguyen CT, Mestman JH. Graves' hyperthyroidism in pregnancy. *Curr Opin Endocrinol Diabetes Obes*. 2019;26(5):232–240.
88. Tozzoli R, D'Aurizio F, Villalta D, Giovanella L. Evaluation of the first fully automated immunoassay method for the measurement of stimulating TSH receptor autoantibodies in Graves' disease. *Clin Chem Lab Med*. 2017;55(1):58–64.
89. Kotwal A, Stan M. Thyrotropin receptor antibodies—an overview. *Ophthalmic Plast Reconstr Surg*. 2018; 34(4S Suppl 1):S20–S27.
90. Clementi M, Di Gianantonio E, Cassina M, et al. Treatment of hyperthyroidism in pregnancy and birth defects. *J Clin Endocrinol Metab*. 2010;95(11):E337–E341.

91. Clementi M, Di Gianantonio E, Pelo E, Mammi I, Basile RT, Tenconi R. Methimazole embryopathy: delineation of the phenotype. *Am J Med Genet.* 1999;83(1):43–46.
92. Wolf D, Foulds N, Daya H. Antenatal carbimazole and choanal atresia: a new embryopathy. *Arch Otolaryngol Head Neck Surg.* 2006;132(9):1009–1011.
93. Tajiri J, Noguchi S, Murakami T, Murakami N. Antithyroid drug-induced agranulocytosis. The usefulness of routine white blood cell count monitoring. *Arch Intern Med.* 1990;150(3):621–624.
94. Williams KV, Nayak S, Becker D, Reyes J, Burmeister LA. Fifty years of experience with propylthiouracil-associated hepatotoxicity: what have we learned? *J Clin Endocrinol Metab.* 1997;82(6):1727–1733.

PART 9

Immunotherapy–Associated Endocrinopathies

CHAPTER 24

Endocrinopathies Associated With Immune Checkpoint Inhibitors

Monica Girotra

CHAPTER OUTLINE

Immune checkpoint inhibition has transformed cancer treatment and has improved long-term survival in patients with advanced malignancies. Antibodies that block cytotoxic T-lymphocyte antigen 4 (CTLA-4) and programmed death 1 (PD1) or its ligand (PD-L1) are now used routinely for cancer treatment. Autoimmune toxicities, known as immune-related adverse events (IRAEs), are seen with these therapies, including endocrine IRAEs. Hypophysitis, thyroid dysfunction, and insulin-dependent diabetes mellitus (IDDM) following immune checkpoint inhibition are seen with distinct clinical presentations.

Mechanism of Action of Anti-cytotoxic T-Lymphocyte Antigen 4 and Anti-programmed Death 1/or Its Ligand for Cancer Therapy

CTLA-4 is a glycoprotein expressed by T-cells and is the first immune checkpoint receptor to be targeted clinically. CTLA-4 controls the scale of early T-cell activation by inhibiting T-cell activity. CTLA-4 counteracts the activity of the T-cell costimulatory receptor, CD28.[1–3] During an immune response, when the T-cell receptor (TCR) recognizes its cognate antigen, CD28 amplifies TCR signaling to activate T-cells. CD28 and CTLA4 share the same B7 ligands.[4–7] CTLA-4 has a higher affinity for B7 and is thought to dampen T-cell activation by outcompeting CD28, as well as delivering inhibitory signals to the T cell.[8–13] CTLA-4 binding inhibits interleukin-2

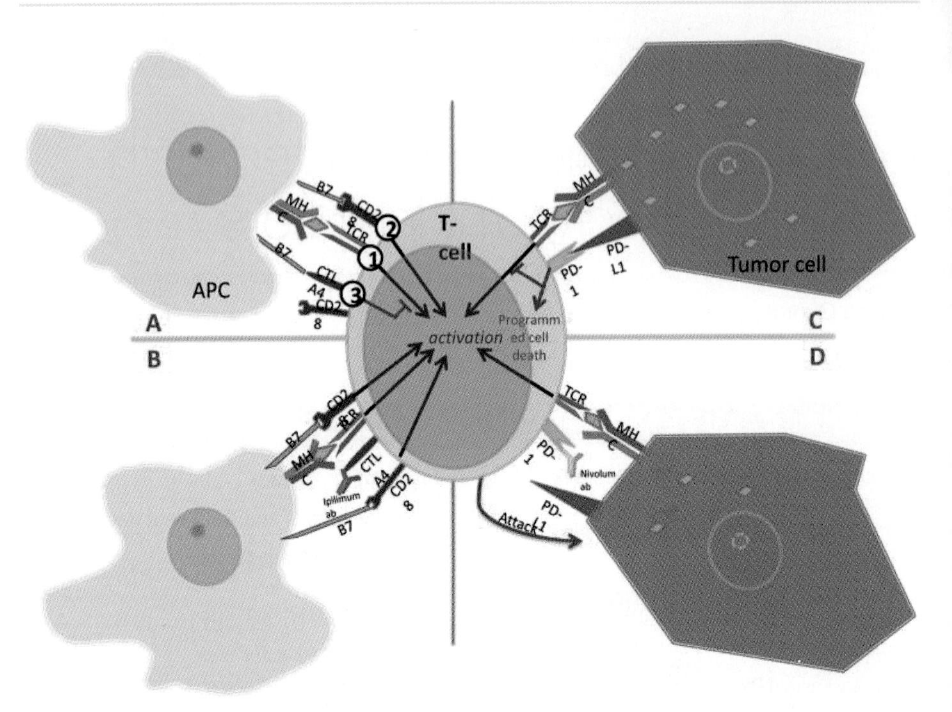

Fig. 24.1 (A) Normal CTLA4 interaction with B7 costimulatory ligand. *1* First activation signal is initiated when T-cell receptor *(TCR)* binds to the antigen presenting cell's *(APC)* major histocompatibility complex (MHC), presenting an antigen. *2* Second activation signal is fired when CD28 receptor binds to B7 costimulatory ligand on the APC. *3* CTLA4 receptors present on T-cell act as a checkpoint, and inhibits T-cell activation by outcompeting CD28 receptors to bind to B7 ligand. This negates the effect of second activation signal. (B) Ipilimumab, an anti-CTLA4 antibody, indirectly increases T-cell activity by binding to the CTLA4 receptor. Second activation signal via B7 and CD28 connection is reactivated. (C) By blocking either programmed death 1 *(PD-1)* or its ligand *(PD-L1)* protein, nivolumab enables the T-cell to detect tumor cells. (D) By blocking either PD-1 or PD-L1 protein, nivolumab enables the T-cell to detect tumor cells. (From Byun DJ, Wolchok JD, Rosenberg LM, Girotra M. Cancer immunotherapy – immune checkpoint blockade and associated endocrinopathies. *Nat Rev Endocrinol.* 2017;13(4):195–207. https://www.ncbi.nlm.nih.gov/pmc/articles/PMC5629093/)

production and cell cycle progression of activated T-cells and prevents T-cell activation.[3,14] The inhibitory role of CTLA-4 in T-cell activation in check is shown by the lethal immune activation phenotype of CTLA-4-knockout mice.[15,16]

Ipilimumab, a monoclonal antibody that binds to CTLA-4 and prevents B7 binding, is effective in the treatment of some malignancies (Fig. 24.1).[17] With B7 now accessible, CD28 binding upregulates T-cell activity.[18–21] By blocking CTLA-4, activated T-cells proliferate and are persistently activated, which allows the targeting of previously poorly immunogenic tumor antigens to cancer cells.[22]

PD-1 is a receptor on immune cells and its ligands, PDL1 and PDL2, are on a variety of cells, including antigen-presenting cells and tumor cells.[23–28] Immune cell activity is reduced when PD1 binds to its ligand. The upregulation of PDL1 expression is seen in some tumor cells, which inhibits T-cell activation and increases cancer cell survival.[29,30] Monoclonal antibodies against PD-1 or its ligands, PDL1 and PDL2, upregulate the immune response and can inhibit tumor cell proliferation.[31–34] Current agents that target these pathways are shown in Table 24.1.

TABLE 24.1 ■ **Common Drugs for Medical Treatment**

Drug Class	Name
CTLA-4 Blockade	Ipilimumab Tremelimumab
PD-1 Blockade	Nivolumab Pembrolizumab
PD-L1 Blockade	Atezolizumab Durvalumab Avelumab

Specific Endocrinopathies Associated With Immune Checkpoint Inhibitor Therapy

HYPOPHYSITIS

Hypophysitis, inflammation of the pituitary gland or pituitary stalk, has increased in incidence after being recognized as a complication from immune checkpoint inhibitor (ICI) therapy. The reported incidence of hypophysitis from anti-CTLA4 therapy has varied greatly from 0.4% to 17%.[35] Tremelimumab has a lower reported incidence compared with ipilimumab (0.4% to 2.6% vs. 0.7% to 18.1%).[35–49] More recent studies with an increased recognition of hypophysitis as a potential complication described incidence rates from 7.4% to 16.3 % following ipilimumab.[38,50,51] Hypophysitis induced by anti-PD1/PDL1 monotherapy is less common (estimated at 1% or less), although more cases may be described as these agents become more widely used and studied more extensively.[35,52–56]

Hypophysitis related to anti-CTLA4 therapy is an urgent endocrine condition, and most frequently presents with nonspecific symptoms such as headache, fatigue, and weakness.[38,56,57] Other, less common symptoms can be nausea, poor appetite, weight loss, vision or mental status changes, temperature intolerance, and arthralgias.[38,40,57] It may also be more common in men.[38] However, this has been suggested to be related to the increased prevalence of men with melanoma in the trials examined. Age may also be a risk factor for hypophysitis after ICI therapy.[38]

Inflammation and subsequent damage to the pituitary gland can manifest in a variety of hormonal deficiencies, the most dangerous being ACTH and TSH deficiency, which leads to secondary adrenal insufficiency and secondary hypothyroidism, respectively. ACTH and TSH deficiency are the most common pituitary hormone deficiency reported after anti-CTLA4–associated hypophysitis (CTLA4-H). Diabetes insipidus or posterior pituitary compromise is rare in these cases.[35,38,40,57] Hypophysitis from ICI therapy can be associated with clinically significant morbidity thought to be largely related to secondary adrenal insufficiency, with an incidence reported at approximately 6% across studies.[35] Adrenal insufficiency and subsequent adrenal crisis can be life-threatening if left untreated/unrecognized. Symptoms of adrenal insufficiency can rapidly improve after steroid replacement with or without thyroid hormone.[38,40] Fifty percent of subjects can have hyponatremia that improves after hormone replacement.[38,57] Hypogonadism from pituitary damage may also occur. Insulin growth factor-1 (IGF-1) levels can be low but are measured less frequently, as growth hormone therapy is contraindicated in active malignancy.[35,38] Both elevated and decreased prolactin levels have been described after hypophysitis related to ICI therapy.[38,54,57,58]

The secondary adrenal insufficiency that results from CTLA4-H is rarely reversible. Long-term glucocorticoid replacement is typically required.[54,57] Recovery from secondary hypothyroidism has been reported from 6% to 64%[38,54]; reports of resolution from secondary hypogonadism vary from 12% to 57%.[38,58,59] Thyroid and gonadotropin function assessment in ill patients can be complex as thyroid and gonadal laboratory tests during sickness can be similar to results seen in pituitary insufficiency (i.e., sick euthyroid syndrome/sickness-induced hypogonadism). Subsequently, differentiating recovery after illness from true recovery from CTLA4-H–induced thyroid or gonadal hormone deficiency may be challenging. However, with respect to cortisol levels, these values typically rise during illness.

In CTLA-4H, pituitary magnetic resonance imaging (MRI) can show mild to moderate diffuse enlargement of the pituitary gland with homogenous or heterogeneous appearance after contrast in 75% to 100% of patients.[35,38] Thickening of the pituitary stalk can be seen. Optic nerve compression is uncommon. The time frame of the MRI with respect to the diagnosis of hypophysitis and the radiologist's experience with this entity may result in a lower possibility of positive findings on MRI. Pituitary enlargement has been shown to precede the clinical diagnosis of CTLA4-H, with the median time to onset of pituitary enlargement appearing 1 week before biochemical evidence of hormone deficiency.[38,54] An enlarged pituitary has been shown to decrease in size over 4 to 12 weeks, and subsequent atrophy of the gland can be seen.[35,54,59,60] Headache and pituitary enlargement may occur less commonly in nivolumab/pemrolizumab patients with hypophysitis (23% in one study).[56]

CTLA4-H has been related to the ICI dose received, although there have been conflicting studies regarding this finding.[38,40,54] Symptom onset has ranged from 6 to 14 weeks after anti-CTLA4 therapy, often occurring after the third treatment.[38,57] As described in one study, hypophysitis from anti-PD1 therapy without CTLA-4 blockade may occur later after therapy (median: 25.8 weeks, interquartile range [IR]: 18.4–44.0) compared with ipilimumab alone (9.3, IR: 7.2–11.1) or patients treated with a combination of both of these agents (12.5, IR: 7.4–18.6).[56]

High-dose steroids have been used to try to reduce pituitary inflammation from CTLA4-H in the hopes of also preserving or reversing pituitary damage; however, they do not appear to improve the course of hormonal recovery.[40,54,57] In addition, there is a concern that the immunosuppressant effect of high-dose steroids could negatively affect the antitumor efficacy of immune checkpoint inhibition.[61] Accordingly, high-dose steroids should be reserved for those with clinically significant illness, hyponatremia, severe headache, or marked pituitary enlargement that approaches the optic apparatus.[15,34]

PRIMARY THYROID DYSFUNCTION

Primary thyroid dysfunction is related to a thyroid gland abnormality, in contrast to secondary hypothyroidism that is related to hypophysitis/pituitary dysfunction. Primary thyroid dysfunction after ICI therapy is usually from thyroiditis and may be seen as diffuse uptake on a positron emission tomography (PET) scan.[62] Thyroiditis can present first as thyrotoxicosis due to thyroid hormone release from inflamed thyroid tissue, which can then result in hypothyroidism. Graves' disease is less common in these patients. Anti-CTLA4 and anti-PD1/PDL1 therapy can result in primary thyroid dysfunction; however, it may be more common with PD1/PDL1 blockade.[40,63] Studies of primary hypothyroidism after ipilimumab reported rates of approximately 5% to 6% occurring from 5 months to 3 years after treatment.[38,40]

In initial studies, the overall rate was approximately 5% to 8% for hypothyroidism and approximately 3% for hyperthyroidism after PD1 inhibition.[35] In thyroiditis, thyrotoxicosis can precede hypothyroidism in the same patient, as described previously. Subsequent studies looking specifically for primary thyroid dysfunction note that the rates could be as high as 14% to 20% after PD1 inhibition, particularly after combination ICI therapy.[63,64] Hypothyroidism onset can be as early as 3 weeks after treatment and up to 10 months following therapy; however, the majority of cases occur within the first 1 to 3 months of ICI treatment.[45,63,64] Up to 50% of the cases of thyrotoxicosis may be transient, with patients subsequently returning to a euthyroid state.[30] If primary hypothyroidism develops following anti-PD1 therapy, it is often permanent.[30,31,62] A previous history of hypothyroidism or a high titer of thyroid peroxidase antibodies at baseline may predict a higher risk of worsening or recurrent hypothyroidism after anti-PD1 treatment.[63] An 8.6% of incidence of hypothyroidism was reported after a trial with atezolizumab, an anti-PDL1 therapy.[65] Additional clinical studies will be required to investigate whether the endocrine adverse events of anti-PDL1 therapy will be comparable with those seen with other ICI treatments.

PRIMARY ADRENAL INSUFFICIENCY

Case reports of adrenalitis have been published, and overall, the incidence of primary adrenal insufficiency appears rare.[66–68] Ipilimumab, pembrolizumab, and nivolumab have been reported to result in primary adrenal insufficiency. Antiadrenal antibodies have been reported in a couple of studies.[69,70] Adrenal inflammation has also been described,[66,67] as well as diffuse increased uptake of bilateral adrenals on PET scan.[67,71] Adrenal atrophy has also been also reported in a subject.[72] The adrenal insufficiency described in these reports is consistent with ICI-induced autoimmune destruction of the adrenal glands.[68,72]

INSULIN-DEPENDENT DIABETES

Insulin-dependent diabetes following anti-PD-1/PD-L1 therapy (ICI-DM) is uncommon (less than 1% incidence).[73,74] ICI-DM typically presents with marked hyperglycemia or diabetic ketoacidosis (DKA) with low C-peptide levels, and appears irreversible. Patients can present with DKA or marked hyperglycemia as early as 1 week and up to 12 months following therapy initiation, with a median of 8.5 weeks with median glucose of 530 mg/dL.[75] Symptoms of DKA or hyperglycemia include polyuria, polydipsia, blurred vision, and malaise. Positive autoantibodies to diabetic autoantigens can be seen with ICI-DM, as well as upregulation of CD8+ T-cell activity.[75,76] Serum glucose is often measured during standard laboratory monitoring during ICI therapy, and practitioners should follow glucose patterns. Aggressive management of DKA and individualized insulin regimens are required to manage ICI-DM. There are rare cases of IDDM following anti-CTLA4 therapy in the literature.[74]

Combination Therapy

Combining CTLA4 and PD1 blockade can result in an additive benefit with respect to cancer therapy.[77–79] However, combination therapy can increase the rate of adverse events. Additive benefits and increased adverse events with combination therapy were reported after trials of nivolumab/ipilimumab combination versus monotherapy. Approximately 59% of the combination arm had grade III–IV toxicities, in comparison with the monotherapy arm (nivolumab or ipilimumab, 21% and 28%, respectively).[78] With respect to endocrinopathies in the combination arm, the trial reported a 17% incidence of hypothyroidism (nivolumab only 11%, ipilimumab only 5%); 11% incidence of hyperthyroidism (nivolumab 4%, ipilimumab 1.0%), and 7% incidence hypophysitis (nivolumab 1%, ipilimumab 4%). Also, a retrospective study showed that the rate of melanoma patients presenting with any type of thyroid abnormalities may be as high as 50% after anti-CTLA4/PD1 combination therapy.[80]

Endocrinopathies and Treatment Response

An association between clinical response and IRAEs from ICI therapy has been reported in trials.[81] In particular, in patients with ipilimumab-related hypophysitis, a prolonged median survival time (19.4 months vs. 8.8 months in patients without hypophysitis) was reported.[38] Extended survival has been reported with anti-PD1 therapy and the development of thyroid dysfunction; however, studies have been conflicting.[64,82] In a study of patients receiving pembrolizumab for non–small cell lung cancer, the median overall survival in those who had thyroid dysfunction was significantly longer than in those without (median = 40 vs, 14 months, $P = 0.029$),[64] although a possible lead time bias could also occur when studying these outcomes, as only those patients benefiting from prolonged survival from ICI therapy may be followed long enough to record the development of adverse events.

Diagnosis and Management

HYPOPHYSITIS

Hypophysitis has mainly been described after anti-CTLA4 therapy, either alone or in combination with anti-PD1/PDL1 agents. It is rare with anti-PD1/PDL1 therapy alone (1% or less), as described previously. Routine screening during therapy with CTLA4 and/or PD1/PDL1 blockade has included baseline and follow-up thyroid function tests (TFTs) but not adrenal function testing. It is important to consider monitoring morning ACTH and cortisol levels during treatment with CTLA4 blockade given that adrenal insufficiency can be life-threatening (Fig. 24.2). Patients who have symptoms suggestive of hypophysitis should have a prompt evaluation for hypopituitarism. Initial evaluation involves morning ACTH and cortisol levels (ideally at or before 8:00 a.m.) as well as TSH and FT4. If hypophysitis is suspected, pituitary imaging with MRI can be performed. A formal visual field examination may be needed for patients who note visual field changes or have evidence of optic chiasm compression on imaging.

Laboratory evaluation can be considered monthly for the first 6 months on therapy given that hypophysitis tends to occur early in treatment after CTLA4 blockade (Fig. 24.2). If laboratory tests are normal and a patient is asymptomatic, the interval could decrease to every 3 months for the following 6 months and further to every 6 to 12 months thereafter (Fig. 24.2). If TFTs show low or low-normal TSH and low free T4, surveillance brain imaging shows an enlarged pituitary, or symptoms consistent with hypophysitis develop; morning (8:00 a.m.) paired ACTH and cortisol levels should be measured. Patients with secondary adrenal insufficiency from CTLA4-H often have a very low 8:00 a.m. cortisol (less than 3 mcg/dL) with a low ACTH (less than 5 pg/mL).[57] Normal subjects have serum cortisol levels in the early morning (at or before 8:00 a.m.) in the 10 to 20 mcg/dL range.[83] Random ACTH and cortisol levels can be measured if early morning laboratory testing is not possible or there is an urgent need at a clinical visit. These values can be frankly low for any time of day in patients with CTLA4-H. Clinicians should confirm that a patient has not been receiving exogenous steroids for a different indication, as this can influence ACTH and cortisol levels. Patients taking exogenous dexamethasone can have a low ACTH and cortisol level because of hypothalamic–pituitary-adrenal (HPA) axis suppression. However, a patient actively taking prednisone or hydrocortisone may have a low ACTH but a normal or high cortisol, as these medications can be picked up in the assay for cortisol. In contrast, dexamethasone is not detected in the cortisol assay. Long-term steroid use can result in suppression of the HPA axis. Corticosteroid administration for another IRAE can also mask the presentation of ICI-induced adrenal insufficiency or hypophysitis. ACTH-stimulation testing is not as useful in detecting early secondary adrenal insufficiency. This is because, initially, in pituitary injury, the adrenal glands may respond to ACTH stimulation because they have not atrophied from the long-term absence of pituitary ACTH

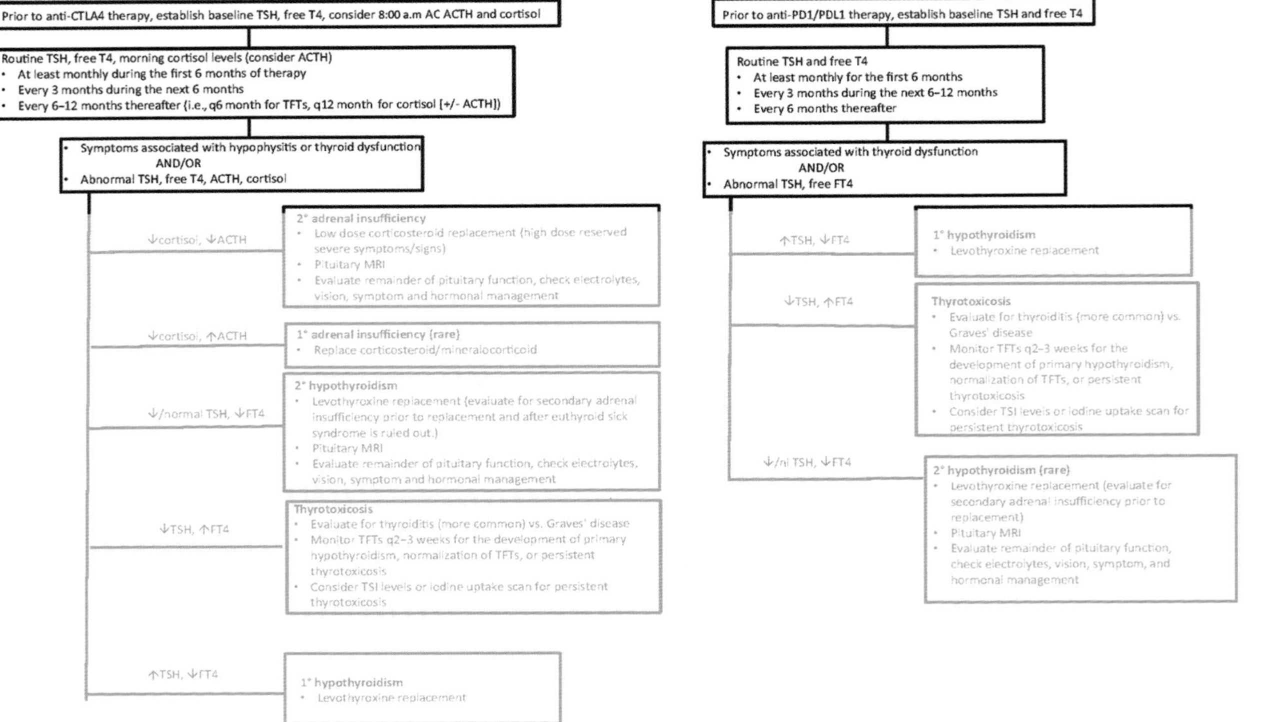

Fig. 24.2 Algorithm for hormonal testing. *ACTH,* Adrenocorticotropic hormone; *CTLA4,* cytotoxic T-lymphocyte antigen 4; *FT4,* free T4; *MRI,* magnetic resonance imaging; *PD1,* programmed death 1; *PDL1,* programmed death 1 ligand; *q,* every; *TFT,* thyroid function test; *TSH,* thyroid-stimulating hormone; *TSI,* thyroid-stimulating immunoglobulin. (From Girotra M, Hansen A, Farooki A, et al. The current understanding of the endocrine effects from immune checkpoint inhibitors and recommendations for management. *JNCI Cancer Spectr.* 2018;2(3):pky021. https://www.ncbi.nlm.nih.gov/pmc/articles/PMC6054022/.)

stimulation.[84] Gonadotropins, testosterone (in males), and estrogen (in premenopausal females) levels should be assessed in those diagnosed with hypophysitis. In those with secondary hypogonadism, prolactin levels can be measured, as hyperprolactinemia can result in hypogonadotropic hypogonadism. There is also a high incidence of hyponatremia in patients with CTLA4-H, which may be due to secondary adrenal insufficiency and/or secondary hypothyroidism.[35] Diabetes insipidus is uncommon in CTLA4-H.[38,57] Growth hormone and IGF1 levels do not necessarily need to be assessed, as growth hormone replacement is contraindicated in patients with active cancer. If CTLA4 and PD1/PDL1 blockade is used, monitoring thyroid function and adrenal function following the recommendation algorithm for anti-CTLA4 monotherapy can be performed as in Fig. 24.2.

In ICI-related hypophysitis, patients can have isolated hormonal deficiency or multiple pituitary hormone deficiencies.[38,57] Therapy goals include hormone replacement and symptom management. Acetaminophen, nonsteroidal antiinflammatories, or steroids can be used to manage headaches. To replace central/secondary adrenal insufficiency, hydrocortisone at approximately 10 mg/m^2 (i.e., 10 to 15 mg in the morning and 5 to 10 mg in the afternoon) or the equivalent dose of daily prednisone can be used.[57] After hormonal replacement is initiated, ICI therapy typically can continue uninterrupted. High-dose steroids can be reserved for critical illness, significant hyponatremia, severe headache, visual disturbances or other neurologic symptoms, or marked pituitary enlargement that is close to the optic chiasm. ICI treatment may be withheld until the patient is stable on hormonal replacement in these more severe clinical situations. Glucocorticoid treatment can decrease pituitary enlargement to help ameliorate associated symptoms; however, high-dose steroids do not appear to reverse hypopituitarism.[54,57–59] Patients with adrenal insufficiency should receive education regarding the need to increase steroids during illness or surgical procedures and should have a medical alert bracelet. Evaluation for pituitary-adrenal axis recovery may be performed every 3 to 6 months for the first year and then every 6 to 12 months, although secondary adrenal insufficiency from CTLA4-H is typically permanent.[57]

Levothyroxine should be used to treat central hypothyroidism after nonthyroidal illness is ruled out. Glucocorticoid replacement should be started before or simultaneously with thyroid hormone replacement in order to prevent precipitating adrenal crisis in those with both ACTH and TSH deficiency.[85] Prolactin can be measured in patients with hypogonadism, as an elevated prolactin can cause secondary hypogonadism. Testosterone replacement may be used to treat male hypogonadism after ruling out hyperprolactinemia and eugonadal sick syndrome. Testosterone replacement therapy should track the Endocrine Society guidelines.[86] If clinically indicated, estrogen replacement can be used in premenopausal women who have hypogonadotropic hypogonadism. Evaluation for pituitary-thyroid and pituitary-gonadal axis recovery may be performed in 3 to 6 months for the first year and subsequently every 6 to 12 months thereafter, as recovery of secondary hypothyroidism and secondary hypogonadism has been reported.[38] Hyponatremia is typically transient and improves following hormonal replacement.

PRIMARY THYROID DYSFUNCTION

Hypothyroidism is the most common endocrine abnormality following either anti-CTLA4 or anti-PD1/PDL1 treatments. Baseline TSH and free T4 can be performed prior to either CTLA4 or PD1/PDL1 blockade and then at least monthly for the first 6 months. If the laboratory tests are normal and the patient is asymptomatic, TFTs can be checked quarterly for months 6 to 12 and about every 6 months thereafter. If a patient has any symptoms or signs of thyroid dysfunction in between visits, TFTs should be measured. Thyroid autoantibodies can be checked if a patient has primary hypothyroidism or thyrotoxicosis.[87]

Clinical and biochemical abnormalities may improve in 2 to 4 weeks in those initially with thyrotoxicosis from thyroiditis, although prolonged thyrotoxicosis has been described.[82] TFTs should be monitored at least every 2 to 3 weeks in those with thyrotoxicosis, as they can progress to hypothyroidism.

Graves' hyperthyroidism and ophthalmopathy are rare after ICI therapy.[88,89] In those with prolonged thyrotoxicosis, goiter, or ophthalmopathy, TSIs, TRAb, or a thyroid uptake scan can be done to evaluate for Graves' hyperthyroidism. One would expect a high iodine uptake in the thyroid gland in Graves' hyperthyroidism. In thyroiditis, one characteristically sees a low iodine uptake. Radioactive iodine uptake scans in cancer patients can be inaccurate given their exposure to imaging using iodinated contrast, which lowers the thyroid's iodine uptake.[90]

Symptom management with a beta-blocker may be used for transient thyrotoxicosis from thyroiditis. Many patients with thyrotoxicosis from thyroiditis are relatively asymptomatic. Glucocorticoid treatment is rarely needed and may be considered in those with heart disease and/or severe symptoms who could warrant withholding of ICI treatment. An ATD, such as methimazole, can be used for Graves' hyperthyroidism. However, these agents are ineffective for thyrotoxicosis from thyroiditis, which causes the majority of cases of ICI-thyrotoxicosis.

Levothyroxine should be started and titrated up every 4 to 6 weeks to normalize TFTs for primary hypothyroidism.[91] Patients can be closely followed without thyroid hormone replacement if asymptomatic with an elevated TSH lower than 10 and normal free T4.[92] In secondary hypothyroidism from pituitary dysfunction (low free T4 with a low or low-normal TSH), secondary adrenal insufficiency should be ruled out before giving thyroid hormone to avoid causing adrenal crisis. A low replacement dose of levothyroxine should be started and increased slowly in elderly patients or those with cardiac disease.[91] Immunotherapy can be withheld in severe symptomatic cases of thyroid dysfunction, although this is uncommon.

PRIMARY ADRENAL INSUFFICIENCY

Monitoring guidelines have not been established for ICI-related primary adrenal insufficiency given its rare occurrence. If adrenal enlargement or atrophy is seen on routine scans, it is important to evaluate adrenal function by measuring ACTH and cortisol levels, as well as a cosyntropin stimulation test, to assess for primary adrenal insufficiency. Both corticosteroid and mineralocorticoid replacement are used to treat primary adrenal insufficiency.

INSULIN-DEPENDENT DIABETES

Even though IDDM is rare during ICI therapy, practitioners should be familiar with the signs and symptoms of DKA or hyperglycemia (polyuria, polydipsia, blurred vision, malaise), as missing this diagnosis can be life-threatening. Serum glucose is often measured during standard laboratory monitoring during ICI therapy, and practitioners should follow glucose patterns. Tests for autoantibodies (glutamic acid decarboxylase/GAD65 Abs, insulin Abs, islet cell Abs, zinc transporter 8/Zn-T8 Abs) and endogenous insulin secretion (C-peptide and insulin levels) can differentiate between insulin-dependent and non–insulin-dependent diabetes. Aggressive management of DKA and individualized insulin regimens are required to manage ICI-DM.

COMBINATION THERAPY

For patients on combined therapy with CTL4 and PD1/PDL1 blockade, clinicians can follow the suggested testing for monotherapy (Fig. 24.2) and be mindful of the potential increased risk of endocrinopathies with combination ICI therapy.

Conclusions

Endocrinopathies induced by immune checkpoint blockade have been reported with increasing detail as indications for these agents expands across all fields of oncology. Even though the precise mechanisms are not known, increased activity of the immune system induced by ICI therapy can result in autoimmunity against normal tissue. Anti-CTLA4 treatment is associated with hypophysitis and primary thyroid dysfunction. PD1/PDL1 blockade is predominantly linked to primary thyroid dysfunction from thyroiditis. Combination CTLA4 and PD1 blockade therapies appear to confer an increased risk for both thyroid dysfunction and hypophysitis compared with monotherapy. Fulminant IDDM has been reported after PD1/PDL1 blockade, with only a few cases reports after CTLA4 blockade. Reports suggest that particular IRAEs can be associated with a superior response to cancer therapy. Additional studies are needed to fully describe this relationship. The overall frequency of endocrinopathies may not be fully appreciated given that earlier clinical trials may not have thoroughly monitored for endocrine adverse events. Clinicians need to be aware of these endocrinopathies as some can be life-threatening if undiagnosed. Fortunately, there are effective screening methods and hormonal replacement therapies for ICI-associated endocrinopathies. If detected and treated early, the morbidity associated with these disorders can be reduced, as well as limit the interruption of life-saving immunotherapy.

References

1. Schwartz RH. Costimulation of T lymphocytes: the role of CD28, CTLA-4, and B7/BB1 in interleukin-2 production and immunotherapy. *Cell.* 1992;71:1065–1068.
2. Lenschow DJ, Walunas TL, Bluestone JA. CD28/B7 system of T cell costimulation. *Annu Rev Immunol.* 1996;14:233–258.
3. Rudd CE, Taylor A, Schneider H. CD28 and CTLA-4 coreceptor expression and signal transduction. *Immunol Rev.* 2009;229:12–26.
4. Freeman GJ, Gribben JG, Boussiotis VA, et al. Cloning of B7-2: a CTLA-4 counter-receptor that costimulates human T cell proliferation. *Science.* 1993;262:909–911.
5. Azuma M, Ito D, Yagita H, et al. B70 antigen is a second ligand for CTLA-4 and CD28. *Nature.* 1993;366:76–79.
6. Linsley PS, Clark EA, Ledbetter JA. T-cell antigen CD28 mediates adhesion with B cells by interacting with activation antigen B7/BB-1. *Proc Natl Acad Sci USA.* 1990;87:5031–5035.
7. Linsley PS, Brady W, Urnes M, Grosmaire LS, Damle NK, Ledbetter JA. CTLA-4 is a second receptor for the B cell activation antigen B7. *J Exp Med.* 1991;174:561–569.
8. Linsley PS, Greene JL, Brady W, Bajorath J, Ledbetter JA, Peach R. Human B7-1 (CD80) and B7-2 (CD86) bind with similar avidities but distinct kinetics to CD28 and CTLA-4 receptors. *Immunity.* 1994;1:793–801.
9. Riley JL, Mao M, Kobayashi S, et al. Modulation of TCR-induced transcriptional profiles by ligation of CD28, ICOS, and CTLA-4 receptors. *Proc Natl Acad Sci USA.* 2002;99:11790–11795.
10. Schneider H, Downey J, Smith A, et al. Reversal of the TCR stop signal by CTLA-4. *Science.* 2006;313:1972–1975.
11. Egen JG, Allison JP. Cytotoxic T lymphocyte antigen-4 accumulation in the immunological synapse is regulated by TCR signal strength. *Immunity.* 2002;16:23–35.
12. Parry RV, Chemnitz JM, Frauwirth KA, et al. CTLA-4 and PD-1 receptors inhibit T-cell activation by distinct mechanisms. *Mol Cell Biol.* 2005;25:9543–9553.
13. Schneider H, Mandelbrot DA, Greenwald RJ, et al. Cutting edge: CTLA-4 (CD152) differentially regulates mitogen-activated protein kinases (extracellular signal-regulated kinase and c-Jun N-terminal kinase) in CD4+ T cells from receptor/ligand-deficient mice. *J Immunol.* 2002;169:3475–3479.
14. Hathcock KS, Laszlo G, Dickler HB, Bradshaw J, Linsley P, Hodes RJ. Identification of an alternative CTLA-4 ligand costimulatory for T cell activation. *Science.* 1993;262:905–907.
15. Tivol EA, Borriello F, Schweitzer AN, Lynch WP, Bluestone JA, Sharpe AH. Loss of CTLA-4 leads to massive lymphoproliferation and fatal multiorgan tissue destruction, revealing a critical negative regulatory role of CTLA-4. *Immunity.* 1995;3:541–547.

16. Waterhouse P, Penninger JM, Timms E, et al. Lymphoproliferative disorders with early lethality in mice deficient in CTLA-4. *Science*. 1995;270:985–988.
17. Hodi FS, O'Day SJ, McDermott DF, et al. Improved survival with ipilimumab in patients with metastatic melanoma. *N Engl J Med*. 2010;363:711–723.
18. Pandolfi F, Cianci R, Lolli S, et al. Strategies to overcome obstacles to successful immunotherapy of melanoma. *Int J Immunopathol Pharmacol*. 2008;21:493–500.
19. Gabrilovich DI, Nagaraj S. Myeloid-derived suppressor cells as regulators of the immune system. *Nat Rev Immunol*. 2009;9:162–174. doi:10.1038/nri2506.
20. Stewart TJ, Smyth MJ. Improving cancer immunotherapy by targeting tumor-induced immune suppression. *Cancer Metastasis Rev*. 2011;30:125–140. doi:10.1007/s10555-011-9280-5.
21. Linsley PS, Brady W, Grosmaire L, Aruffo A, Damle NK, Ledbetter JA. Binding of the B cell activation antigen B7 to CD28 costimulates T cell proliferation and interleukin 2 mRNA accumulation. *J Exp Med*. 1991;173:721–730.
22. Zou W. Regulatory T cells, tumour immunity and immunotherapy. *Nat Rev Immunol*. 2006;6:295–307.
23. Topalian SL, Sznol M, McDermott DF, et al. Survival, durable tumor remission, and long-term safety in patients with advanced melanoma receiving nivolumab. *J Clin Oncol*. 2014;32:1020–1030. doi:10.1200/JCO.2013.53.0105.
24. Topalian SL, Hodi FS, Brahmer JR, et al. Safety, activity, and immune correlates of anti-PD-1 antibody in cancer. *N Engl J Med*. 2012;366:2443–2454.
25. Latchman Y, Wood CR, Chernova T, et al. PD-L2 is a second ligand for PD-1 and inhibits T cell activation. *Nat Immunol*. 2001;2:261–268.
26. Freeman GJ, Long AJ, Iwai Y, et al. Engagement of the PD-1 immunoinhibitory receptor by a novel B7 family member leads to negative regulation of lymphocyte activation. *J Exp Med*. 2000;192:1027–1034.
27. Topalian SL, Drake CG, Pardoll DM. Targeting the PD-1/B7-H1(PD-L1) pathway to activate anti-tumor immunity. *Curr Opin Immunol*. 2012;24:207–212.
28. Agata Y, Kawasaki A, Nishimura H, et al. Expression of the PD-1 antigen on the surface of stimulated mouse T and B lymphocytes. *Int Immunol*. 1996;8:765–772.
29. Dong H, Strome SE, Salomao DR, et al. Tumor-associated B7-H1 promotes T-cell apoptosis: a potential mechanism of immune evasion. *Nat Med*. 2002;8:793–800. doi:10.1038/nm730.
30. Yamazaki T, Akiba H, Iwai H, et al. Expression of programmed death 1 ligands by murine T cells and APC. *J Immunol*. 2002;169:5538–5545.
31. Okazaki T, Honjo T. PD-1 and PD-1 ligands: from discovery to clinical application. *Int Immunol*. 2007;19:813–824. doi:10.1093/intimm/dxm057.
32. Zou W, Chen L. Inhibitory B7-family molecules in the tumour microenvironment. *Nat Rev Immunol*. 2008;8:467–477. doi:10.1038/nri2326.
33. Taube JM, Anders RA, Young GD, et al. Colocalization of inflammatory response with B7-h1 expression in human melanocytic lesions supports an adaptive resistance mechanism of immune escape. *Sci Transl Med*. 2012;4. doi:10.1126/scitranslmed.3003689 127ra137.
34. Chow LQ. Exploring novel immune-related toxicities and endpoints with immune-checkpoint inhibitors in non-small cell lung cancer. *Am Soc Clin Oncol Educ Book*. 2013. doi:10.1200/EdBook_AM.2013.33.e280.
35. Byun DJ, Wolchok JD, Rosenberg LM, et al. Cancer immunotherapy—immune checkpoint blockade and associated endocrinopathies. *Nat Rev Endocrinol*. 2017;134:195–207.
36. Albarel F, Gaudy C, Castinetti F, et al. Long-term follow-up of ipilimumab-induced hypophysitis, a common adverse event of the anti-CTLA-4 antibody in melanoma. *Eur J Endocrinol*. 2015;1722:195–204.
37. Ansell SM, Hurvitz SA, Koenig PA, et al. Phase I study of ipilimumab, an anti-CTLA-4 monoclonal antibody, in patients with relapsed and refractory B-cell non-Hodgkin lymphoma. *Clin Cancer Res*. 2009;1520:6446–6453.
38. Faje AT, Sullivan R, Lawrence D, et al. Ipilimumab-induced hypophysitis: a detailed longitudinal analysis in a large cohort of patients with metastatic melanoma. *J Clin Endocrinol Metab*. 2014;9911:4078–4085.
39. Royal RE, Levy C, Turner K, et al. Phase 2 trial of single agent ipilimumab (anti-CTLA-4) for locally advanced or metastatic pancreatic adenocarcinoma. *J Immunother*. 2010;338:828–833.

40. Ryder M, Callahan M, Postow MA, et al. Endocrine-related adverse events following ipilimumab in patients with advanced melanoma: a comprehensive retrospective review from a single institution. *Endocr Relat Cancer*. 2014;212:371–381.
41. Yang JC, Hughes M, Kammula U, et al. Ipilimumab (anti-CTLA4 antibody) causes regression of metastatic renal cell cancer associated with enteritis and hypophysitis. *J Immunother*. 2007;308:825–830.
42. Attia P, Phan GQ, Maker AV, et al. Autoimmunity correlates with tumor regression in patients with metastatic melanoma treated with anti-cytotoxic T-lymphocyte antigen-4. *J Clin Oncol*. 2005;2325:6043–6053.
43. Downey SG, Klapper JA, Smith FO, et al. Prognostic factors related to clinical response in patients with metastatic melanoma treated by CTL-associated antigen-4 blockade. *Clin Cancer Res*. 2007;13(22 Pt 1): 6681–6688.
44. Hersh EM, O'Day SJ, Powderly J, et al. A phase II multicenter study of ipilimumab with or without dacarbazine in chemotherapy-naïve patients with advanced melanoma. *Invest New Drugs*. 2011;293:489–498.
45. Ku GY, Yuan J, Page DB, et al. Single-institution experience with ipilimumab in advanced melanoma patients in the compassionate use setting: lymphocyte count after 2 doses correlates with survival. *Cancer*. 2010;1167:1767–1775.
46. Chung KY, Gore I, Fong L, et al. Phase II study of the anti-cytotoxic T-lymphocyte-associated antigen 4 monoclonal antibody, tremelimumab, in patients with refractory metastatic colorectal cancer. *J Clin Oncol*. 2010;2821:3485–3490.
47. Kirkwood JM, Lorigan P, Hersey P, et al. Phase II trial of tremelimumab (CP-675,206) in patients with advanced refractory or relapsed melanoma. *Clin Cancer Res*. 2010;163:1042–1048.
48. Ralph C, Elkord E, Burt DJ, et al. Modulation of lymphocyte regulation for cancer therapy: a phase II trial of tremelimumab in advanced gastric and esophageal adenocarcinoma. *Clin Cancer Res*. 2010;165:1662–1672.
49. Ribas A, Camacho LH, Lopez-Berestein G, et al. Antitumor activity in melanoma and anti-self responses in a phase I trial with the anti-cytotoxic T lymphocyte-associated antigen 4 monoclonal antibody CP-675,206. *J Clin Oncol*. 2005;2335:8968–8977.
50. Ryder M, Callahan M, Postow MA, et al. Endocrine-related adverse events following ipilimumab in patients with advanced melanoma: a comprehensive retrospective review from a single institution. *Endocr Relat Cancer*. 2014;212:371–381.
51. Eggermont AM, Chiarion-Sileni V, Grob JJ, et al. Prolonged survival in stage III melanoma with ipilimumab adjuvant therapy. *N Engl J Med*. 2016;37519:1845–1855.
52. Brahmer JR, Tykodi SS, Chow LQ, et al. Safety and activity of anti-PD-L1 antibody in patients with advanced cancer. *N Engl J Med*. 2012;36626:2455–2465.
53. Herbst RS, Soria JC, Kowanetz M, et al. Predictive correlates of response to the anti-PD-L1 antibody MPDL3280A in cancer patients. *Nature*. 2014;5157528:563–567.
54. Min L, Hodi FS, Giobbie-Hurder A, et al. Systemic high-dose corticosteroid treatment does not improve the outcome of ipilimumab-related hypophysitis: a retrospective cohort study. *Clin Cancer Res*. 2015;214:749–755.
55. Topalian SL, Hodi FS, Brahmer JR, et al. Safety, activity, and immune correlates of anti-PD-1 antibody in cancer. *N Engl J Med*. 2012;36626:2443–2454.
56. Faje A, Reynolds K, Zubiri L, et al. Hypophysitis secondary to nivolumab and pembrolizumab is a clinical entity distinct from ipilimumab-associated hypophysitis. *Eur J Endocrinol*. 2019;181(3):211–219.
57. Sinha AG, Zheng J, Girotra M. Pituitary dysfunction after CTLA-4 blockade: time course and hypothalamic-pituitary-adrenal (HPA) axis recovery. Abstract and oral presentation in: Endocrine Society 100th Annual Meeting, Chicago, IL. *Endocr Rev*. 2018:392.
58. Blansfield JA, Beck KE, Tran K, et al. Cytotoxic T-lymphocyte-associated antigen-4 blockage can induce autoimmune hypophysitis in patients with metastatic melanoma and renal cancer. *J Immunother*. 2005;286:593–598.
59. Min L, Vaidya A, Becker C. Association of ipilimumab therapy for advanced melanoma with secondary adrenal insufficiency: a case series. *Endocr Pract*. 2012;183:351–355.
60. Carpenter KJ, Murtagh RD, Lilienfeld H, et al. Ipilimumab-induced hypophysitis: MR imaging findings. *Am J Neuroradiol*. 2009;309:1751–1753.
61. Faje AT, Lawrence D, Flaherty K, et al. High-dose glucocorticoids for the treatment of ipilimumab-induced hypophysitis is associated with reduced survival in patients with melanoma. *Cancer*. 2018; 124(18):3706–3714.

62. de Filette J, Jansen Y, Schreuer M, et al. Incidence of thyroid-related adverse events in melanoma patients treated with pembrolizumab. *J Clin Endocrinol Metab*. 2016;10111:4431–4439.
63. Delivanis DA, Gustafson MP, Bornschlegl S, et al. Pembrolizumab-induced thyroiditis: comprehensive clinical review and insights into underlying involved mechanisms. *J Clin Endocrinol Metab*. 2017;1028:2770–2780.
64. Osorio JC, Ni A, Chaft JE, et al. Antibody-mediated thyroid dysfunction during T-cell checkpoint blockade in patients with non-small-cell lung cancer. *Ann Oncol*. 2017;283:583–589.
65. McDermott DF, Sosman JA, Sznol M, et al. Atezolizumab, an anti-programmed death-ligand 1 antibody, in metastatic renal cell carcinoma: long-term safety, clinical activity, and immune correlates from a phase Ia study. *J Clin Oncol*. 2016;348:833–842.
66. Min L, Ibrahim N. Ipilimumab-induced autoimmune adrenalitis. *Lancet Diabetes Endocrinol*. 2013;13:e15.
67. Bacanovic S, Burger IA, Stolzmann P, et al. Ipilimumab-induced adrenalitis: a possible pitfall in 18F-FDG-PET/CT. *Clin Nucl Med*. 2015;40(11):e518–e519.
68. Castinetti F, Albarel F, Archambeaud F, et al. French Endocrine Society guidance on endocrine side effects of immunotherapy. *Endocr Relat Cancer*. 2019;26(2):G1–G18 Feb.
69. Paepegaey A-C, Lheure C, Ratour C, et al. Polyendocrinopathy resulting from pembrolizumab in a patient with a malignant melanoma. *J Endocrine Soc*. 2017;1:646–649. doi:10.1210/js.2017-00170.
70. Hescot S, Haissaguerre M, Pautier P, Kuhn E, Schlumberger M, Berdelou A. Immunotherapy-induced Addison's disease: a rare, persistent and potentially lethal side-effect. *Eur J Cancer*. 2018;97:57–58.
71. Trainer H, Hulse P, Higham CE, Trainer P, Lorigan P. Hyponatraemia secondary to nivolumab-induced primary adrenal failure. *Endocrinol Diabetes Metab Case Rep*. 2016;2016:16–0108. doi:10.1530/EDM-16-0108.
72. Hescot S, Haissaguerre M, Pautier P, Kuhn E, Schlumberger M, Berdelou A. Immunotherapy-induced Addison's disease: a rare, persistent and potentially lethal side-effect. *European Journal of Cancer*. 2018;97:57–58. doi:10.1016/j.ejca.2018.04.001.
73. Perdigoto AL, Quandt Z, Anderson M, Herold KC. Checkpoint inhibitor-induced insulin-dependent diabetes: an emerging syndrome. *Lancet Diabetes Endocrinol*. 2019;7(6):421–423. doi:10.1016/S2213-8587(19)30072-5.
74. Stamatouli AM, Quandt Z, Perdigoto AL, et al. Collateral damage: insulin-dependent diabetes induced with checkpoint inhibitors. *Diabetes*. 2018;67980:1471–1480. doi:10.2337/dbi18-0002.
75. Gauci ML, Laly P, Vidal-Trecan T, et al. Autoimmune diabetes induced by PD-1 inhibitor-retrospective analysis and pathogenesis: a case report and literature review. *Cancer Immunol Immunother*. 2017;66(11):1399–1410.
76. Hughes J, Vudattu N, Sznol M, et al. Precipitation of autoimmune diabetes with anti-PD-1 immunotherapy. *Diabetes Care*. 2015;384:e55–e57.
77. Postow MA, Chesney J, Pavlick AC, et al. Nivolumab and ipilimumab versus ipilimumab in untreated melanoma. *N Engl J Med*. 2015;37221:2006–2017.
78. Wolchok JD, Chiarion-Sileni V, Gonzalez R, et al. Overall survival with combined nivolumab and ipilimumab in advanced melanoma. *N Engl J Med*. 2017;37714:1345–1356.
79. Hodi FS, Chesney J, Pavlick AC, et al. Combined nivolumab and ipilimumab versus ipilimumab alone in patients with advanced melanoma: 2-year overall survival outcomes in a multicentre, randomised, controlled, phase 2 trial. *Lancet Oncol*. 2016;1711:1558–1568.
80. Morganstein DL, Lai Z, Spain L, et al. Thyroid abnormalities following the use of cytotoxic T-lymphocyte antigen-4 and programmed death receptor protein-1 inhibitors in the treatment of melanoma. *Clin Endocrinol (Oxf)*. 2017;864:614–620.
81. Weber JS, Kähler KC, Hauschild A. Management of immune-related adverse events and kinetics of response with ipilimumab. *J Clin Oncol*. 2012;3021:2691–2697.
82. Orlov S, Salari F, Kashat L, et al. Induction of painless thyroiditis in patients receiving programmed death 1 receptor immunotherapy for metastatic malignancies. *J Clin Endocrinol Metab*. 2015;1005:1738–1741.
83. Hägg E, Asplund K, Lithner F. Value of basal plasma cortisol assays in the assessment of pituitary-adrenal insufficiency. *Clin Endocrinol (Oxf)*. 1987;262:221–226.
84. Suliman AM, Smith TP, Labib M, et al. The low-dose ACTH test does not provide a useful assessment of the hypothalamic-pituitary-adrenal axis in secondary adrenal insufficiency. *Clin Endocrinol (Oxf)*. 2002;564:533–539.

85. Smith JC. Hormone replacement therapy in hypopituitarism. *Expert Opin Pharmacother*. 2004;55:1023–1031.
86. Seftel AD, Kathrins M, Niederberger C. Critical update of the 2010 Endocrine Society clinical practice guidelines for male hypogonadism: a systematic analysis. *Mayo Clin Proc*. 2015;908:1104–1115.
87. Sinclair D. Clinical and laboratory aspects of thyroid autoantibodies. *Ann Clin Biochem*. 2006;43(Pt 3): 173–183.
88. Min L, Vaidya A, Becker C. Thyroid autoimmunity and ophthalmopathy related to melanoma biological therapy. *Eur J Endocrinol*. 2011;1642:303–307.
89. Borodic G, Hinkle DM, Cia Y. Drug-induced Graves' disease from CTLA-4 receptor suppression. *Ophthal Plast Reconstr Surg*. 2011;274:e87–e88.
90. Hamnvik OP, Larsen PR, Marqusee E. Thyroid dysfunction from antineoplastic agents. *J Natl Cancer Inst*. 2011;10321:1572–1587.
91. Jonklaas J, Bianco AC, Bauer AJ, et al. Guidelines for the treatment of hypothyroidism: prepared by the American Thyroid Association task force on thyroid hormone replacement. *Thyroid*. 2014;2412:1670–1751.
92. Pearce SH, Brabant G, Duntas LH, et al. 2013 ETA guideline: management of subclinical hypothyroidism. *Eur Thyroid J*. 2013;24:215–228.

PART 10

Endocrine Responses in Critically Ill Trauma Patients: Nuclear Emergency

CHAPTER 25

Endocrine Responses in Critically Ill and Trauma Patients

Lane L. Frasier ■ Jane J. Keating ■ Adam Michael Shiroff

CHAPTER OUTLINE

Introduction

The human body maintains homeostasis via multiple regulatory systems that exert tight control over every organ system, with continuous regulation via negative feedback mechanisms. These systems often have overlapping and complementary effects leading to coordinated changes across multiple body systems in response to a stimulus or stressor. Heart rate, blood pressure, and systemic venous and arterial tone are controlled via the sympathetic and parasympathetic nervous systems, interfacing closely with renin, aldosterone, angiotensin, and arginine vasopressin (AVP) to regulate intravascular volume and osmolality. The hypothalamus–pituitary–adrenal axis is responsible for ensuring appropriate adrenergic and glucocorticoid responses to stress, with downstream effects on metabolisms, glycolysis, gluconeogenesis, and immune function. These systems work in concert to maintain homeostasis in response to stressors including exercise, illness, and injury. Under ideal conditions, with resolution of the external stressor, these systems return to baseline function and homeostasis is restored.

Critical illness, by definition, is any life-threatening condition that would result in death without support of one or more organ systems.[1] During critical illness, homeostasis is severely disrupted, and one or more regulatory systems are unable to compensate for the inciting event. When regulatory mechanisms are inadequate or, conversely, inadequately regulated, they can cause or exacerbate critical illness. For example, sepsis is defined as a dysregulated host response to infection[2] resulting in end organ dysfunction. Additionally, critical illness, especially when prolonged, can result in uncoupling of normal stimulus-response homeostatic mechanisms, resulting in prolonged derangement in physiologic parameters and the inability to return to a baseline state of health, described as chronic critical illness. Although a consensus definition for chronic critical illness does not yet exist, it includes patients with a prolonged (more than 7 days[3]) illness who suffer ongoing organ dysfunction, cognitive decline, malnutrition and an ongoing catabolic state, recurrent or persistent infections, and profound persistent weakness.[3–6]

In this chapter we provide an overview of the normal (expected) response to critical illness and trauma, review what is known about endocrine systems and regulation during chronic critical illness, and discuss specific systems which are impacted during these events. Understanding normal and dysregulated host responses to critical illness and trauma is a vital part of providing critical care, and investigation into the mechanisms underlying chronic critical illness represents a rich target for future interventions in patients with this condition.

Normal Response to Stress

SYMPATHETIC NERVOUS SYSTEM

Stimulation of the sympathetic nervous system due to pain, fever, injury, and illness results in stimulation of the adrenal medulla, which releases epinephrine, and post-ganglionic cells of the sympathetic nervous system, which release norepinephrine. Levels of these hormones can rise 10- to 100-fold in the setting of an acute stress response.[7] Norepinephrine primarily stimulates α-receptors, whereas epinephrine stimulates both β- and α-receptors, with multiple effects throughout the body.[7] Alpha-receptor activation results in vasoconstriction and increased vascular tone and relaxation of smooth muscle of the gastrointestinal tract. Beta-receptor activation results in bronchodilation, as well as increased heart rate (chronotropy) and contractility (inotropy), which work in concert to increase cardiac output. Collectively, these actions work to increase oxygen delivery and vascular tone.

Some patients exhibit a reduced response to increases in epinephrine and norepinephrine in acute illness or trauma. This is especially common in elderly adults and is multifactorial in nature. Resting sympathetic tone increases with increasing age,[8] concomitant with decrease sensitivity of α- and β-receptors, resulting in decreased response to elevated sympathetic nervous system output. Arterioles in older adults are less responsive to α-adrenergic stimulation,[9] and older adults have a reduced maximal heart rate. In addition, older patients are more likely to be prescribed medications such as beta-blockers and calcium channel blockers that prevent increased vasoconstriction and chronotropy. In these patients, the pulse may be inappropriately normal, and early signs of hypovolemia and/or sepsis may be easily missed. Additionally, these patients have reduced physiologic reserve, as they are unable to mount an adrenergic response commensurate with an inciting stressor and can quickly develop hypotension and malperfusion as a result of vasoplegia and hypovolemia. Clinicians should have a high index of suspicion when evaluating these patients and be alert for signs of hypovolemia, hemorrhage, and sepsis.

RENIN–ANGIOTENSIN–ALDOSTERONE SYSTEM

In concert with tight management of serum osmolality and total body volume, regulated by AVP (see later), the renin-angiotensin-aldosterone system is responsible for managing sodium balance and extracellular sodium levels via several mechanisms. Renin is secreted by juxtaglomerular cells in the afferent arteriole of the kidney in response to decreased perfusion pressure, activation of sympathetic nerve fibers in the afferent arterioles, and decreased NaCl delivery to the macula densa.[10] Renin then activates angiotensinogen, produced in the liver, to yield angiotensin I, which moves through the circulation where it is converted to angiotensin II by angiotensin-converting enzyme by pulmonary and renal endothelial cells. Angiotensin II stimulates aldosterone release by the adrenal cortex which enhances NaCl reabsorption throughout the proximal and distal tubule and collecting duct,[10] increases arteriolar vascular tone, which acts to increase blood pressure, and stimulates AVP secretion and decreases urine water losses to increase circulating volume.

ARGININE VASOPRESSIN

The pituitary is closely coupled with the renal system to maintain water balance, serum osmolarity, and intravascular volume. AVP is responsible for regulating the amount of water excreted into urine, therefore maintaining appropriate body water volume and serum osmolality. The strongest mediator of AVP secretion is serum osmolality.[11] In the setting of appropriate serum osmolality, serum AVP levels are low, and the renal collecting duct excretes high volumes of water, resulting in urine with low osmolality. However, as the serum osmolality climbs, relatively small changes in serum osmolality substantially increase AVP secretion.[11] Cells of the anterior hypothalamus called osmoreceptors sense the rising osmolality and signal production of AVP in the supraoptic and paraventricular nuclei of the hypothalamus, which is transported in granules to the posterior pituitary before being released. Serum AVP travels to the renal system where it induces the retention of free water, reducing urine production and returning serum osmolality to normal levels, and returning AVP production to baseline levels.

AVP is also regulated to a lesser extent by decreased blood pressure or blood volume.[11] This is driven by baroreceptors in both low-pressure left atrium and pulmonary artery, which respond to changes in vascular volume, and high-pressure baroreceptors in the aortic arch and carotid sinus, which respond to changes in arterial pressure. Signals from these baroreceptors are relayed to the supraoptic and paraventricular nuclei of the hypothalamus, resulting in AVP production and release. However, these baroreceptors are less sensitive than the osmoreceptors regulating serum osmolality, and a 5% to 10% decrease in blood volume or blood pressure is required before AVP will be released by this mechanism.[11] Additionally, changes in blood pressure and blood volume alter the hypothalamus's response to changes in serum osmolality. With hypovolemia, small changes in osmolality will cause AVP release at osmolalities previously within the normal range. This will result in the conservation of intravascular volume at the expense of decreased serum osmolality. Conversely, with blood volume overload, the serum osmolality set point shifts in the opposite direction, and a higher osmolality is required before AVP will be secreted, resulting in increased water diuresis.

Critically ill patients may develop two conditions involving dysregulation of AVP and serum osmolality. Patients may over-secrete AVP in syndrome of inappropriate anti-diuretic hormone, or SIADH, resulting in inappropriate water retention, low urine output, and hyponatremia. This condition can be caused by malignancy, trauma including intracranial hemorrhage, pulmonary conditions including pneumonia, and medications including selective serotonin reuptake inhibitors (SSRIs), thiazide diuretics, and antiepileptic medications including carbamazepime and oxcarbazepine. Diagnostic criteria include serum Na less than 135 mmol/L, serum osmolality less than 275 mOsm/kg, and spontaneous urine osmolality greater than 100 mOsm/kg.[12] Treatment typically consists of fluid restriction and addressing the underlying etiology causing SIADH.

Conversely, central diabetes insipidus (DI) results from the lack of production and release of AVP. When this occurs, there is minimal water reabsorption in the renal collecting ducts and patients can produce up to 20 L of dilute urine per day, resulting in substantial hypovolemia and hypernatremia. Central DI is commonly caused by traumatic brain injury, central nervous system infections, and tumors. Diagnosis is obtained by performing a water deprivation test, with measurement of serum and urine osmolality before and after water deprivation.[13] Treatment involves reversing inciting causes, when possible, and administration of desmopressin, a vasopressin analogue, to stimulate renal water reabsorption.

In addition to its role in regulating serum osmolality and intravascular volume, AVP also plays a key role in maintaining vascular tone under normal conditions and when patients are in shock. Several conditions, including sepsis and hemorrhagic shock, disrupt normal vasomotor tone, resulting in vasoplegia, hypotension, and hypoperfusion. This can occur despite activation of catecholamine release and activation of the renin-angiotensin system[14] and is mediated at least in part due to increased production of nitric oxide.[15,16] Vasopressin levels would be expected to increase with hypovolemia and hypotension; however, as shock worsens, plasma vasopressin levels decrease,[15,17] perhaps due to depletion of vasopressin stores in the neurohypophysis.[15] Restoration of normal vasopressin levels may improve outcomes in patients with shock: in a recent randomized clinical trial, Sims et al. found that low-dose supplementation of AVP in patients with traumatic hemorrhage had decreased transfusion requirements.[18] A separate randomized controlled trial (RCT) by Gorden et al. found that patients with septic shock required less renal replacement therapy when randomized to vasopressin (0.06 units/minute) versus epinephrine, but no difference in survival.[19]

GROWTH HORMONE

Growth hormone (GH) is released by the anterior pituitary in a pulsatile fashion in response to hypothalamic release of growth hormone-releasing hormone (GHRH). GH has complex effects on multiple peripheral tissues, but in general promotes protein anabolism by increasing amino acid uptake and increased protein synthesis, and utilization of fat stores by stimulating triglyceride breakdown. Regulation of GH release is complex and can be stimulated by hormones other than GHRH, including ghrelin, and inhibited by somatostatin and insulin-like growth factor 1 (IGF-1).[20–23] In critical illness, GH secretion increases, with higher peaks and more frequent pulses of hormone secretion,[20] stimulating release of IGF-1 and inducing lipolysis and hepatic gluconeogenesis.[24]

In chronic critical illness, GH release pulsatility is suppressed, correlating with low levels of IGF-1, and appears to contribute to muscle and bone loss seen in chronic critical illness.[20,25]

HYPOTHALAMIC–PITUITARY–ADRENAL AXIS

Stressful stimuli activate the hypothalamic–pituitary–adrenal (HPA) axis. The hypothalamus releases corticotropin-releasing hormone (CRH), which stimulates the pituitary to release adrenocorticotropic hormone (ACTH). ACTH in turn stimulates the adrenal cortex to release cortisol, a steroid hormone with numerous effects throughout the body. Both cortisol and cortisone have a much higher affinity for mineralocorticoid receptors than glucocorticoid receptors, and at baseline levels of hormone, largely bind to mineralocorticoid receptors.[26] However, with stress, glucocorticoid levels increase and begin occupying glucocorticoid receptors as well. Glucocorticoids, after binding to their receptors in the cellular cytosol,[27] pass into the cell nucleus to regulate transcription of genes related to metabolism, inflammation, and the immune response.

Regulation of the HPA Axis

Under normal circumstances, the HPA axis operates via negative feedback. Elevations in ACTH and cortisol result in decreased secretion of CRH and ACTH, respectively. With acute critical illness, cortisol concentrations are elevated substantially above baseline and remain elevated for several days. With moderate and short episodes of stress and subsequent glucocorticoid secretion, negative feedback inhibition of the HPA axis is rapid (minutes to hours).[27] Several studies have found that ACTH levels in critically ill patients were substantially lower than baseline, consistent with negative feedback. Despite this, cortisol levels remain elevated, due in part to decreased cortisol degradation.[1,28,29] In experimental studies, critically ill patients had a cortisol half-life five times longer than non-critically ill patients.[1,30] Interpretation of serum cortisol levels is complicated by the fact that most cortisol is bound to cortisol-binding globulin and therefore not biologically active; furthermore, stress states appear to impact the availability of glucocorticoid receptors, further modulating the effects of the elevated cortisol levels seen in illness and injury.[1]

With ongoing illness and glucocorticoid production, inhibition of the HPA axis decreases[27] and the normal circadian variation of cortisol is flattened, promoting skeletal muscle catabolism and muscle wasting with fat redistribution, central adiposity, and development of metabolic syndrome and insulin resistance or type 2 diabetes. With prolonged use, corticosteroids also decrease osteoblast number and function resulting in decreased bone formation, osteopenia and osteoporosis, and frequently results in hypertension by causing increased vascular tone in response to baseline levels of endogenous vasoactive agents.[27]

Glucocorticoids in Acute Critical Illness

Glucocorticoids play several critical roles in the normal stress response. They increase vascular reactivity to other vasoactive agents, including norepinephrine and angiotensin II. Glucocorticoids also decrease overall inflammation via several mechanisms. They reduce cell apoptosis at sites of injury and inflammation while simultaneously inducing apoptosis of inflammatory immune cells, including eosinophils, thymocytes, mast cells, and antigen-presenting cells such as dendritic cells.[27] Inhibition of antigen presentation results in a lymphocyte shift from T helper 1 (Th1) to T helper 2 (Th2) cells,[31] shifting cytokine production away from interferon (IFN)-γ, interleukin (IL)-2, and tumor necrosis factor (TNF)-β and encouraging production of IL-4, IL-5, IL-6, IL-10, and IL-13. Overall, this dampens the adaptive immune response and works to prevent an over exuberant host immune response to infection, which could result in excessive hypotension, inflammation, and end-organ dysfunction, which contribute to sepsis. Concomitant with this dampening effect, hematopoietic stem cells are induced by IL-1, IL-6, and other cytokines to produce populations of immature myeloid cells.[4] This myelopoiesis seems to balance the dampening of the adaptive immune response by bolstering the innate immune system.

Glucocorticoids also regulate metabolism via several mechanisms. Glucocorticoids induce inhibition of glucose uptake in peripheral tissues including skin, fibroblasts, white blood cells, and adipocytes, resulting in peripheral hyperglycemia and relative insulin resistance.[27] Glucocorticoids also stimulate lipolysis and muscle cell release of amino acids and activate glucose-6-phosphatase. Together, these effects result in increased hepatic gluconeogenesis by making substrates for gluconeogenesis available and increasing the enzymes necessary for this process. Finally, glucocorticoids induce hepatic liver glycogen synthesis via increased synthesis and activation of hepatic glycogen synthase. This mechanism can be interpreted as preparation for rapid production of glucose on demand from glycogen stores. Overall, these metabolic changes result in decreased lipogenesis and muscle anabolism and increased gluconeogenesis and glycogen storage, resulting in the increased glucose availability for tissues during times of stress.[27]

Glucocorticoids in Chronic Critical Illness

In chronic critical illness, ACTH levels remain suppressed, but cortisol levels remain persistently elevated due to reduced degradation and loss of binding proteins, including albumin, resulting in ACTH-cortisol dissociation. With minimal ACTH stimulation, adrenal tissue atrophies, resulting in depletion of cholesterol esthers and the enzymes necessary for epinephrine and norepinephrine production.[20]

Ongoing glucocorticoid-driven myelopoiesis results in ongoing immunosuppression, which is perpetuated by myeloid-derived suppressor cells that secrete antiinflammatory cytokines IL-10 and transforming growth factor (TGF)-β, antagonize clonal lymphocyte expansion,[4] and decrease T-lymphocyte responsiveness, the persistence of which is associated with poor outcomes in patients with sepsis,[16,26,32,33] including increased risk of nosocomial infection, prolonged intensive care unit (ICU) stay, and mortality. Ongoing marrow production of myeloid cell populations comes at the expense of lymphopoiesis and erythropoiesis, resulting in immunosuppression and anemia or chronic disease. This prolonged state of simultaneous immunosuppression and inflammation has been termed the “Persistent Inflammation-Immunosuppression

Catabolism Syndrome"[3] and is typified by a patient admitted with sepsis or severe injury who has ongoing organ failure, persistent malnutrition and protein catabolism despite appropriate supplementation of macronutrients and calories, poor wound healing, and ongoing functional decline.

Inappropriate or Inadequate Response to Stress

ADRENAL INSUFFICIENCY

Humans and animals without functional adrenal glands are unable to cope with increased metabolic demands from acute illness or injury. Animals and human patients with adrenal insufficiency demonstrate reduced efficacy in the setting of vasoactive medications, which resolves with administration of exogenous glucocorticoids.[34]

Absolute adrenal insufficiency can result from bilateral adrenalectomy, adrenal hemorrhage or trauma, autoimmune conditions, and metastases to the adrenal glands with tissue destruction and subsequent loss of function. These patients frequently have symptoms of adrenal insufficiency in day-to-day life requiring steroid supplementation. More commonly in the ICU, critically ill patients demonstrate a relative adrenal insufficiency in which they are unable to respond appropriately to an acute stressor with an appropriate increase in cortisol production. Relative adrenal insufficiency should be suspected in patients receiving prolonged glucocorticoid therapy due to chronic suppression of ACTH and subsequent adrenal atrophy and in patients with peripheral vascular collapse despite appropriate volume resuscitation. Acute adrenal insufficiency is discussed further in Chapter 14.

THYROIDAL DISEASE

The thyroid is controlled by the hypothalamic–pituitary–thyroid (HPT) axis and feedback loop. The hypothalamus releases thyrotropin-releasing hormone (TRH), which stimulates the secretion of thyroid-stimulating hormone (TSH) by the anterior pituitary. TSH then causes release of thyroid hormones from the thyroid gland. Thyroxine (T4) is converted to the active hormone triiodothyronine (T3). Studies have shown that serum concentrations of these hormones are adaptive and respond to certain environmental factors, and therefore are impacted by critical illness.[36]

Patients hospitalized in the ICU often have low serum concentrations of T4 and T3. In this patient population, despite low T3 and T4, TSH is typically maintained within normal range or is slightly decreased. This is a deviation from the typical negative feedback regulation in the HPT axis, which in primary hypothyroidism would result in an increase in serum TSH. These laboratory value changes found in patients with critical illness are referred to as nonthyroidal illness syndrome (NTIS).[32]

Evidence suggests that sickness, including both acute and chronic illnesses, result in a decrease in serum T3 concentration. As disease progresses, serum T3 further decreases, and is associated with prognosis. NTIS is thought to be present in the majority of critically ill patients. Debate exists as to whether this hypothyroidism is protective or harmful to their recovery. For example, many patients in the ICU seem to display the signs and symptoms classic to patients with hypothyroidism, including hypothermia, muscle weakness, impaired consciousness, and depressed myocardial function. On the other hand, the patient may benefit from depressed metabolism in order to avoid uncontrolled catabolism.[33]

The pathogenesis of NTIS is not entirely understood. The HPT axis is downregulated by severe illness at both the hypothalamic and pituitary level, causing subsequent changes to the negative feedback regulation in the HPT axis. Additionally, liver metabolism of thyroid hormone, as well as the enzymatic processes associated with thyroid hormone metabolism, are altered. Likewise, the proinflammatory cytokines involved in the acute phase response of critical illness directly affect thyroid hormone metabolism.[36] Unlike T4, which is produced only in the thyroid, 80% of T3 is produced by the peripheral 5′-doidination of T4 to T3 in muscle, liver, and kidney by 5′-monodeiodinases (D1 and D2). During critical illness, T3 production decreases. Several mechanisms are thought to inhibit D1 and D2, such as high serum cortisol concentration, high circulating free fatty acid, treatment with drugs that inhibit 5′-monodeiodinase activity, like amiodarone and propranolol, and elevated levels of cytokines.[37]

An additional factor affecting thyroid function in the ICU is poor oral and enteral intake, resulting in malnutrition. Decreased caloric intake during critical illness is thought to contribute to the development of NTIS. Serum thyroid hormones are decreased during a period of fasting and during decreased caloric intake in patients with critical illness.[38] Likewise, many of the drugs commonly used in critical illness result in decreased thyroid function. For example, patients receiving high-dose glucocorticoids (greater than 20 mg/day prednisone), dopamine, or dobutamine often have suppressed TSH. However, in patients with hyperthyroidism, TSH is classically less than 0.01, whereas patients receiving the medications listed above typically have values in the range of 0.08 to 0.4. Therefore, a sensitive TSH assay can be useful. Other frequently used medications, including furosemide, nonsteroidal antiinflammatory drugs (NSAIDs), heparin, anticonvulsants, and metformin, can alter thyroid function tests by mechanisms that are not completely understood.[39]

Patients who take levothyroxine for known hypothyroidism should have it continued during their hospitalization. Likewise, patients with long-standing hypothyroidism and new-onset critical illness are at increased risk of the development of myxedema coma. Given the prevalence of NTIS in patients with critical illness and the decrease of serum thyroid hormones (especially T3) in this patient population, the diagnosis of untreated hypothyroidism can be challenging. In patients suspected to have primary hypothyroidism, the most useful test is measurement of plasma TSH. This is because a normal plasma TSH will rule out primary hypothyroidism. Patients with NTIS who also have primary hypothyroidism will have a high serum TSH. Of note, patients with acute illness and primary hypothyroidism may have a decrease in the typical rise in TSH. Therefore, in this patient population, a high serum TSH and low serum T4 is indicative of hypothyroidism; however, these laboratory abnormalities have been seen in patients recovering from NTIS. Primary hypothyroidism is also supported by a high serum T3 to T4 ratio and typically this ratio is reversed in NTIS. The treatment of hypothyroidism and myxedema coma is to replace thyroid hormone, treat underlying illnesses, and provide supportive care.[32,37]

Diagnosis of hyperthyroidism in patients with NTIS is important and can be difficult, as patients in the ICU are not immune to thyrotoxicosis or thyroid storm. Furthermore, surgery and infection are known precipitating factors of thyroid storm, and therefore patients in the ICU are at increased risk. The combination of decreased TSH, high T4, and normal T3 may suggest a combination of thyrotoxicosis and NTIS but are not specific. Symptoms of thyroid storm, including arrhythmias, fever, and altered mental status, should raise the suspicion of hyperthyroidism in the critically ill. Patients with presumed thyrotoxicosis and thyroid storm in the ICU should be treated aggressively with supportive measures, beta-blockers, intravenous glucocorticoids, and antithyroid drugs.[40] Thyrotoxicosis is discussed further in Chapters 1 and 2.

The outcomes of critically ill patients with abnormal thyroid function tests have been studied but are largely inconclusive. For example, a low serum T3 is associated with increased hospital stay and need for mechanical ventilations for patients with acute heart failure.[41] Additionally, low serum T3 is predictive of a 30-day mortality in patients with community-acquired pneumonia.[42] Low serum T4 values are also associated with increased mortality in critically ill patients. However, additional evidence suggests that low serum T3 levels may be beneficial in the critically ill.[43]

As mentioned previously, the treatment of NTIS is the ICU is controversial. Only a few, small RCTs have studied the effects of treatment with thyroid hormones on patients with NTIS, and there is little consistency regarding treatment choice, as both T3 and levothyroxine have been studied. Additionally, it is noteworthy that normalizing serum thyroid hormone concentrations do not necessarily result in normal tissue concentrations of thyroid hormones in the critically ill. One subset of patients who may benefit from thyroid hormone treatment is patients with heart failure. Although there has been largely inadequate study on this subject, the results are encouraging. An RCT of patients with dilated cardiomyopathy showed positive effects of levothyroxine treatment on cardiac function. In general, there is no conclusion regarding the effectiveness of thyroid hormone treatment of patients in the ICU with NTIS.[37]

In chronic critical illness, hypothalamic TRH is decreased, TSH secretion pulsaltility is lost, and patients demonstrate low plasma T4 and T3. Although the exact mechanism driving TRH suppression is unclear, it appears to be due to an altered set point for feedback inhibition within the hypothalamus.[20] Multiple animal and human studies demonstrate peripheral tissue adaptation by increasing thyroid hormone transporters and increasing peripheral activation of thyroid hormone.[20] These low peripheral T3 levels correlate with muscle and bone anabolism, contributing to the ongoing metabolic wasting seen in the chronically critically ill.[20,30]

GLYCEMIC DYSREGULATION

Glycemic dysregulation, often referred to as "stress hyperglycemia" in the critically ill and trauma population, is common and associated with many factors. The pathophysiology is multifactorial and only partially understood. During critical illness, complex interactions between counterregulatory hormones and cytokines cause excessive production of glucose, which is also coupled with insulin resistance. Stress increases glycogenolysis and gluconeogenesis. Glycogenolysis is triggered by increased catecholamines, whereas gluconeogenesis is triggered by an increase in stress response glucagon. Additionally, insulin resistance exacerbates hyperglycemia and is described as the inability of muscle and adipocyte tissue to take up glucose, which is caused by an alteration of insulin signaling and the downregulation of type 4 glucose transporters (GLUT-4) during critical illness. Likewise, post injury or postoperatively, the influence of cytokines can induce insulin resistance.[44] Additionally, increased glucose reabsorption and decreased renal glucose clearance has been described.[45] All of these factors together lead to glycemic dysregulation and hyperglycemia in the trauma and critically ill patient population.

In the past, hyperglycemia was not routinely treated in the ICU, as it was considered an essential adaptive response to critical illness.[44] However, uncontrolled hyperglycemia has been studied extensively and is associated with poor outcomes. As a result, greater attention is paid to the correction of hyperglycemia in the ICU. In a large RCT of 1826 patients, patients in the ICU with hyperglycemia had a higher mortality that those who were normoglycemic.[46] Several subgroups of critically ill patients have been studied as well. For example, hyperglycemic patients following trauma have increased mortality, length of stay, and incidence of infection.[47,48] Similarly, patients with isolated traumatic brain injury and hyperglycemia have worse neurologic outcomes and increased intracranial pressure.[49]

Although it is clear that preventing uncontrolled hyperglycemia in the critically ill and trauma population is desirable, the optimal blood glucose range remains controversial. A single-center RCT of 1548 ICU patients known as the Leuven surgical trial compared conventional blood glucose management (targeted blood glucose of 180 to 200 mg/dL) with intention-to-treat (IIT) (targeted blood glucose of 80 to 110 mg/dL) and found that overall mortality was improved in the IIT group.[50] However, this study was never able to be replicated and received criticism for an abnormally high mortality rate among the control group. In a later large, multicenter trial, the Normoglycemia in Intensive Care Evaluation Survival Using Glucose Algorithm Regulation (NICE-SUGAR) trial, surgical patients treated with IIT (target blood glucose level of 81 to 108 mg/dL) had significantly increased risk of severe hypoglycemia and increased 90-day mortality when compared with the conventional glucose control group (target blood glucose of less than

180 mg/dL).[51] In addition, the Volume Substitution and Insulin Therapy in Severe Sepsis (VISEP) trial was a multicenter trial that found that ITT (target blood glucose level of 80 to 110 mg/dL) significantly increased the rates of hypoglycemia as well as serious adverse events when compared with conventional glucose control (target blood glucose level of 180 to 200 mg/dL).[52]

In support of this evidence, as well as additional studies in critically ill patients, a targeted blood glucose of 140 to 180 mg/dL in most critically ill adult patients is recommended, rather than a more stringent target of 80 to 110 mg/dL or a more liberal target of 180 to 200 mg/dL. In order to achieve this target, intravenous fluids containing glucose should be minimized. Additionally, attempts should be made to avoid prolonged hypoglycemia. Short-acting insulin and insulin infusions should commonly be employed in the ICU to avoid this complication.[53,54]

Summary

Patients with chronic critical illness experience derangements in multiple endocrine signaling pathways. Clinicians caring for these patients must have a firm understanding of the normal endocrine responses to critical illness and injury, as well as the ability to identify when these derangements are inadequate, maladaptive, and require additional therapy. The remainder of this book will expand on these conditions, providing a framework for diagnosis and management.

Substantial work remains to be done to improve our understanding of both normal endocrine feedback loops as well as the role of endocrine dysregulation in the development of chronic critical illness. Future work must identify the mechanisms that allow some patients to recover from critical illness and injury while others remain susceptible to ongoing infection, inflammation, and ongoing decline. Ultimately, intervening in these system derangements offers the possibility of improving outcomes for patients who survive their acute illness, decreasing the incidence of chronic critical illness and persistent inflammation-immunosuppression catabolism syndrome.

References

1. Boonen E, Bornstein SR, van den Berghe G. New insights into the controversy of adrenal function during critical illness. *The Lancet Diabetes and Endocrinology*. 2015;3(10):805–815. doi:10.1016/S2213-8587(15)00224-7.
2. Gül F, Arslantaş MK, Cinel İ, Kumar A. Changing definitions of sepsis. *Turk Anesteziyoloji ve Reanimasyon Dernegi Dergisi.* 2017;45(3):129–138. doi:10.5152/TJAR.2017.93753.
3. Mira JC, Gentile LF, Mathias BJ, et al. Sepsis pathophysiology, chronic critical illness, and persistent inflammation-immunosuppression and catabolism syndrome. *Critical Care Medicine*. 2017;45(2):253–262. doi:10.1097/CCM.0000000000002074.
4. Efron PA, Mohr AM, Bihorac A, et al. Persistent inflammation, immunosuppression, and catabolism and the development of chronic critical illness after surgery. *Surgery*. 2018;164(2):178–184.
5. Kahn JM, Le T, Angus DC, et al. The epidemiology of chronic critical illness in the United States. *Critical Care Medicine*. 2015;43(2):282–287. doi:10.1097/CCM.0000000000000710.
6. Lamas D. Chronic critical illness. *New England Journal of Medicine*. 2014;370(2):175–177. doi:10.1056/NEJMms1310675.
7. Westfall TC. Sympathomimetic drugs and adrenergic receptor antagonists. *Encyclopedia of Neuroscience*. 2009;685–695. doi:10.1016/B978-008045046-9.01156-6.
8. Hotta H, Uchida S. Aging of the autonomic nervous system and possible improvements in autonomic activity using somatic afferent stimulation. *Geriatrics and Gerontology International*. 2010;10(1). doi:10.1111/j.1447-0594.2010.00592.x SUPPL.
9. Moore A, Mangoni AA, Lyons D, Jackson SHD. The cardiovascular system in the ageing patient. *British Journal of Clinical Pharmacology*. 2003;56(3):254–260. doi:10.1046/j.0306-5251.2003.01876.x.
10. Koeppen BM, Stanton BA. Regulation of extracellular fluid volume and NaCl balance. In: Koeppen BM, Stanton BA, eds. *Renal Physiology*. 6th ed. St. Louis: Elsevier; 2018:84–102. https://www.clinicalkey.com/#!/content/book/3-s2.0-B9780323595681000068.

11. Koeppen BM, Stanton BA. Regulation of body fluid osmolality: regulation of water balance. In: Koeppen BM, Stanton BA, eds. *Renal Physiology*. 6th ed. St Louis: Elsevier; 2018:66–83. https://www.clinicalkey.com/#!/content/book/3-s2.0-B9780323595681000056.
12. Gross P. Clinical management of SIADH. *Therapeutic Advances in Endocrinology and Metabolism*. 2012;3(2):61–73. doi:10.1177/2042018812437561.
13. Seay NW, Lehrich RW, Greenberg A. Diagnosis and management of disorders of body tonicity—hyponatremia and hypernatremia: Core Curriculum 2020. *American Journal of Kidney Diseases*. 2020;75(2):272–286. doi:10.1053/j.ajkd.2019.07.014.
14. Sylvester JT, Scharf SM, Gilbert RD, Fitzgerald RS, Traystman RJ. Hypoxic and CO hypoxia in dogs: hemodynamics, carotid reflexes, and catecholamines. *Am J Physiol*. 1979;236(1):H22-8.
15. Landry DW, Oliver JA. The pathogenesis of vasodilatory shock. *N Engl J Med*. 2001;345(8):588–595.
16. Thiemermann C, Szab C, Mitchell JA. Vascular hyporeactivity. *Pharmacology*. 1993;90:267–271.
17. Errington ML, Rocha M, Silva E. Vasopressin clearance and secretion during haemorrhage in normal dogs and in dogs with experimental diabetes insipidus. *J Physiol*. 1972;227(2):395–418.
18. Sims CA, Holena D, Kim P, et al. Effect of low-dose supplementation of arginine vasopressin on need for blood product transfusions in patients with trauma and hemorrhagic shock: a randomized clinical trial. *JAMA Surgery*. 2019;154(11):994–1003. doi:10.1001/jamasurg.2019.2884.
19. Gordon AC, Mason AJ, Thirunavukkarasu N, et al. Effect of early vasopressin vs norepinephrine on kidney failure in patients with septic shock: the VANISH randomized clinical trial. *JAMA*. 2016;316(5):509–518. doi:10.1001/jama.2016.10485.
20. van den Berghe G. On the neuroendocrinopathy of critical illness: perspectives for feeding and novel treatments. *American Journal of Respiratory and Critical Care Medicine*. 2016;194(11):1337–1348. doi:10.1164/rccm.201607-1516CI.
21. Kojima M, Hosoda H, Date Y, Nakazato M, Matsuo H, Kangawa K. Ghrelin is a growth-hormone-releasing acylated peptide from stomach. *Nature*. 1999;402(656-660).
22. Cowley MA, Smith RG, Diano S, et al. The distribution and mechanism of action of ghrelin in the CNS demonstrates a novel hypothalamic circuit regulating energy homeostasis. *Neuron*. 2003;37(4):649–661.
23. Lechan RM. Neuroendocrinology. In: Melmed S, Koenig R, Rosen C, Auchus R, Goldfine A, eds. *Williams Textbook of Endocrinology*. 14th ed. St. Louis: Elsevier; 2019:114–183. e17.
24. Elijah IE, Branski LK, Finnerty CC, Herndon DN. The GH/IGF-1 system in critical illness. *Best Practice and Research: Clinical Endocrinology and Metabolism*. 2011;25(5):759–767. doi:10.1016/j.beem.2011.06.002.
25. van den Berghe G, Wouters P, Weekers F, et al. Reactivation of pituitary hormone release and metabolic improvement by infusion of growth hormone-releasing peptide and thyrotropin-releasing hormone in patients with protracted critical illness. *J Clin Endocrinol Metab*. 1999;84:1311–1323. https://academic.oup.com/jcem/article-abstract/84/4/1311/2864259.
26. Chrousos GP. Glucocorticoid Action: Physiology. In: Jameson JL, de Groot L, eds. *Endocrinology: Adult and Pediatric*. 7th ed. St. Louis: Elsevier; 2015:1727–1740.e5. https://www.clinicalkey.com/#!/content/book/3-s2.0-B9780323189071000998.
27. Cidlowski JA, Malchoff CD, Malchoff DM. Glucocorticoid receptors, their mechanisms of action, and glucocorticoid resistance. In: Jameson JL, de Groot L, eds. *Endocrinology: Adult and Pediatric*. 7th ed. St. Louis: Elsevier; 2016:1717–1726.e4. https://www.clinicalkey.com/#!/content/book/3-s2.0-B9780323189071000986.
28. Vassiliadi DA, Dimopoulou I, Tzanela M, et al. Longitudinal assessment of adrenal function in the early and prolonged phases of critical illness in septic patients: relations to cytokine levels and outcome. *Journal of Clinical Endocrinology and Metabolism*. 2014;99(12):4471–4480. doi:10.1210/jc.2014-2619.
29. Boonen E, Vervenne H, Meersseman P, et al. Reduced cortisol metabolism during critical illness. *New England Journal of Medicine*. 2013;368(16):1477–1488. doi:10.1056/NEJMoa1214969.
30. van den Berghe G, de Zegher F, Baxter RC, et al. Neuroendocrinology of prolonged critical illness: effects of exogenous thyrotropin-releasing hormone and its combination with growth hormone secretagogues. *J Clin Endocrinol Metab*. 1998;83:309–319. https://academic.oup.com/jcem/article-abstract/83/2/309/2865096.
31. Elenkov IJ, Papanicolaou DA, Wilder RL, Chrousos GP. Modulatory effects of glucocorticoids and catecholamines on human interleukin-12 and interleukin-10 production: clinical implications. *Proceedings of the Association of American Physicians*. 1996;108(5):374–381.

32. Wiersinga WM, van den Berghe G. Nonthyroidal illness syndrome. In: Braverman LE, Cooper D, eds. *Ingbar's the Thyroid: A Fundamental and Clinical Text*. 10th ed. Philadelphia: Lippincott Williams & Wilkins (LWW); 2012:203–217.
33. Utiger RD. Altered thyroid function in nonthyroidal illness and surgery—to treat or not to treat? *New England Journal of Medicine*. 1995;333(23):1562–1563. doi:10.1056/NEJM199512073332310.
34. Annane D, Cavaillon J-M. Corticosteroids in sepsis: from bench to bedside? *Shock*. 2003;20(3):197–207. doi:10.1097/01.shk.0000079423.72656.2f4.
35. Alkemade A, Friesema EC, Unmehopa UA, et al. Neuroanatomical pathways for thyroid hormone feedback in the human hypothalamus. *Journal of Clinical Endocrinology and Metabolism*. 2005;90(7):4322–4334. doi:10.1210/jc.2004-2567.
36. Fekete C, Lechan RM. Negative feedback regulation of hypophysiotropic thyrotropin-releasing hormone (TRH) synthesizing neurons: role of neuronal afferents and type 2 deiodinase. *Frontiers in Neuroendocrinology*. 2007;28(2-3):97–114. doi:10.1016/j.yfrne.2007.04.002.
37. Fliers E, Bianco AC, Langouche L, Boelen A. Thyroid function in critically ill patients. *The Lancet Diabetes and Endocrinology*. 2015;3(10):816–825. doi:10.1016/S2213-8587(15)00225-9.
38. Boelen A, Wiersinga WM, Fliers E. Fasting-induced changes in the hypothalamus-pituitary-thyroid axis. *Thyroid*. 2008;18(2):123–129. doi:10.1089/thy.2007.0253.
39. Haugen BR. Drugs that suppress TSH or cause central hypothyroidism. *Best Practice and Research: Clinical Endocrinology and Metabolism*. 2009;23(6):793–800. doi:10.1016/j.beem.2009.08.003.
40. Ringel MD. Management of hypothyroidism and hyperthyroidism in the intensive care unit. *Critical Care Clinics*. 2001;17(1):59–74. doi:10.1016/S0749-0704(05)70152-4.
41. Rothberger GD, Gadhvi S, Michelakis N, Kumar A, Calixte R, Shapiro LE. Usefulness of serum triiodothyronine (T3) to predict outcomes in patients hospitalized with acute heart failure. *American Journal of Cardiology*. 2017;119(4):599–603. doi:10.1016/j.amjcard.2016.10.045.
42. Liu J, Wu X, Lu F, Zhao L, Shi L, Xu F. Low T3 syndrome is a strong predictor of poor outcomes in patients with community-acquired pneumonia. *Scientific Reports*. 2016;6. doi:10.1038/srep22271.
43. Casaer MP, Mesotten D, Hermans G, et al. Early versus late parenteral nutrition in critically ill adults. *New England Journal of Medicine*. 2011;365(6):506–517. doi:10.1056/NEJMoa1102662.
44. Dungan KM, Braithwaite SS, Preiser JC. Stress hyperglycaemia. *The Lancet*. 2009;373(9677):1798-1807. doi:10.1016/S0140-6736(09)60553-5.
45. Sicardi Salomón Z, Rodhe P, Hahn RG. Progressive decrease in glucose clearance during surgery. *Acta Anaesthesiologica Scandinavica*. 2006;50(7):848–854. doi:10.1111/j.1399-6576.2006.01066.x.
46. Krinsley JS. Association between hyperglycemia and increased hospital mortality in a heterogeneous population of critically ill patients. *Mayo Clinic Proceedings*. 2003;78(12):1471–1478. doi:10.4065/78.12.1471.
47. Laird AM, Miller PR, Kilgo PD, Meredith JW, Chang MC. Relationship of early hyperglycemia to mortality in trauma patients. *Journal of Trauma: Injury, Infection and Critical Care*. 2004;56(5):1058–1062. doi:10.1097/01.TA.0000123267.39011.9F.
48. Bochicchio G v, Sung J, Joshi M, et al. Persistent hyperglycemia is predictive of outcome in critically ill trauma patients. *The Journal of Trauma: Injury, Infection, and Critical Care*. 2005;58(5):921–924. doi:10.1097/01.TA.0000162141.26392.07.
49. Jeremitsky E, Omert LA, Dunham CM, Wilberger J, Rodriguez A. The impact of hyperglycemia on patients with severe brain injury. *The Journal of Trauma: Injury, Infection, and Critical Care*. 2005;58(1):47–50. doi:10.1097/01.TA.0000135158.42242.B1.
50. van den Berghe G, Wouters P, Weekers F, et al. Intensive insulin therapy in critically ill patients. *New England Journal of Medicine*. 2001;345(19):1359–1367. doi:10.1056/NEJMoa011300.
51. Finfer S, Bellomo R, Blair D, et al. Intensive versus conventional glucose control in critically ill patients. *New England Journal of Medicine*. 2009;360(13):1283–1297. doi:10.1056/NEJMoa0810625.
52. Brunkhorst FM, Engel C, Bloos F, et al. Intensive insulin therapy and pentastarch resuscitation in severe sepsis. *New England Journal of Medicine*. 2008;358(2):125–139. doi:10.1056/NEJMoa070716.
53. Heyland DK, Dhaliwal R, Drover JW, Gramlich L, Dodek P. Canadian clinical practice guidelines for nutrition support in mechanically ventilated, critically ill adult patients. *Journal of Parenteral and Enteral Nutrition*. 2003;27(5):355–373. doi:10.1177/0148607103027005355.
54. Nutrition Critical Care. Systematic Reviews 10.4a. Optimal glucose control: insulin therapy. *Critical Care Nutrition*. 2018. www.criticalcarenutrition.com.

CHAPTER 26

Use of Potassium Iodide in a Nuclear Emergency

Daniel J. Toft ■ Arthur B. Dr. Schneider

CHAPTER OUTLINE

Preamble

In contrast to other chapters in this volume, the emergency reviewed here arises from an external event. It is also different in the paucity of risk factors associated with a nuclear emergency. In fact, one could say that the only risk factor is living or spending time in the vicinity of an operating nuclear energy facility.

The goal of this chapter is to discuss how to avert the thyroid-related consequences of a radiologic emergency, not how to diagnosis and treat a medical emergency. Therefore, even though this chapter focuses on the role of potassium iodide (KI), it is important to remember that it is only one part in the response. Of equal or greater importance, depending on the circumstances, are evacuation and dietary measures, especially the control of the milk pathway (see later).

This chapter mainly emphasizes medically related issues. It is based on the authoritative guidelines from the following organizations: Center for Disease Control and Prevention (CDC), U.S. Food and Drug Administration (FDA), World Health Organization, American Thyroid Association, and U.S. Department of Health and Human Services (Box 26.1). For the most part, this chapter is directed to the use of KI in the United States, since variations in other countries are minimal. The guidelines listed in Box 26.1 should be consulted for a wider geographic perspective.

How Does Potassium Iodide Protect the Thyroid?

Many sources, including those directed to the general population, state that the protective effect of KI is a result of the dilution of radioactive iodine. Although this is correct and intuitively clear, dilution is not the only mechanism. The well-known (but incompletely understood) Wolff-Chaikoff effect may play an even more important role.[1,2] Two recent studies shed light on this incompletely understood phenomenon.[3,4] These studies, one using experimental studies in rats[4] and the other using analytical methods (a systems biology approach),[3] indicate that the thyroid

BOX 26.1 ■ Guidelines from Reliable Sources That Formed the Basis for This Chapter

Centers for Disease Control and Prevention

Potassium Iodide (KI)
https://www.cdc.gov/nceh/radiation/emergencies/ki.htm
(Page last reviewed: 4/4/2018 [accessed 11/19/2019])
Content source: National Center for Environmental Health (NCEH), Agency for Toxic Substances and Disease Registry (ATSDR), National Center for Injury Prevention and Control (NCIPC)

U.S. Food and Drug Administration

Guidance. Potassium Iodide as a Thyroid Blocking Agent in Radiation Emergencies, 2001 https://www.fda.gov > media > download
Accessed 11/19/2019
https://www.fda.gov/drugs/bioterrorism-and-drug-preparedness/frequently-asked-questions-potassium-iodide-ki
Content current as of: 10/14/2016
Accessed 11/19/2019

World Health Organization

Iodine thyroid blocking Guidelines for use in planning for and responding to radiological and nuclear emergencies, 2017
Available at https://www.who.int/ionizing_radiation/pub_meet/iodine-thyroid-blocking/en/
Accessed 11/19/2019

American Thyroid Association

Leung AM, Bauer AJ, Benvenga S, et al. American Thyroid Association scientific statement on the use of potassium iodide ingestion in a nuclear emergency. *Thyroid*. 2017;27(7):865–877.

U.S. Department of Health and Human Services

Radiation Emergency Medical Management
Potassium iodide (KI)
Available at https://www.remm.nlm.gov/potassiumiodide.htm
Updated 6/26/2019
Accessed 12/8/2019

is protected by the downregulation of the sodium-iodide symporter (NIS), thyroid peroxidase (TPO), and monocarboxylate transporter 8 (MCT8). KI ingestion thus limits radiation exposure to the thyroid by preventing radioiodine entry and organification.

What Are the Sources of Exposure to Radioactive Iodine?

The most likely source of exposure to radioactive iodine is from an accident at an operating nuclear power plant. A decommissioned or off-line nuclear facility does not retain significant amounts of ^{131}I, given its half-life of about 8 days. A "dirty bomb" usually refers to a conventional explosion with the aim of spreading radioactivity. Such a bomb could contain ^{131}I stolen from a medical facility (an unlikely occurrence), but the amount of ^{131}I exposure to any person would be very low. A 2019 episode in northern Russia, presumably related to a missile development accident, released radioactivity into the air, but the presence of radioactive iodine in the release has not been substantiated; nevertheless, local supplies of KI around the site were reportedly quickly sold out.[5] Research reactors, academic or otherwise, are also subject to potential accidents. However, the amount of radioactive iodine from these potential sources, except in the immediate vicinity, is unlikely to reach the level where KI is advised.

KI is also used in the nuclear medicine setting. It is administered to protect the thyroid when a radioactive iodine–containing agent, such as ^{131}I-labeled MIGB (metaiodobenzylguanidine), is used for diagnostic or therapeutic purposes. (The recommended amounts and duration of administration are outside the scope of this chapter.)

Nuclear bombs are more complex. In the past, before the harmful effects of radiation were fully realized, inadequately protected facilities making fissionable materials were a source of environmental radioactive contamination (e.g., the Hanford, Washington reactors released an estimated 685,000 curies (Ci) of radioactive iodine into the atmosphere in the 1940s[6]), but this is no longer the case. Similarly, in the era of above-ground nuclear testing, radioactive iodine was released into the upper atmosphere. The two bombs used in 1945 over Hiroshima and Nagasaki exploded at high altitude, and the resulting radioactive iodine did not concentrate in a localized area.

What Are the Risks of Exposure to Radioactive Iodine?

The majority of what is known about the relationship between radiation exposure and thyroid cancer comes from studies of external radiation. The relationship between dose and the excess relative risk of thyroid cancer is essentially linear in the dose ranges that potentially occur after a nuclear power plant accident.[7,8] The lowest dose where there is a demonstrable risk of thyroid cancer is 50 mCi (5 rads).[9] This dose limit informs the guidelines for the response to radioactive iodine exposure, as discussed below. At the higher thyroid doses typically experienced during many types of cancer therapy, the risk reaches a plateau, then subsides, but does not disappear. The risk rises over decades before decreasing, but never returning to background levels. In addition to dose, age at exposure is strongly related to risk, with children at much higher risk than adults.[9] This also informs the KI guidelines, which emphasize that in the event of a radiation emergency the use of KI should be prioritized for children under the age of 18 and pregnant women.[10]

Any doubt about the carcinogenic effects of radioactive iodine (predominantly ^{131}I) were dispelled in the aftermath of the Chernobyl accident.[11,12] Prospective studies conducted in Ukraine, Belarus, and the Bryansk Oblast of Russia have been largely concordant.[13–15] A clinically important observation was that thyroid cancers could be evident as early as about 5 years after the exposure. It should be noted that several factors affected the outcome of the Chernobyl accident. Most of the region surrounding the site of the accident was, at the time of the accident, iodine insufficient. This would have enhanced the uptake of radioactive iodine into the thyroid and could have affected the clinical course of the subsequent thyroid cancers. Aggravating the effects of the accident was the delay in making the at-risk population aware of the accident and the delay in controlling the intake of radioactive iodine through the dietary pathway (especially though the milk pathway).

For many years, it was assumed that internal radiation was less carcinogenic than external radiation. Importantly for the development of the KI guidelines, the Chernobyl experience has called that view into doubt. The risk estimates (expressed as excess relative risk; ERR) and behavior over time for Chernobyl-related thyroid cancer are similar to those after external radiation exposure, so it is now likely that the effects are essentially the same.[16,17]

Availability of Potassium Iodide in the United States

The seminal study of Blum and Eisenbud investigated the effectiveness of KI with respect to interval between radioactive iodine exposure and the time of KI ingestion.[18] This publication led to the potentially amusing conclusion that the best time to take KI is before the accident. Subsequent events in Fukushima show why this cannot be considered humorous. In Fukushima, the major releases did not occur immediately after the accident began. Rather the major releases of radioactive elements, including iodine, began when explosions destroyed the reactor containment measures. In other words, there was time between the start of the accident and the start of major radioactivity releases into the atmosphere. Presumably, in future accidents, KI could be taken before exposure. The protective effect of KI falls rapidly. Some estimates are that protection is less than 50% at 8 hours[18,19] and other estimates is that protection at 8 hours is even less.[20,21]

As a result of these time-related factors, it is widely accepted in the United States and internationally that to be effective, potassium iodide needs to be pre-distributed to people in the vicinity of operating nuclear power plants. An American Thyroid Association statement lists the factors supporting and opposing pre-distribution.[10] In the United States, KI is pre-distributed to households within 10 miles of an operating nuclear power plant and to locations such as schools and hospitals within that limit.

Only FDA-approved KI products may be marketed legally in the United States.[22] As of October 2016, the KI products that are FDA-approved and available are: iOSAT tablets (130 mg, from Anbex, Inc.), ThyroSafe tablets (65 mg, from Recipharm AB), ThyroShield oral solution (65 mg/mL, from Arco Pharmaceuticals, LLC), and Potassium Iodide Oral Solution USP (65 mg/mL, from Mission Pharmacal Company). Directions for preparing a KI solution from tablets, required to protect infants and very young children, are available.[23] No prescription is needed to obtain KI. Other iodine-containing tablets can be found on the internet, including one with the dangerously named "Potassium Iodate Nuclear Anti-Radiation" pills. In addition to its lack of FDA approval, calling it an antiradiation pill can lead the unaware to tragically misguided decisions, for example, to remain in place when evacuation is preferable or mandated. The appellations "anti-radiation pills," "anti-nuke tablets," and similar ones are all too common. Potassium iodate is available in other countries.

The FDA-approved shelf life of KI is 7 years. If a state follows certain storage guidelines, the shelf life can be extended. For those whose only access is to KI tablets that have expired, it is safe to take them.[24] The method for distributing KI within the 10-mile radius varies from place to place. There is little known about the effectiveness of pre-distribution of KI with respect to percent coverage and public awareness about proper KI storage and administration. In the United States, what little is known shows substantial shortcomings that need to be addressed.[25–27] In France, it has been reported that 60% of eligible homes within 10 km of active nuclear reactors have obtained KI.[28]

Guidelines for Use

Age and dose: The guidelines developed by the CDC regarding the radiation exposure above which KI is recommended are shown in Table 26.1. There are age-specific thresholds because the susceptibility of the thyroid to develop cancer decreases markedly with age. In fact, for the oldest category, KI is advised only as a means to avoid hypothyroidism.

Time-limited exposure to radioactive iodine: The recommended amount of KI is based on the pharmacokinetics of KI. In the event of a time-limited exposure, KI should not be taken if 12 hours have passed since the cessation of the exposure.[21] During the first 12 hours, radioactive iodine will be incorporated into thyroid proteins and KI taken after that will delay its release, potentially increasing, rather than decreasing thyroid exposure (an action of high-dose KI that is used in the treatment of thyroid storm).

Prolonged exposure: The aim of public health measures after an accident is to avoid prolonged exposure to all radioactivity. If high levels of radioactivity continue to be present beyond 1 day, it is likely that evacuation will be advised. If evacuation is not possible and exposure to radioactive iodine continues, then KI should be taken daily.

Pregnancy and breastfeeding [Figs. 26.1 **and** 26.2]**:** According to the American Academy of Pediatrics (AAP) guidelines, pregnant women at risk for internal radiation exposure should take KI to protect themselves and their fetus, but KI should only be taken once because continued excess iodine may adversely affect the fetus' thyroid function.[29] For this reason, other means of protection from continued radiation exposure such as evacuation should be prioritized for pregnant women. For fetuses exposed to one or more doses of KI (in the case where continued maternal radiation exposure is unavoidable), as neonates their thyroid function should be monitored and hypothyroidism treated as necessary.

TABLE 26.1 ■ **Threshold Thyroid Radioactive Exposures and FDA-Recommended Doses of KI for Different Risk Groups**

	Predicted Thyroid Exposure	KI dose (mg)	# of 130-mg Tablets[a]	mL oral solution of 65 mg/mL[b]
Adults over 40 years	>500 cGy	130	1	2
Adults over 18 through 40 years	>10 cGy	130	1	2
Pregnant or lactating women	>5 cGy	130	1	2
Adolescents over 12 through 18 years[c]	>5 cGy	65	1/2	1
Children over 3 through 12 years	>5 cGy	65	1/2	1
Over 1 month through 3 years	>5 cGy	32	1/4 (see liquid option)	0.5
Birth through 1 month	>5 cGy	16	1/8 (see liquid option)	0.25

[a]Double for 65-mg tablets
[b]30-mL bottles with dropper marked for 1, 0.5, and 0.25 mL
[c]Adolescents approaching adult size (>70 kg) should receive the full adult dose (130 mg).
FDA, Food and Drug Administration; *KI,* potassium iodide.

Breastfeeding women should take KI only once and consider substituting formula (made with radiation-free water) or uncontaminated milk for their child. There is insufficient KI in breast milk to protect nursing infants. The infant should receive KI in liquid form according to the guidelines. Mothers should pump breast milk so that their supply remains intact so that nursing may resume following the resolution of the radiation emergency. If breast milk is the only source of nutrition, nursing should continue, and the infant subsequently monitored for hypothyroidism.

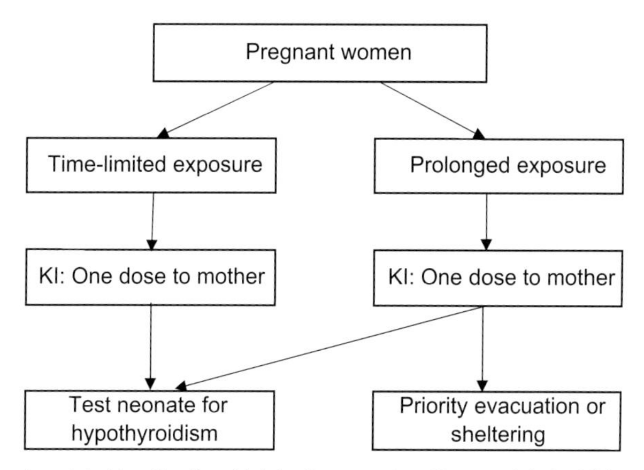

Fig. 26.1 Algorithm for minimizing the thyroid risk of pregnant mothers and their children during a radiation emergency. *KI,* Potassium iodine.

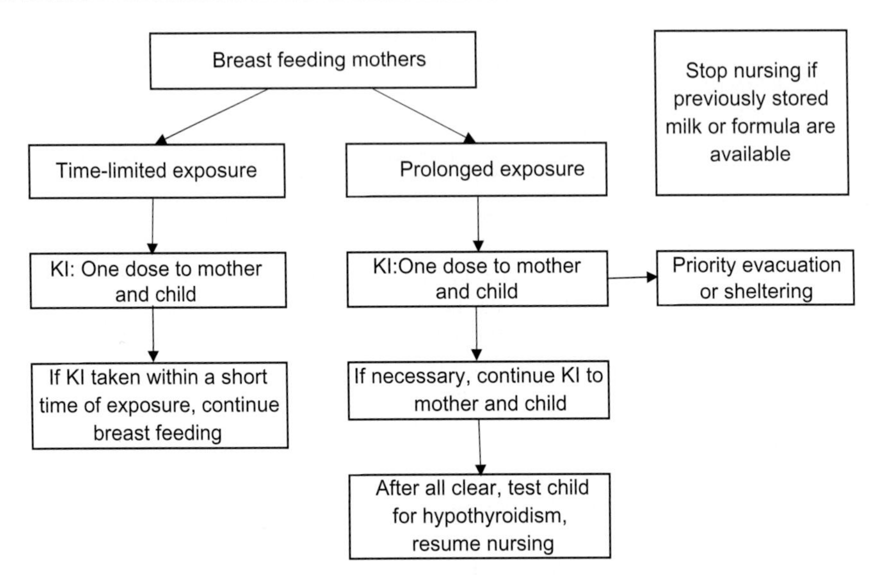

Fig 26.2 Algorithm for minimizing thyroid risk of breastfeeding mothers and their infants during a radiation emergency. *KI,* Potassium iodine.

Public health communications in times of risk: It is difficult to imagine a completely effective communication of risk to the thyroid in the midst of responding to a nuclear power plant accident. First, the precision of predicting the potential thyroid exposure is limited, as seen in the Fukushima accident aftermath. Some people were inadvertently evacuated to an area where the exposure was greater than the evacuation zone. Second, thyroid protection will be only one concern among several, some with higher visibility, for example, evacuation. Third, among the population, radiation risk is poorly understood and usually substantially overestimated. As was reported, following the Fukushima accident, concerns of people on the west coast of the United States led to exhaustion of KI supplies (it is not clear how much was actually consumed).

An important role of physicians practicing in the area of a nuclear power facility should be to provide continuing education about KI to their patients (in addition to in coordination with efforts sponsored by the government). In addition, they should identify patients at risk for possible side effects of KI.

Safety and Possible Side Effects of Potassium Iodide

Virtually all that is known about the safety and potential risks of giving KI to a large population comes from a study in Poland following the Chernobyl accident.[30] This study included about 35,000 people, about 12,000 children among them. No adverse effects on thyroid function were found. In newborns who received a high dose of KI, a transient increase in thyroid-stimulating hormone was observed, with resolution by the 16th to 20th day of life. A small number of extrathyroidal side effects were reported, particularly vomiting and skin rashes, with 286 and 129 reports, respectively, in 11,482 KI-treated children.

Fetuses are at risk of neonatal goiter if exposure to KI is prolonged. People with preexisting thyroid disease, particularly nontoxic multinodular goiter, are at risk of developing hyper- or hypothyroidism. People who are sensitive to iodine may develop immune-related angioedema, arthralgia, eosinophilia, urticaria, and rashes. Specifically, according to the package insert for iOSAT, contraindications include known sensitivity to iodides or any ingredient in the formulation, dermatitis herpetiformis, hypocomplementemic vasculitis, and nodular thyroid disease (e.g., multinodular goiter) with heart disease.

Additional Measures to Protect the Thyroid

Radioactive iodine is released into the atmosphere where it can spread over long distances. Precipitation brings the radioactive iodine down to earth where it can be consumed by goats and cows eating the radioactive grass. The ingested radioactive iodine is concentrated into the animal's milk. When the milk is consumed by people, the radioactive iodine is concentrated in the thyroid gland. This is most pronounced in children, whose iodine uptake is high and their glands are small, accentuating the risk. The milk pathway was responsible for the largest fraction of thyroid exposure after releases from the Hanford facility in the 1940s and after the Chernobyl accident. Therefore, controlling the milk supply is of utmost importance. Of course, milk produced prior to the accident is safe.

Even if the milk pathway is completely controlled, the airway pathway (direct inhalation) remains of concern, and KI tablets are still advisable. In the immediate area, iodine isotopes in addition to ^{131}I may be present, and these other isotopes have a less well-defined risk profile. If evacuation is advised or mandated, car windows and fan intake should be closed. If evacuation is not undertaken, staying indoors with windows closed is best. Later, as occurred at Chernobyl, cleanup workers are at risk for accumulating substantial doses of ^{131}I through the inhalation pathway.

The Aftermath

Although not an "emergency," it is relevant to think about the role of endocrinologists in monitoring thyroid health after a nuclear accident. This topic has been considered in detail by the International Agency for Research on Cancer (IARC).[31,32] There is little monitoring that is universally agreed upon. One area of agreement is to monitor the thyroid function of fetuses and neonates who were exposed to KI and are at risk for transient hypothyroidism. Similarly, it is generally agreed that people with goiters who took KI, especially multiple times, should be monitored for hypo- and hyperthyroidism.

Little else about monitoring is clear-cut because it is monitoring for thyroid cancer. The experiences after Chernobyl and Fukushima are far from instructive. After Chernobyl, the ^{131}I doses were high and thousands of thyroid cancers were diagnosed in people exposed during childhood. It is unlikely that the conditions during the Chernobyl accident will occur again. After Fukushima, the thyroid doses of radioactive iodine were well below those that have been associated with a risk of thyroid cancer. Nevertheless an extensive ultrasound-based monitoring program for all children in the Fukushima area was initiated.[33] Although the exact reason why this was started is somewhat contentious, it is clear that public demand was a predominant factor. The IARC Expert Group "recommends against population based thyroid screening after a nuclear accident, because the harms outweigh the benefits at the population level."[31] Of the 324,301 children screened in the first 5 years following the Fukushima accident, 187 cases of thyroid cancer have been found.[34] For children who receive a very high dose (100 to 500 mGy), the IARC recommendation is similar to those in the recent report from the International Late Effects of Childhood Cancer Guideline Harmonization Group,[35] and are based on the dearth of evidence to support or reject monitoring. Both groups suggest what is generally referred to as informed "shared decision making." A technical guideline for methods of monitoring the thyroid dose after a nuclear incident, prepared by the Open Project for European Radiation Research Area, is available.[36]

References

1. Leung AM, Braverman LE. Consequences of excess iodine. *Nat Rev Endocrinol.* 2014;10(3):136–142.
2. National Research Council (U.S.). Committee to Assess the Distribution and Administration of Potassium Iodide in the Event of a Nuclear Incident., National Research Council (U.S.). Board on Radiation Effects Research. *Distribution and administration of potassium iodide in the event of a nuclear incident.* Washington, DC: National Academies Press; 2004.
3. Cohen DPA, Lebsir D, Benderitter M, Souidi M. A systems biology approach to propose a new mechanism of regulation of repetitive prophylaxis of stable iodide on sodium/iodide symporter (NIS). *Biochimie.* 2019;162:208–215.
4. Lebsir D, Manens L, Grison S, et al. Effects of repeated potassium iodide administration on genes involved in synthesis and secretion of thyroid hormone in adult male rat. *Mol Cell Endocrinol.* 2018;474:119–126.
5. Balmforth T, Kiselyova M. (2019, August 9). *Russians rush to buy iodine after blast causes radiation spike: reports.* Reuters. Retrieved February 15, 2020, from https://www.reuters.com/article/us-russia-blast/russians-rush-to-buy-iodine-after-blast-causes-radiation-spike-reports-idUSKCN1UZ0ZT.
6. Heeb CM. *Iodine-131 releases from the Hanford Site, 1944–1947.* Technical report, United States; 1993.
7. Ron E, Lubin JH, Shore RE, et al. Thyroid cancer after exposure to external radiation: a pooled analysis of seven studies. *Radiat Res.* 1995;141(3):259–277.
8. Veiga LH, Holmberg E, Anderson H, et al. Thyroid cancer after childhood exposure to external radiation: an updated pooled analysis of 12 studies. *Radiat Res.* 2016;185(5):473–484.
9. Lubin JH, Adams MJ, Shore R, et al. Thyroid cancer following childhood low-dose radiation exposure: a pooled analysis of nine cohorts. *J Clin Endocrinol Metab.* 2017;102(7):2575–2583.
10. Leung AM, Bauer AJ, Benvenga S, et al. American Thyroid Association scientific statement on the use of potassium iodide ingestion in a nuclear emergency. *Thyroid.* 2017;27(7):865–877.
11. Baverstock K, Egloff B, Pinchera A, Ruchti C, Williams D. Thyroid cancer after Chernobyl. *Nature.* 1992;359(6390):21–22.
12. Kazakov VS, Demidchik EP, Astakhova LN. Thyroid cancer after Chernobyl. *Nature.* 1992;359(6390):21.
13. Tronko MD, Howe GR, Bogdanova TI, et al. A cohort study of thyroid cancer and other thyroid diseases after the Chornobyl accident: thyroid cancer in Ukraine detected during first screening. *J Natl Cancer Inst.* 2006;98(13):897–903.
14. Astakhova LN, Anspaugh LR, Beebe GW, et al. Chernobyl-related thyroid cancer in children of Belarus: a case-control study. *Radiat Res.* 1998;150(3):349–356.
15. Jacob P, Bogdanova TI, Buglova E, et al. Thyroid cancer among Ukrainians and Belarusians who were children or adolescents at the time of the Chernobyl accident. *J Radiol Prot.* 2006;26(1):51–67.
16. Brenner AV, Tronko MD, Hatch M, et al. I-131 dose response for incident thyroid cancers in Ukraine related to the Chornobyl accident. *Environ Health Perspect.* 2011;119(7):933–939.
17. Ron E. Thyroid cancer incidence among people living in areas contaminated by radiation from the Chernobyl accident. *Health Phys.* 2007;93(5):502–511.
18. Blum M, Eisenbud M. Reduction of thyroid irradiation from 131-I by potassium iodide. *JAMA.* 1967;200(12):1036–1040.
19. Zanzonico PB, Becker DV Effects of time of administration and dietary iodine levels on potassium iodide (KI) blockade of thyroid irradiation by 131I from radioactive fallout. *Health Phys.* 2000;78(6):660–667.
20. Hanscheid H, Reiners C, Goulko G, et al. Facing the nuclear threat: thyroid blocking revisited. *J Clin Endocrinol Metab.* 2011;96(11):3511–3516.
21. U.S. Department of Health & Human Services REMM. (2019, November 26). *Potassium Iodide (KI).* Retrieved December 8, 2019, from https://www.remm.nlm.gov/potassiumiodide.htm.
22. U.S. Food and Drug Administration. (2016, October 14). *Frequently Asked Questions on Potassium Iodide (KI).* Retrieved February 8, 2020, from https://www.fda.gov/drugs/bioterrorism-and-drug-preparedness/frequently-asked-questions-potassium-iodide-ki.
23. U.S. Food and Drug Administration. (2018, March 8). *Potassium iodide ("KI"): instructions to make potassium iodide solution for use during a nuclear emergency (liquid form).* Retrieved February 8, 2020, from https://www.fda.gov/drugs/bioterrorism-and-drug-preparedness/potassium-iodide-ki.
24. U.S. Nuclear Regulatory Comission. (2016, March 3). *What is the shelf life of KI tablets?* Retrieved February 8, 2020, from https://www.nrc.gov/about-nrc/emerg-preparedness/about-emerg-preparedness/potassium-iodide/ki-faq.html#shelflife.

25. Blando J, Robertson C, Pearl K, Dixon C, Valcin M, Bresnitz E. Evaluation of potassium iodide prophylaxis knowledge and nuclear emergency preparedness: New Jersey. *Am J Public Health*. 2007;97(Suppl 1): S100–S102.
26. Blando J, Robertson C, Pearl K, Dixon C, Valcin M, Bresnitz E. Assessment of potassium iodide (KI) distribution program among communities within the emergency planning zones (EPZ) of two nuclear power plants. *Health Phys*. 2007;92(Suppl 2):S18–S26.
27. Zwolinski LR, Stanbury M, Manente S. Nuclear power plant emergency preparedness: results from an evaluation of Michigan's potassium iodide distribution program. *Disaster Med Public Health Prep*. 2012;6(3):263–269.
28. Le Guen B, Stricker L, Schlumberger M. Distributing KI pills to minimize thyroid radiation exposure in case of a nuclear accident in France. *Nat Clin Pract Endocrinol Metab*. 2007;3(9):611.
29. Linet MS, Kazzi Z, Paulson JA. Council On Environmental H. Pediatric considerations before, during, and after radiological or nuclear emergencies. *Pediatrics*. 2018;142(6):e20183001.
30. Nauman J, Wolff J. Iodide prophylaxis in Poland after the Chernobyl reactor accident: benefits and risks. *Am J Med*. 1993;94(5):524–532.
31. Togawa K, Ahn HS, Auvinen A, et al. Long-term strategies for thyroid health monitoring after nuclear accidents: recommendations from an Expert Group convened by IARC. *Lancet Oncol*. 2018;19(10):1280–1283.
32. IEGoTHMaN Accidents. *Thyroid Health Monitoring After Nuclear Accidents*: Lyon, France: International Agency for Research on Cancer; 2018.
33. Yasumura S, Hosoya M, Yamashita S, et al. Study protocol for the Fukushima Health Management Survey. *J Epidemiol*. 2012;22(5):375–383.
34. Ohtsuru A, Midorikawa S, Ohira T, et al. Incidence of thyroid cancer among children and young adults in Fukushima, Japan, screened with 2 rounds of ultrasonography within 5 years of the 2011 Fukushima Daiichi nuclear power station accident. *JAMA Otolaryngol Head Neck Surg*. 2019;145(1):4–11.
35. Kremer LC, Mulder RL, Oeffinger KC, et al. A worldwide collaboration to harmonize guidelines for the long-term follow-up of childhood and young adult cancer survivors: a report from the International Late Effects of Childhood Cancer Guideline Harmonization Group. *Pediatr Blood Cancer*. 2013;60(4):543–549.
36. Etherington G, Marsh J, Gregoratto D, et al. *CAThyMARA report: Technical guidelines for radioiodine in thyroid monitoring. OPERRA Deliverable D5.31.*2017.

INDEX

Page numbers followed by "*f*" indicate figures; "*t*" indicate tables; and "*b*" indicate boxes.